Ethics and Health Policy

Ethics and Health Policy

Edited by

Robert M. Veatch
*Associate for Medical Ethics,
Institute of Society, Ethics
and the Life Sciences*

and

Roy Branson
*Senior Research Scholar
Center for Bioethics
Kennedy Institute
Georgetown University*

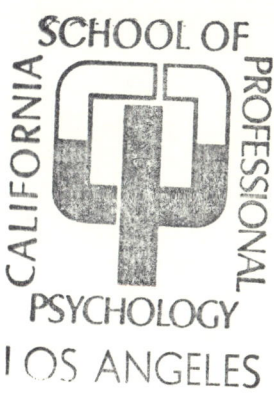

Ballinger Publishing Company • Cambridge, Massachusetts
A Subsidiary of J.B. Lippincott Company

 This book is printed on recycled paper.

Copyright © 1976 by Ballinger Publishing Company. All rights reserved. No part of this publication may be reproduced, stored in a retrieval system, or transmitted in any form or by any means, electronic, mechanical photocopy, recording or otherwise, without the prior written consent of the publisher.

International Standard Book Number: 0-88410-137-1

Library of Congress Catalog Card Number: 76-3741

Library of Congress Cataloging in Publication Data

Main entry under title:
  Ethics and health policy.

  Bibliography: p.
  Includes index.
  1. Medical ethics. 2. Medical care—United States. 3. Medical policy—United States. I. Veatch, Robert M. II. Branson, Roy. [DNLM: 1. Ethics, Medical. 2. Health and welfare planning—U.S. 3. Delivery of health care—U.S. W50 E84]
R724.E82   174'.2   76-3741
ISBN 0-88410-137-1

Contents

List of Figures	xi
List of Tables	xiii
Contributors	xv
Introduction	xix

Part One
Health Care Delivery: Fundamental Ethical Conflicts

Section A: The Patient and Society	3
Preamble	3

Chapter One
The Scope of Bioethics: Individual and Social
by *Roy Branson* — 5

Chapter Two
Conceptual Foundations for an Ethics of Medical Care
by *Albert F. Jonsen and André E. Hellegers* — 17

Chapter Three
Conceptual Foundations for an Ethics of Medical Care:
A Response
by *Paul Ramsey*   35

Chapter Four
Self-Reliance and the Collective Good: Medicine in China
by *Victor W. Sidel and Ruth Sidel*   57

Urban Health Care	59
Maoist Principles	65
The Role of the Mass	67
The Role of Indigenous Health Personnel	70
The Role of the Professional	71
The Role of the Patient	72
Summary	74

Section B: Justice and Health Care Delivery   77

Preamble   77

Chapter Five
Social Justice and Equal Access to Health Care
by *Gene Outka*   79

To Each According to his Merit or Desert	81
To Each According to his Societal Contribution	85
To Each According to his Contribution in Satisfying Whatever is Freely Desired by Others in the Open Marketplace of Supply and Demand	87
To Each According to his Needs	89
Similar Treatment for Similar Cases	91

Chapter Six
Ethics and Health Care Delivery: Computers and Distributive Justice
by *Joseph Fletcher*   99

Distributive Justice	101
Telescopes, Not Only Microscopes	104
Quantifying Qualities (Values)	106

Contents vii

Chapter Seven
Health Care and Justice in Contract Theory Perspective
by *Ronald M. Green* 111

Chapter Eight
What Is a "Just" Health Care Delivery?
by *Robert M. Veatch* 127

Theories of Justice in Health Care 128
Remaining Special Problems 136
Justice in National Health Insurance Proposals 142

Section C: The Right to Health Care 155

Preamble 155

Chapter Nine
Biomedical Progress and the Limits of Human Health
by *Daniel Callahan* 157

Chapter Ten
The Right to Health Care and the Anxiety of Liberalism: A Reply to Daniel Callahan
by *Peter Steinfels* 167

Chapter Eleven
Freedoms and Utilities in the Distribution of Health Care
by *Peter Singer* 175

Health Care as a Right 176
Distributive Justice 177
Intrinsic Evil 178
Freedom 178
Utility 186
A National Health Service? 188

Part Two
Ethics and Allocating Scarce Medical Resources

Preamble 197

Chapter Twelve
Who Shall Live When Not All Can Live?
by *James F. Childress* — 199

Analogous Conflict Situations — 200
Criteria of Selection for SLMR — 202
The Values of Random Selection — 205

Chapter Thirteen
The Selection Process as Viewed from Within: A Reply to Childress
by *Frederic B. Westervelt* — 213

Chapter Fourteen
The Totally Implantable Artificial Heart: Economic, Ethical, Legal, Medical, Psychiatric, and Social Implications
by the *Artificial Heart Assessment Panel, National Heart and Lung Institute* — 219

The Panel and the Problem — 219
Issues in the Use of the Clinically Acceptable Device:
 Alternative Power Sources — 232
Issues in the Use of the Clinically Acceptable
 Artificial Heart: Allocation and Regulation — 236

Chapter Fifteen
Separate Views on the Artificial Heart
by *Clark C. Havighurst* — 247

Utilitarianism and Justice — 248
The Nuclear-Powered Artificial Heart — 250
Financing and Patient Selection — 253

Part Three
Ethics and Health Policy Planning

Preamble — 259

Chapter Sixteen
On Measuring Economic Benefits of Health Programs
by *Rashi Fein* — 261

Early History	261
Recent Developments	269
Conceptual Issues	273
Conclusions	282

Chapter Seventeen
Community Participation in Health Care Decisions
by *Laurelyn Veatch* — 289

Five Claims to Policy-Making Authority	290
The Beginnings of the Community Boards	293
A Middle-Class Community Board	295
A Chronic-Care Facility	296
A Community Board with Staff	297
Patronage	298
Board Members' Roles	298
Issues	299
Achieving Goals	300
The Future of Community Boards	302

Chapter Eighteen
Technology Assessment and Genetics
by *LeRoy Walters* — 307

Concept of Technology Assessment	307
Assessment of Biomedical Technology	311
Assessment of Genetic Technology	313
A Theoretical Perspective on Technology Assessment	316

Index — 325

List of Figures

4-1	Organization of Cities in the PRC	60
4-2	Instructions Posted at a Lane Health Station in Peking: Working Responsibilities for Red Medical Workers	63
4-3	Family Planning Chart in the Silvery Lane Health Station, Hangchow, Serving 2700 People, September 1971	65
8-1	Bases of Distribution	131
14-1	Expected Mortality Within Ten Years for 1,000 Persons With An Artificial Heart Compared to 1,000 Persons in the General Population	225
18-1	Overall Impacts of an Assessed Technology	318

List of Tables

8-1	Day Limits of National Health Insurance Proposals, 93rd Congress (Listed from most limited to most inclusive in-patient hospital coverage)	144
14-1	Potential Candidates for an Artificial Heart Among Persons Dying of Heart Disease, United States, 1967	223
14-2	Prevalence of Chronic Disabling Conditions By Age	224
18-1	Key Impact Questions	309

Contributors

(The) Artificial Heart Assessment Panel of the National Heart and Lung Institute was formed to assess artificial heart devices and their clinical application. Its purpose was to explore the implications of the totally implantable artificial heart that warranted research, study and discussion, to investigate the effects of these devices on the individual's quality of life, and to identify the ethical issues involved in the use of this technology. Reprinted here are excerpts from the June 1973 report.

Roy Branson is a Senior Research Scholar at the Joseph and Rose Kennedy Institute for the Study of Human Reproduction and Bioethics, Georgetown University. He holds a Ph.D. in Religious Ethics from Harvard University. He has published in journals such as *Encounter, Journal of Religious Ethics* and the *Hastings Center Report.*

Daniel Callahan is Director of the Institute of Society, Ethics and the Life Sciences. He holds a Ph.D. in philosophy from Harvard University. He is author of *The Tyranny of Survival* and *Abortion: Law, Choice and Morality*. His essay is also included in a forthcoming book edited by Florian Stuber and Michael Mooney. To be published by Columbia University Press.

James F. Childress is Joseph P. Kennedy, Sr. Professor of Christian Ethics in the Center for Bioethics of the Kennedy Institute at Georgetown University. He holds a Ph.D. degree from Yale University and was formerly Chairman of the Department of Religious Studies at the University of Virginia. He is the author of *Civil Disobedience and Political Obligation* and co-editor of *Secularization and the Protestant Prospect*. His essay is reprinted, with permission, from *Soundings* 43 (Winter, 1970), pp. 339-55.

Rashi Fein, Professor of the Economics of Medicine, is a staff member at the Center for Community Health and Medical Care, Harvard Medical School. He has a Ph.D. degree from The Johns Hopkins University and is the author of *Economics of Mental Illness; The Doctor Shortage: An Economic Diagnosis; Financing Medical Education: An Analysis of Alternative Policies and Mechanisms* (with Gerald Weber); and *A Right to Health: The Problem of Access to Primary Medical Care* (with Charles Lewis and David Mechanic, in press). His essay originally appeared in Gordon McLachlon and Thomas McKeown (eds.), *Medical History and Medical Care* (London: Oxford University Press, 1971, pp. 181-217) and is reprinted with permission from Nuffield Provincial Hospitals Trust, London, England.

Joseph Fletcher is Robert Treat Paine Professor, Emeritus, Episcopal Theological School, and Visiting professor, Medical Ethics at the University of Virginia and the Graduate School of Biomedical Sciences, University of Texas. He has an S.T.D. degree from Kenyon College and is the author of *Morals and Medicine* and *The Ethics of Genetic Control.*

Ronald M. Green is Assistant Professor in the Department of Religion at Dartmouth College. He holds a Ph.D. in Religious Ethics from Harvard University and is the author of *Population Growth and Justice.*

Clark C. Havighurst is Professor of Law and Director of the Program on Legal Issues in Health Care, Duke University School of Law, and was a member of the Artificial Heart Assessment Panel. His comments on the Artificial Heart Assessment Panel's report are included in that volume.

André E. Hellegers, M.D., is Professor of Obstetrics-Gynecology and Physiology-Biophysics, Georgetown University Medical School; and is Director, The Joseph and Rose Kennedy Institute for the Study of Human Reproduction and Bio-ethics, Georgetown University. Dr. Hellegers has published extensively in the area of obstetrics, physiology, demography and bioethics. His essay, co-authored with Albert R. Jonsen, originally appeared in the volume *Ethics of Health Care*, edited by Laurence R. Tancredi, (Washington, D.C.: National Academy of Sciences, 1974, pp. 3-20) and is reprinted with permission.

Albert R. Jonsen is Associate Professor of Bioethics, Health Policy Program and Departments of Medicine and Pediatrics, School of Medicine, University of California at San Francisco. He is a member of the National Commission on the Protection of Human Subjects and was a member of the Artificial Heart Assessment Panel. He holds a Ph.D. degree from Yale University. His essay co-authored with André E. Hellegers originally appeared in the volume *Ethics of Health Care*, edited by Laurence R. Tancredi, (Washington, D.C.: National Academy of Sciences, 1974, pp. 3-20) and is reprinted with permission.

Gene Outka is Associate Professor of Religious Ethics in the Department of Religious Studies and in the Divinity School, Yale University. He holds a B.D. and a Ph.D. from Yale University. He is the author of *Agape: An Ethical Analysis* and co-editor of *Norm and Context in Christian Ethics* and of *Religion and Morality*. His essay is reprinted, with permission, from the *Journal of Religious Ethics* 2 (Spring, 1974), pp. 11-32.

Paul Ramsey is Harrington Spear Paine Professor of Religion at Princeton University. He holds a B.D. and a Ph.D. from Yale University. He is author of *The Patient as Person: Explorations in Medical Ethics, The Ethics of Fetal Research,* and *Fabricated Man: The Ethics of Genetic Control.* An abbreviated version of his essay originally appeared in the volume *Ethics of Health Care,* Laurence R. Tancredi (ed.), (Washington, D.C.: National Academy of Sciences, 1974, pp. 21-29) and is reprinted with permission.

Ruth Sidel is a psychiatric social worker and is author of *Women and Child Care in China* and *Families of Fengsheng: Urban Life in China.* She has an M.S.W. degree from the Boston University School of Social Work. Her essay, co-authored with Victor Sidel, first appeared under the title "Medicine in China: Individual and Society" in the *Hastings Center Studies* 2 (No. 3, September 1974), pp. 23-36.

Victor Sidel is Chairman, Department of Social Medicine, Montefiore Hospital and Medical Center and Professor of Community Health, Albert Einstein College of Medicine. He holds an M.D. degree from Harvard University, and is author (with Ruth Sidel) of *Serve the People: Observations on Medicine in the People's Republic of China.*

Peter Singer is Senior Lecturer in the Department of Philosophy at La Trobe University in Australia. He holds a B. Phil. degree from Oxford and an M.A. from the University of Melbourne. His essay, included here, is also forthcoming in a volume to be released by Battelle Institute entitled

Peter Steinfels is Associate for the Humanities at the Institute of Society, Ethics and the Life Sciences and Editor of its journal, the *Hastings Center Report*. He is co-editor of *Death Inside Out*.

Laurelyn Veatch holds an M.A. in political science from the University of California, Berkeley, and an M.A. in sociology from the New School for Social Research. Her essay first appeared under the title "Community Boards in Search of Authority" in the *Hastings Center Report* 5 (No. 5, October 1975), pp. 23-30.

Robert M. Veatch is Associate for Medical Ethics at the Institute of Society, Ethics and the Life Sciences. He has an M.S. in pharmacology from the University of California Medical Center, San Francisco, and a Ph.D. in medical ethics from Harvard University. He is the editor (with Willard Gaylin and Councilman Morgan) of *The Teaching of Medical Ethics* and (with Peter Steinfels) of *Death Inside Out*.

LeRoy Walters is Director of the Center for Bioethics of the Joseph and Rose Kennedy Institute for the Study of Human Reproduction and Bioethics, Georgetown University, and a member of Georgetown's Department of Philosophy. He holds a Ph.D. in ethics from Yale University and is editor of the annual *Bibliography of Bioethics*. He has published essays on medical confidentiality, fetal research, and the just-war tradition. His essay in this volume is reprinted, with permission, from *Theological Studies* 33 (No. 4, December 1972), pp. 666-683.

Frederic B. Westervelt is Chief, Renal Division, Department of Medicine, University of Virginia School of Medicine, and Director, Renal Unit, University of Virginia Medical Center. He holds an M.D. degree from the University of Virginia. His essay is reprinted, with permission, from *Soundings* 43 (Winter, 1970), pp. 356-362.

Introduction

In the Hippocratic Oath the physician pledges that he will benefit the patient according to his ability and judgment. Even if the modern physician has not read the oath since medical school, that aggressive commitment to the individual patient has remained dominant in the modern Western medicine, especially in its American expression. This is not to say that commitment to the patient has always remained first on the mind of every physician, but it has continued to be the ethical ideal by which physicians and others have judged medical care. This has tended to make medical ethics, especially physician ethics, focus on the problems of the individual patient-physician relationship. What the patient should be told; when, if ever, treatment should be stopped on a terminally ill patient; when, if ever, a confidence should be broken; whether it is acceptable to perform an abortion—these have been core problems.

While this focus on the ethical problems of the individual patient-physician relationship has a certain compatibility with the individualism of American society, several forces have recently made us reexamine and broaden our concern for ethics in a medical context. First, in the past several decades medicine has really begun to potently affect people's health in a positive and predictable way. This has meant that the stakes have become much higher. The public is now aggressively interested in how and to whom health care gets delivered. Second, with the evolution of systematic medical research, individuals were, for the first time, receiving medical attention for the good of others. An old ethic which said that the physician's duty was to benefit the patient was incompatible with research designed to gain knowledge primarily for the benefit of others. Third, systematic health planning began to emerge, if not as a science, at least as an organized effort by academics and government officials. Growing out of

McNamara's Defense Department policy analysis in the 1960s, cost-benefit analysis has been used increasingly in health policy planning at the federal level. Based on the conviction that cost-benefit ratios are always estimated, at least intuitively, and ought to be as accurate as possible, elaborate techniques for policy comparisons have emerged. The premises of government officials calculating the benefits and costs of alternative health policies for a society are radically different from those of the individual patient or physician choosing among alternative courses of treatment. The Hippocratic injunction that the physician should benefit his patient can be of little help to the health planner at the National Institutes of Health. Fourth, and perhaps most significant, there has been a fundamental change in American society. An interest in human rights and social justice, kindled first by the issues of race and war, has spread to other areas of social policy including health. The public concern for questions of justice and welfare has led us to challenge traditional assumptions and traditional ethical premises. The questions now being asked are more health policy questions, questions of distribution and priority. They are fundamentally questions of social and political ethics, not those of the individual patient-physician relationship, and they are more and more being asked by patients, citizens, and governmental officials who have never shared the values of the Hippocratic tradition. The movement toward national health insurance is one example of health-policy questioning focusing upon ethical questions that cannot be avoided. Planning for national policies on hemodialysis machines and artificial hearts is another.

Those who have explored the borders between ethics and health policy have had to adjust. For some it was a major shift of attention, for others it has been a readjustment of interests in disciplines that were already social in nature: social ethics, economics, law, and the other social and policy sciences. The Institute of Society, Ethics and the Life Sciences, in an effort to respond to this shift, established a Research Group on Ethics and Health Policy under a grant from the Robert Wood Johnson Foundation. One of our first discoveries was that there was virtually no source where the ethical problems of health policy were discussed systematically. Some articles were beginning to appear, but these often dealt only with special issues, and were difficult to obtain. One of our first efforts has been to collect together in one accessible source a wide-ranging group of explorations of the ethical problems of health-policy planning and health-care delivery. This collection, together with several of the original essays in the volume—those by Branson, Fletcher, Green, Callahan, Steinfels, and Robert and Laurelyn Veatch—were prepared with the support of the Johnson Foundation, which is gratefully acknowledged. We also appreciate the help of Patricia Pierce and Nancy Taylor in the preparation of the manuscript.

Robert M. Veatch and Roy Branson

**Part I:
Health Care Delivery:
Fundamental Ethical
Conflicts**

Section A:
The Patient and Society

PREAMBLE

Medicine has traditionally been aggressively patient centered. The physician's duty (whether or not he lives up to it) is thought to be to do what he thinks will benefit the patient—in the singular. That physician is not only permitted, he is really obligated to ignore the interests of the greater society. The physician, qua physician, ought not to mix social, political, and economic considerations with his care for his patient. Yet in a complex and expensive national health care system the social impact cannot be ignored. Research requires using normal volunteer research subjects for the interests of society; national policy-makers cannot write a blank check.

The four chapters in this section offer four serious but radically different approaches to this classical conflict in political philosophy between the individual and society. In the first, Roy Branson introduces the debate, revealing that medical- and bioethics has traditionally been locked into an individualistic perspective because of the individualistic perspective of those who have defined the problems in medical ethics: physicians and other health care professionals. In the second chapter, Albert Jonsen and André Hellegers argue that medical ethics has focused almost exclusively on the virtues of the good doctor, to the exclusion of what they call a theory of duties and a theory of justice. They maintain that these are essential to any complete ethical stance. To ignore them is to ignore many of the social conflicts of health care. Paul Ramsey, in a rebuttal to Jonsen and Hellegers, stands as a defender of the more traditional approach of medical ethics. He argues that an ethic for health care can, at least in large part, be derived from "that quite personal situation of one qualified practitioner in relation to one other, suffering human being." In the final chapter of this section Victor and Ruth Sidel give us a glimpse of medicine in a society with a radically different political philosophy. Medicine in China, they reveal, has addressed the question of the relation between the individual and society and come up with some fascinating and provocative answers.

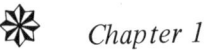 *Chapter 1*

The Scope of Bioethics: Individual and Social

Roy Branson

Bioethics must identify issues and problems according to the full range of considerations appropriate to ethics. Like other disciplines outside the natural sciences concerned with medicine, such as the history of medicine and sociology of medicine, bioethics can become preoccupied with questions about individual, personal behavior typically and understandably raised by physicians and researchers. However, if bioethics is clear that it includes social ethics, it will feel obligated to deal with questions of how medical institutions ought to be organized; how they should relate to one another and to other institutions in society.

The fields of history of medicine and sociology of medicine provide models for the evolution of bioethics. For years a debate has raged within the history of medicine about the appropriate scope of its subject matter. Despite the social concerns during the thirties and forties of Henry Sigerist, the prominent director of the influential Johns Hopkins Institute of the History of Medicine, much of medical history has been written by physicians recounting the exploits of individual scientists or clinicians.

But certain physician-historians are clear that the history of medicine should be intimately involved in social history. Edwin C. Clarke in a summary essay to his *Modern Methods in the History of Medicine*, argues that science is not the sole focus of the historian of medicine, because medicine's purpose is finally not scientific, but the health of man.

> As all of medicine and its associated technologies are directed towards man in health and disease, it would seem to follow naturally that the history of

medicine should have the same nucleus. This in essence means that medical history proper should be compounded of all the scientific and social aspects of human health and of disease.[1]

Agreeing that the history of medicine must expand into the history of health, John C. Greene, a social historian, insists that the historian of medicine has gone well beyond recounting the achievements of individual physicians. It is imperative that "the medical historian studies the history of a social institution or complex of social institutions."[2]

The debate concerning the proper scope of the history of medicine began in the late thirties and forties. In the fifties a similar debate started when the sociology of medicine began to organize itself in the United States, and has continued to this day.

Eliot Freidson, founding editor of the *Journal of Health and Social Behavior*, argues strenuously that the sociologist should not limit himself to the perspective of medicine for at least two reasons. First, "while medicine has a foundation in scientific knowledge, its characteristics as a social institution lead it inevitably to have a distorted view of itself, its knowledge, and its mission." Secondly, the sociologist should not get trapped in "the characteristic emphasis of medical science on the biological process taking place within the individual organism and the characteristic common-sense individualism that lies at the heart of the approach of the medical profession to itself."[3]

Sociology of medicine is most distinctly functioning as sociology when it takes as its prime unit of analysis, not the individual body, mind, or even whole person, but those structures of organized interrelationships called "institutions." As a result, Freidson insists that for him "the organization of medical care is to be considered to be the central issue for a sociological analysis of medicine."[4]

Twenty years after the history of medicine "came of age" and ten years after the formal organization of the sociology of medicine, ethics also found itself facing new and urgent problems in relating a humanistic discipline to medicine and the natural sciences. Not that there had been no medical ethics before the sixties, of course. There had been, and it was dominated by physicians. For centuries physicians assumed that they would draw up codes of ethics for themselves. From Hippocrates (400 B.C.) to the Principles of Medical Ethics of the American Medical Association (1957) physicians have articulated sets of specific rules governing the doctor's relationship to his patient and to other physicians. In the nineteenth and twentieth centuries physicians wrote essays and books on a topic they called "medical ethics," though some others have said that much of their work might more accurately be called "medical etiquette." Except for certain religiously sponsored medical schools, references to medical ethics in the medical school curriculum typically concentrated on physicians' own understanding of their obligations to each other and their individual patients. The codes of medical ethics specified how a doctor should act; but, even more, what kind of person he should be. Jonsen and Hellegers argue that in the long tradition of ethical codes in medicine, the "vision of the 'upright man instructed in the art of healing' predominates"; that indeed "exhortations to virtue constitute the heart of code ethics."[5]

When Van Rensselaer Potter, a cancer researcher who claimed he "invented a new word and a new scholastic enterprise called Bioethics"[6] by writing a book with that title in 1971, explained the focus he wanted for the new discipline of bioethics, he made it clear that he expected it to carry on the traditional task of medical ethics: to help individual scientists to be better men. "The individual physician who's doing clinical experimentation needs help and he wants help in arriving at a personal ethic that will help him to be able to live with himself." He ends his book with a "Bioethical Creed for individuals," which includes six beliefs and commitments. He hoped that "if the Bioethical Creed as individual belief were acceptable to a substantial fraction of influential scientists in different parts of the world, others would perhaps gain the courage to join in a worldwide movement," which would in turn support efforts to convert "the proposed mores into rational action."[7]

For all his possible differences with Potter, Daniel Callahan, director of the Institute for Society, Ethics, and the Life Sciences, sometimes sounds as though he also wants the scope of bioethics to remain what it has always been: medical ethics to aid the physician trying to decide how he should relate to individual patients. Callahan recounts with chagrin the time a group of physicians asked for a quick, definite answer to a difficult case, and he found that as an ethicist "when faced with an actual case ... there was nothing whatever in my philosophical training which had prepared me to make a flat, clear-cut ethical decision at a given hour on a given afternoon."[8] He wants to make sure that bioethics "enables those who employ it to reach reasonably specific, clear decisions in those instances which require them—in the case of what is to be done about Mrs. Jones by four o'clock tomorrow afternoon, after which she will either live or die depending upon the decision made."[9]

Paul Ramsey, one of the country's best known ethicists, in his now standard work, *The Patient as Person*, assumes that the scope of topics bioethics analyzes will remain limited to the sphere of the physician and research scientist. The ethicist should reflect on basic principles, but on principles relevant to "the question, What ought the doctor to do?"[10] While Ramsey wants bioethics to retain its autonomy, he is willing for physicians and scientists to select the topics for theoretical reflection.

As in history or sociology of medicine, focusing on the problems of the physician seems inevitably to limit ethics to the personal. As an ethicist, Ramsey is concerned to isolate and refine from a variety of medical settings a more accurate understanding of a principle such as informed consent. But these contexts (with an exception that we will examine later) raise the issue of informed consent because the problem is fidelity between individuals: the researcher and an infant subject of an experiment, the physician and a hopelessly dying patient, the surgeon and a potential donor of an organ for a transplant. The title of his book fits its scope perfectly. As he says, his volume "is addressed to patients as persons, to physicians of patients who are persons."[11] Ramsey is not concerned with what ethical principles demand of the structure of health care in the nation. His focus in medicine is individual ethics.

Several ethicists since Ramsey's book appeared have called for bioethics to become involved in social ethics. Richard McCormick complains:

> We have been accustomed to think of "medico-moral problems" in terms of decisions about procedures touching the health and life of individual patients. In this sense medical ethics has suffered from the individualism which has infected ethics in general. It has equivalently excluded a whole crucial domain from the area of ethical concern, or at least it has not given proportionate attention to this area.[12]

Jonsen and Hellegers feel that bioethics as individual ethics might have been adequate when medical practice was "a solo physician diagnosing and treating a single patient," but not when "accepted forms of diagnosis and treatment, of research, of prevention, engage the manufacture of products, the construction of buildings, and the enactment of laws." They insist that "the institutionalization of practice and profession calls for an institutional ethic."[13]

With the awareness increasing that the scope of bioethics should expand beyond studying the obligations of one individual to another, it may be helpful to distinguish between two other categories of ethical reflection: analysis of the responsibilities of institutions to individuals, and analysis of the responsibilities of institutions to other institutions. Certainly more work needs to be done on how not only practicing physicians but hospitals and other medical institutions should guarantee the rights of the individuals they serve. But ethical research on those topics does not reach the issues of how medical institutions ought to relate to one another or to other systems of institutions involved in health care in the nation.

The purpose of distinguishing within bioethics among what might be called individual, institutional, and interinstitutional ethics is not to freeze topics in one category or another. Some problems flow back and forth from the individual to the interinstitutional. But bioethicists should be as ready to consult with policy-makers struggling with questions of fairness in health-care systems as they are with physicians and research scientists.

It is possible to illustrate the differences among individual, institutional, and interinstitutional dimensions in bioethics by studying how a single ethical concept like consent operates in each of the three categories.

Ramsey relates informed consent within the relationship of an individual doctor and an individual patient to basic ethical considerations.

> The principle of an informed consent is a statement of the fidelity between the man who performs medical procedures and the man on whom they are presented.... Fidelity is the bond between consenting man and consenting man in these procedures. The principle of an informed consent is the cardinal *canon of loyalty* joining men together in medical practice and investigation. In this requirement, faithfulness among men—the faithfulness that is normative for all the covenants or moral bonds of life with life—gains specification for the primary relations peculiar to medical practice.[14]

Having done what he understands an academic ethicist should do, relate general ethical theory to a principle in bioethics, Ramsey proceeds to analyze specific ways in which informed consent ought to govern both experimentation and therapy in the doctor-patient relationship. There is a negative aspect and a positive one. Negatively, informed consent is a restraint on the physician. "No man is good enough to experiment upon another without his consent. The same can be said of the doctor-patient relation having treatment in view."[15] Positively, the doctor and patient are embarked on a "joint venture in which patient and physician can say and ideally should both say, 'I cure.' "[16]

Ramsey does go on to describe informed consent in ways that could contribute to a more social ethical analysis within bioethics, but he does not pursue the possibility. He himself does not develop the institutional implications of statements such as "Integrity still needs to be sustained in its setting in a system of medical 'checks and balances' anchored in the requirement of consent,"[17] or "Informed consent alone exhibits and establishes medical practice and investigation as a voluntary association of free men in a common cause."[18]

Since Ramsey's book appeared, others have proceeded to discuss how not only individual physicians but medical institutions can make informed consent more of a reality. The Department of Health, Education and Welfare made a complex set of proposals in 1973 for creating a network of review committees in both university research institutions and the government to protect the right of experimental subjects to informed consent. The Kennedy Institute, Center for Bioethics, in turn, wrote a detailed analysis of whether such institutionalized populations as infants, the mentally retarded, or prisoners could, in fact, give informed consent within DHEW's guidelines, or any others. Its analysis of the institutional checks and balances that are needed to protect any possibility of informed consent recommended a clarification of the power of ethical review boards to overrule a scientific review board's approval of proposed research. The report also suggested that categories of membership on ethical review boards consenting to medical experimentation be reconstituted so that the majority on such panels did not come from the medical community conducting the research but from the nonmedical population providing subjects for experimentation.[19]

Another concrete example of a study exploring how medical institutions might organize themselves more properly to protect the right of individuals to informed consent is Budd Shenkin and David Warner's suggestion to hospitals: "Giving the Patient His Medical Record: A Proposal to Improve the System," which appeared in an issue of the *New England Journal of Medicine*.

> We propose that legislation be passed to require that complete and unexpurgated copy of all medical records both inpatient and outpatient, be issued routinely and automatically to patients as soon as the services provided are recorded. The legislation should also require that physician and hospital qualifications (accreditations, memberships, etc.) and charges for services be recorded. Hospital records should be available regularly to patients on the ward, and copies sent to them upon termination of hospitalization.[20]

Pointing out that only three states now allow patients direct access to their own medical records, they declare that availability of records would enable patients to be much more autonomous in making judgments and choices. Now "patients have little opportunity to exercise informed free choice of physicians in either primary or secondary care.... Adopting the Proposal would free patients to choose and change physicians more easily ... to differentiate legitimate physicians from quacks."[21] But they think that their proposal would not only (negatively) put limits on the physician, it would increase positively the patient's sense of participating and sharing the process of healing with a physician now more trusted because of his candor.

Shenkin and Warner are aware that their proposal fits into a more comprehensive analysis of how the entire institutional structure of health care might be more responsive to the will of patients—actual and potential. They recognize that their proposal goes beyond peer review to public review of a most decentralized sort; that "published guides to medical care would soon flourish, and professional consultant services for records 'translation,' interpretation and evaluation would arise in response to consumer demand."[22] They acknowledge that physicians will immediately fear the greater exposure to malpractice suits, though they are not likely to be exposed to more unjustified litigation. Since, however, they are limiting themselves to a specific proposal for how hospitals might change their policy for writing medical records in order to allow the patient to give a more fully informed and free consent, they do not explore how systems of medical review boards or malpractice compensation ought to be organized in order to make the consent of the public more possible.

The DHEW Secretary's Commission on Medical Malpractice tried to accomplish just that task. Consent is a central consideration throughout the commission's 1973 report. It first of all endorses informed consent as the right of individual patients, then proceeds to endorse one institutional arrangement for protecting that right. "The commission finds that patients have a right to the information contained in their medical records." The commission stops short of Shenkin and Warner's proposal, however, recommending that the records be provided to "legal representative, public or private, without having to file suit."[23]

The commission could not bring itself to recommend another major reordering of the relationship of medical, commercial, and legal institutions to each other: the adoption of a no-fault malpractice compensation system. It cited the difficulty of defining a medical accident, and also the greater cost involved in no-fault malpractice insurance over the present system. It left uncriticized an elaborate proposal for no-fault medical insurance it had itself commissioned. At one point the commission had taken the position that its primary concern was fairness both to patients and to health-care providers, but evidently it concluded that relating that criterion to no-fault malpractice was indeed beyond its competence. In effect, it threw up its hands and said that the issue would have to be decided within the context of debates over the even more comprehensive issue of nation health insurance. "The form that insurance program takes will undoubtedly alter significantly the impact that the malpractice problem has on all concerned. To the degree that it covers the cost of remedial medicine and hospital care, such insurance should help alleviate the problem."[24]

Another way to illustrate the differences among individual, institutional, and interinstitutional dimensions in bioethics is to study how a single scientific subject, such as heart research, brings a variety of ethical principles into the discussion. As one might expect, Paul Ramsey sees transplants as a prismatic problem for ethical theory.

> The chief principle governing in medical investigations is that they shall proceed only after an informed and free consent has been obtained. This means that donor and recipient alike must consent to heart transplant. . . . It is this canon of loyalty between physician-investigator and patient-subject—and not any other that I can think of—which may have been violated in some or many, if not all, of the heart transplants to date.[25]

Ramsey, as an ethicist, relates a problem in medicine to not only a central principle in bioethics, but normative ethics generally.

The issue that precipitated his discussion involved relations between individuals. Although it can be, informed consent is not always a principle that is directly relevant to questions of how institutions should treat patients. For instance, how should specialty groups in hospitals decide who should receive heart transplants or artificial hearts? On this issue Ramsey steps beyond individual ethics into institutional ethics and does not cite informed consent. He (and James Childress independently) developed the principle of random selection. Rejecting suggestions that selection should be on the basis of the patient's social worth, Ramsey argues that "the equal right of every human being to live, and not relative personal or social worth, should be the ruling principle. When not all can be saved and all need not die, this ruling principle can be applied only or best by random choice among equals."[26] When the issue of heart research moves from individual-to-individual relations to questions of how institutions should fairly disburse their resources, Ramsey finds it necessary to broaden his theoretical resources. His discussion shifts from informed consent as a specification of fidelity and loyalty in individual relationships to random selection as a form of equality in an institutional setting.

But Ramsey will go no further. He will not outline an ethical framework within which institutions might relate to each other in a more just system of health care. Indeed, he comes close to saying no one can do so. "The larger questions of medical and social priorities are almost, if not altogether, incorrigible to moral reasoning."[27]

When Albert Jonsen found himself as the one ethicist on a National Heart and Lung Institute panel to study the totally implantable artificial heart, he discovered a consensus supporting random selection of recipients. However, Ramsey's words proved almost prophetic when the panel faced the broader social ethical question of whether to recommend approval of plans by research institutions to develop a convenient, efficient nuclear-powered heart or to set limits on those research institutions because of fears that families of recipients would be exposed to radiation. At this and other critical points Jonsen later complained that "the Panel could not draw on any sustained stream of critical thought on the nature and purpose of technology assessment, especially when it is charged with ethical judgments."[28]

Nevertheless the panel proceeded to suggest methods of evaluating the artificial heart. Although it earlier acknowledged certain limitations to utilitarian philosophy, the panel discussed "methodologies for evaluation and comparison," and relied on a rather obvious utilitarianism. It recognized that other considerations were needed—"Introspection and intuition have been and will continue to be important elements of the evaluation process." What was fundamentally required, however, was a quantification of a population's values.

> Few would disagree that the quality of intuitive judgments can be improved by reliance on additional information gained from non-introspective processes. In particular, there is good reason for seeking information on the value weights that would be assigned to various advantages and disadvantages by the individuals to whom they accrue. The significance of these weights for our decision is that they serve as quantitative measures of the extent to which each advantage (disadvantage) contributes to (detracts from) individual well-being. If the sum of any individual's value weights for the advantages arising from a particular action were greater than the sum of his (negative) value weights for the disadvantages we could conclude that the action will improve his well-being.... The best we can hope for, in considering an issue as complex as the use of artificial hearts, is to obtain some very crude "ballpark" figures.[29]

Jonsen and a minority of the panel vigorously disassociated themselves from this section of the report, saying "they regarded this kind of exercise as a numbers game."[30]

Many ethicists might concur with Jonsen when he concludes after serving on the panel that

> Ethics must learn to speak the language of public policy.... Problems of distributive justice, which this development raises in a vivid way, must be debated in the public forum. As health and health policy become absorbing issues of public interest, the formulation of a "coherent conceptual framework" for ethical analysis and debate become both indispensable and challenging.[31]

Ramsey himself no doubt sees the need for such analysis, but he has been so concerned that ethicists would become involved in balancing rights against benefits for society in a crude utilitarianism that he has shunned the social ethics of biomedicine. He is even wary of utilitarian tendencies when Jonsen and Hellegers call for bioethics to give greater consideration to the justice of networks of health care institutions. He is suspicious of their appeal to justice in terms of the "common good," especially when they contrast a theory of the common good with a theory of duty and obligation.

Ramsey can be no happier than anyone else at the prospect of a range of policies in health care being justified on unsatisfactory ethical grounds—issues like the importation of physicians to the United States from developing countries, or plans for distributing physicians throughout the United States. But he might well feel that there is no point in ethicists exploring the possibility of becoming professional consultants to policy-makers, as some have already begun to do with physicians and research scientists, unless the academic discipline of ethics develops concepts as helpful to interinstitutional analysis as informed consent and random selection have proved to be for the individual and institutional ethics of medicine.

One of Ramsey's colleagues at Princeton, Gene Outka, has taken the occasion of the debate over health maintenance organizations to explore the possibilities of articulating one such principle: equal access to health care.[32] Essential physical needs are understood as given rather than acquired, as fortuitous rather than deserved. Varying needs are appreciated as requiring varying amounts of treatments in order to maintain equality.

On the other hand, similar cases of physical need should receive similar care. Income or geographic distinction do not alter the category of physical need, and are considered irrelevant. Justice, then, requires equal access to similar medical treatment for similar cases of physical need, irrespective of such differences as wealth or place of residence.

Outka draws some general implications of his ethical principle for the issue of health maintenance organizations, and endorses their being at least one of the country's health care systems. Whatever one may think of health maintenance organizations and Outka's defense of them, he has formulated an ethical principle that illuminatingly relates nonutilitarian normative theory to interinstitutional issues in bioethics.

Outka's effort, and other articles in this book, are examples of how ethical theory appears to be providing greater resources for social ethical analysis than that of merely commending the use of a utilitarian calculus.

Professor John Rawls's book *A Theory of Justice*,[33] which proposes an alternative to utilitarianism, has been called "the most substantial and interesting contribution to moral philosophy since the war," and "part of a recent movement of thought among philosophers away from the skepticism about rationality in ethics."[34] Ramsey, welcoming Rawls's book as "a super dreadnought sent out to do battle with the last remnants of Utilitarianism," says "it bids fair to become the outstanding work on ethics published in this century."[35] Essays in this volume debate Rawls's views at length. Whatever their use of or quarrel with his work, they take seriously the priorities he sets out for ethics. If bioethics were to follow Rawls, it would not simply add the interinstitutional concerns of social ethics to its agenda; bioethics would make certain that considerations of social justice at least logically took precedence over analysis of individual obligations.

Rawls clearly states that the basic principles governing society should be established before deciding individual cases.

> The principles for the basic structure of society are to be agreed to first, principles for individuals next.... The important thing is that the various principles are to be adopted in a definite sequence.... The sequence in either case reflects the fact that obligations presuppose principles for social forms.... For this reason, it seems simpler to adopt all principles for individuals after those for the basic structure. That principles for institutions are chosen first shows the social nature of the virtue of justice.... A person's obligations and duties presuppose a moral conception of institutions and therefore that the content of just institutions must be defended before the requirements for individuals can be set out. And this is to say that, in most cases, the principles for obligations and duties should be settled upon after those for the basic structure.[36]

The passage is worth quoting at some length because Rawls remains consistent throughout his book to this method of moral reasoning; a careful movement from general to specific.

Rawls would presumably believe that the first task of bioethics attempting to rely on justice as fairness would be to create a just structure of health care. The institutional and individual obligations would be affected by making particular determinations within such a just framework.

Daniel Callahan has called for a new culture with a fresh ethic "suffusing its laws, customs, institutional arrangements, political life and super-ego." With such an ethic, human beings would be able to live and die "securely, harmoniously and humanely in the presence of constant technological advances in the medical and biological sciences."[37]

Ethics is not creating a culture with a new set of attitudes or behavior patterns, but it is attempting a more modest task: clarifying notions of normative ethics. As this process continues, bioethics will respond to not only problems faced by individual physicians or patients, but also the interinstitutional issues of medicine and health care delivery. As it does so, bioethics will broaden to encompass considerations of social justice, thereby more accurately reflecting the full scope of ethics.

Notes to Chapter One

1. Edwin C. Clarke, Ed., *Modern Methods in the History of Medicine* (London: The Athlone Press of the University of London, 1971), p. 201.

2. John C. Greene, "The History of Medicine as a Part of the University Complex," in *Education in the History of Medicine*, ed. by John B. Blake (New York: Hafner Publishing Co., 1968), p. 97.

3. Eliot Freidson, *Professional Dominance: The Social Structure of Medical Care* (New York: Atherton Press, 1970), p. 55.

4. Ibid., p. 57.

5. Albert Jonsen and André Hellegers, "Conceptual Foundations for an Ethics of Medical Care," Chapter Two of this volume (pp. xx-xx).

6. Van Rensselaer Potter, "Bioethics for Whom?" and "General Discussion II," *Annals of the New York Academy of Science* 196 (1972), pp. 200-05, 243-46.

7. Van Rensselaer Potter, *Bioethics: Bridge to the Future* (Englewood Cliffs, N.J.: Prentice-Hall, 1971), p. 94.

8. Daniel Callahan, "Bioethics as a Discipline," *Hastings Center Studies* 1/1:ix, 66-73 (1973), 68.

9. Ibid., p. 72.

10. Paul Ramsey, *The Patient as Person: Exploration in Medical Ethics* (New Haven: Yale University Press, 1970), p. xi.

11. Ibid.

12. Richard McCormick, "Issue Areas for a Medical Ethics Program," pp. 103-114 in *The Teaching of Medical Ethics*, ed. by Veatch, Gaylin, and Morgan (New York: Institute of Society Ethics and the Life Sciences, 1973), p. 112.

13. Jonsen and Hellegers.

14. Ramsey, p. 69.

15. Ibid., p. 7.

16. Ibid., p. 6.

17. Ibid., p. 8.

18. Ibid., p. 11.

19. Roy Branson, et al., "A Preliminary Analysis of the Draft DHEW Guidelines for the Protection of Special Subjects in Biomedical Research," unpublished paper written at the Joseph and Rose Kennedy Institute for the Study of Human Reproduction and Bioethics, Washington, D.C., 1974.

20. Budd Shenkin and David Warner, "Giving the Patient His Medical Record: A Proposal to Improve the System," *New England Journal of Medicine* 289/13, 688-92 (September 27, 1973), 688.

21. Ibid., p. 689.

22. Ibid.

23. Department of Health, Education and Welfare, "Medical Malpractice: Report of the Secretary's Commission on Medical Malpractice," DHEW Publication No. (OS) 73-88 (January 16, 1973), 74, 77.

24. Ibid., p. 101.

25. Ramsey, p. 222.

26. Ibid., p. 256.

27. Ibid., p. 240.

28. Albert R. Jonsen, "The Totally Implantable Artificial Heart," *Hastings Center Report* 3/5, 1-4 (November 1973), 4.

29. Department of Health, Education and Welfare, "Report of the Artificial Heart Assessment Panel of the National Heart and Lung Institute," DHEW Publication No. (NIH) 74-191 (June 1973), 94, 95.

30. Ibid., p. 94.

31. Jonsen, p. 4.

32. Gene Outka, "Social Justice and Equal Access to Health Care," Chapter Five of this volume, pp. xx-xx.

33. John Rawls, *A Theory of Justice* (Cambridge: Harvard University Press, 1971).

34. Stuart Hampshire, "A New Philosophy of the Just Society," *The New York Review of Books* (February 24, 1972), 34-35.

35. Paul Ramsey, "The Nature of Medical Ethics," 14-28 in *The Teaching of Medical Ethics*, ed. by Veatch, Gaylin, and Morgan (New York: Institute of Society Ethics and the Life Sciences, 1973), p. 27.

36. Rawls, p. 110.

37. Daniel Callahan, *The Tyranny of Survival* (New York: Macmillan, 1973), p. 155.

Chapter 2

Conceptual Foundations for an Ethics of Medical Care

Albert R. Jonsen and André E. Hellegers

Medical ethics is currently a muddle. Many questions are asked, but few are answered. Many anxieties are aired, but few are assuaged. Worst of all, the diversity of subjects discussed and the variety of arguments propounded makes one wonder whether there is any proper subject matter or proper methodology deserving the name "medical ethics."

During July 1973, when this essay was first conceived, the newspapers carried three major (and many minor) stories about "medical ethics." In New York, a respected physician was accused of injecting potassium chloride into his dying cancer patient. In Chicago, the American Medical Association commented on the standards governing the ownership of stock in pharmaceutical companies by individual physicians and by the association itself. In Aiken, South Carolina, three obstetricians refused, for what they called "social reasons," to deliver the babies of welfare mothers unless the mothers submitted to sterilization. All three stories were headlined "medical ethics." Euthanasia, financial investments, sterilization for social reasons: all three concerning behavior by physicians, all three pertaining, immediately or remotely, to the practice of medicine. This may justify the praenomen "medical." But what justifies the surname "ethics"?

This chapter is called "Conceptual Foundations for an Ethics of Medical Care." The title, while rather grandiose, refers to the modest task of stating the propriety of denominating certain sorts of considerations medical "ethics" or the "ethics" of medical care. This chapter was designed as a roadmap for a conference on health care and changing values, to provide to its participants the main features of the topography of that ancient realm of the mind called "ethics," through which modern medicine must travel.

Popularly, ethics seems to mean any body of prescriptions and prohibitions, dos and don'ts, that persons consider to carry uncommon weight in their lives. When their lives are deeply involved in certain activities, ethics can refer to the rules that guide those activities. The *Lexicon* of the Sydenham Society defined "ethics, medical" as "the laws of the duties of medical men to the public, to each other and to themselves with regard to the exercise of their profession."[1] In this purview, euthanasia, financial investments in drugs, and sterilization for social reasons obviously belong to the family of ethics.

However, ethics, at least for most ethicists, means much more than a body of prescriptions and prohibitions. Ethics means the critical assessment and reconstruction of such bodies in the context of a comprehensive theory of human morality. By "morality" the present authors mean the actual behavior of human beings, involving judgments, actions, and attitudes, constructed around rationally conceived and effectively based norms whereby that behavior can be judged right or wrong and around values whereby states affected by that behavior are judged good or bad. By "ethics" the authors mean an academic discipline, a systematic set of propositions that constitute the intellectual instruments for the analysis of morality.

This discipline seeks to elucidate how the norms and values are established and perceived and how the actions are justified. It inquires how one argues or should argue from norms and facts to decisions. It tries to show how values and norms are related to purposes and results. In order to accomplish such analyses, it must elaborate a theory, within which these elements are comprehensively described and coherently articulated. It provides, when rightly done, not only a descriptive discipline of morality, but a normative one as well, for its analysis purports to reveal the roots of obligation and value appreciation, thereby exposing not how men *do in fact* behave, but how *in principle* they *should* behave. Ethics, then, is the normative discipline of morality.[2]

An adequate ethics would be a theoretical system capable of suggesting some answers to the sorts of questions arising about morality. The authors believe that, since there are at least three sorts of questions, an adequate ethics would consist of at least three principle theories, which we call, in reverence to the traditions of the discipline, the theory of virtue, the theory of duties, and the theory of the common good.

In response to questions like "What sort of person can rightly be called a morally good man?" the theory of virtue will expatiate on the character of moral agents, their attitudes, habits, affections, and motives. In response to questions like "What ought I to do in this situation?" the theory of action will discuss the nature of action, its objectives, goals, intentions, consequences, and conditions for freedom, and voluntariety. In response to questions like "What is the best form of human society?" the theory of common good seeks to understand not the good man alone, nor his right actions, but the social institutions that make and are made by good men acting rightly.

Medical ethics is, we believe, a species of the genus "ethics." It should, then, be constructed out of the three essential theories of ethics. We shall contend in this chapter that, traditionally, medical ethics has dwelt mostly within two of those three theories, namely, the theories of virtue and of duty. Both of these theories, while in need of refurbishing and modernization, remain indispensable to medical ethics. But the nature of contemporary medicine demands that they be complemented by the third essential theory, the common good. We shall review two traditional forms of medical ethics, indicating their relationship to the classical ethical theories. We shall then state the condition of modern medicine which calls for the theory of the common good. We suggest that this does not merely add an appendix to medical ethics, but that it can be the source of a new concept of the discipline, which can affect profoundly the more traditional theories of virtue and duty.

The term "medical ethics" is frequently applied to those statements of professional standards which are set forth in "codes." There are many such codes, but we shall select the *Ethical Principles of the American Medical Association* as a paradigm. We believe that our analysis applies generally to what is sometimes called "code ethics."[3]

The A.M.A. code, adopted in 1847 and revised four times (1903, 1912, 1947, 1955), now consists of ten sections in which such subjects as consultations and precedence, scientific competence, professional courtesy, cooperation with nonphysician health personnel, solicitation of patients, fees, conditions of practice, and confidentiality are treated. Some of these subjects are discussed at length but, for the most part, the principles are succinctly expressed. For example, "It is unethical ... for a physician to provide or prescribe unnecessary services or unnecessary ancillary facilities" (Section 4). "The acceptance of rebates on appliances and prescriptions or of commissions from those who aid in the care of patients is unethical" (Section 7). The preamble states that "these principles ... are not immutable laws to govern the physician, for the ethical practitioner needs no such laws; rather they are standards by which he may determine the propriety of his own conduct" (Preamble). The substance of the code, which in its latest edition comes to sixty-seven pages, consists of these standards, which serve to "standardize" the more common transactions, social and economic, between physicians, between physicians and patients, and between physicians and third parties, such as legal authorities, insurance providers, and the press. We call these standards "pragmatic directions."[4]

Interspersed among these pragmatic directions are occasional exhortations to cultivate certain virtues considered proper to the physician. A citation from the Hippocratic literature opens Section One—"[The physician] should be modest, sober, patient, prompt to do his whole duty without anxiety; pious without going so far as superstition, conducting himself with propriety in his profession and in all the actions of his life." Physicians are expected, "in their relationship with patients, with colleagues and with the public, to maintain under God, as they have down the ages, the most inflexible standards of personal honor" (notes, Section Two). At various points, the virtues of fearlessness, benevolence, patience, and delicacy are recommended. The Preamble notes that, while "interpretation of these principles by an appropriate authority will be required at times ... as a rule ... the physician who is capable, honest, decent, courteous, vigilant, and an observer of the Golden Rule, and who conducts his affairs in the light of his own conscientious interpretation of these principles will find no difficulty in the discharge of his professional obligations."[5]

Pragmatic standards for common transactions predominate; exhortations to virtue are sparse and, one might cynically say, perfunctory. The predominance of the pragmatic directions has prompted many to refer to the codes as an "etiquette" rather than an "ethic." One of the first codes is *Decorum*, more literally the *Etiquette*, found in the Hippocratic corpus; during the nineteenth century medical codes were frequently called "etiquettes." Dr. Chauncey Leake writes in the preface to his edition of *Percival's Medical Ethics*, which served as exemplar for the early A.M.A. codes:

> The term "medical ethics" introduced by Percival is a misnomer. Based on Greek traditions of good taste ... it refers chiefly to the rules of etiquette developed in the profession to regulate the professional contacts of its members with each other.... Medical etiquette is concerned with the conduct of physicians toward each other and embodies the tenets of professional courtesy. Medical ethics should be concerned with the ultimate consequences of the conduct of physicians toward their individual patients, and toward society as a whole, and it should include consideration of the will and motive behind this conduct.[6]

The concept of etiquette is enticing because it sidesteps the pitfalls of having to define morality. An etiquette is a set of conventional rules, usually quite arbitrary, that reflect behavior in polite society. With obvious repugnance, but impeccable *noblesse oblige*, Lord Chesterfield admonished his son, "Without hesitation, kiss the Pope's slipper or whatever else the etiquette of that court requires." An etiquette is hardly susceptible to ethical analysis, for it is seldom possible or profitable to attempt to justify its precepts, which are either simply "just done" or devised with a clear view to avoiding arguments about precedence, confusion over procedures, etc.

Etiquette is, then, a set of rules for external behavior that may be presumed to come from an internally virtuous man. Obviously the external behavior may not reflect the internal man. Yet this is not sufficient to become cynical about the rules of etiquette. At best, they will truly reflect virtue. At worst, they are likely to keep the individual on his *qui vive*.

However, the word "etiquette" is a misleading description of the codes. They do consist predominantly of pragmatic and arbitrary standards of behavior. But the sparse, almost perfunctory, exhortations to virtue in the modern codes are the faded tokens of their ancestry as ethics. The immediate progenitor of the American codes, Percival's *"Medical Ethics,"* is a treatise on the "Gentleman Physician." The word "gentleman" denoted, in the eighteenth century, much more than a polite, gracious, considerate man with *savoir faire*; it was a synonym for the virtuous man. A century earlier, Isaac Walton had written, "I would rather prove myself a Gentleman, by being learned and humble, valiant and inoffensive, virtuous and communicable than by a fond ostentation of riches."[7] The long tradition of medicine, from the Hippocratic Corpus through the Admonita and Epistulae of the Middle Ages, the *Medicus Politicus* of the Renaissance, and the eighteenth-century treatises on *Duties* and *Character of the Physician*, is replete with exhortations to virtues proper to those who would practice medicine. This whole tradition mingles these exhortations with pragmatic directions about bedside manners, consultations, and fees; but the vision of the "upright man instructed in the art of healing" predominates.

These exhortations to virtue tend to dwindle, almost disappear, in more recent codes. Apparently, they seem to some superfluous, for they belabor the obvious. To others, they seem futile, for they cannot be enforced. Again, they seem vacuous, for they offer no practical guidance for action. Finally, they might seem embarrassing, for they smack of posturing for public consumption.

However, we suggest that these exhortations to virtue constitute the heart of code ethics. Indeed, they are the justification for calling the codes "ethics" at all. They give to the pragmatic directions a moral substance without which they are merely etiquettes. Their disappearance in current codes is not merely a mildly deplorable withering of a charming, but rather quaint, affirmation of the good, the true, and the beautiful. It reflects fundamental uncertainty about the character desired in the person who would practice medicine.

The theory of virtue is a treatise about moral character. It has always been recognized that moral judgments bear not only on the rightness or wrongness of discrete actions, but also upon the goodness or badness of rather fixed states of persons who perform actions. Although "virtue" and "vice" are words with Victorian tone, great ethicists from Aristotle through Kant to Hartmann have used them to describe rationally intended, affectively rooted attitudes whereby persons consistently seem to incline toward certain sorts of behavior. Terms such as "benevolence," "honesty," "trustworthiness," "sobriety" described particular modes of these states of character.[8]

The great ethicists have always noted that, while a spectrum of virtues should adorn the good man, particular dispositions were proper to certain roles: courage to the soldier, fairness to the judge, discretion to the ruler. A theory of virtue in medical ethics must explore that disposition most proper to the relationship between physician and patient—trust.

The patient approaching the physician suffers from more than his illness; he suffers from significant social disadvantages. He enters a mysterious domain, where arcane knowledge and rare skills rule. He is nervous, fearful, and perhaps even terrified. He places himself in the hands of a fallible human being. The novelist Kurt Vonnegut writes sardonically in *Goodby, Mr. Rosewater*, "The most exquisite pleasure in the practice of medicine comes from nudging a layman in the direction of terror, then bringing him back to safety again." The potential for such sadism, which does lie within any physician's power, must be countered by the bond of trust. This bond, or as Paul Ramsey aptly dubs it, "covenant," arises from more than a contract; it is nourished by the evident trustworthiness of the physician.[9]

Codes do not create virtue. Their pragmatic directions establish certain regularities of procedure that elicit public confidence. But confidence elicited is fulfilled and confirmed only in the personal relationship that Lian de Entralgo calls "the medical friendship," a delicate alliance which must at the same time encourage confidence and discourage dependency.[10] The apparent fading of this friendship, under the cold exigencies of scientific skill, technical expertise, harried services and, frankly, cupidity, has been blamed by many as the major cause of the "dehumanization" of care.

In sum, code ethics, as they presently exist, might be called the archeological ruins of a doctrine of medical virtue. The codes are, in their present form, collections of pragmatic directions that mark the outer limits of the physician-patient covenant. Their inspiration, and the inner confirmation of this covenant, requires the virtue of trustworthiness. Restoration of exhortations to virtue in the codes would not, of course, insure the actual existence of virtue in physicians. This comes from the manner in which the profession selects and socializes its members, from exemplarity and from exercise. Nonetheless, the theory of virtue in medical ethics requires serious reflection on the virtues proper to the physician, and on the obstacles to their realization in contemporary settings and in contemporary men. Multiplication of codes, regulations, statutes, and standards, particularly if they are expected to be self-enforcing, as are most professional codes, is futile unless those to whom they are addressed comprehend and possess the virtues of the physician.

Virtue is the inner spirit of morality; action is its outer manifestation. The virtuous physician without skill may provide comfort, but cold comfort, to one seeking cure. Medicine is a practical science: theory and experience evoked in clinical decision and action. Medical ethics, then, must be concerned about the rightness of acts as about the goodness of the agent. A theory of virtue is a necessary, but not sufficient, part of medical ethics.

Ethics provides a second complementary theory, often called theory of duty, which defines the criteria whereby actions are judged right or wrong. It analyzes the relationship between intentions and consequences, motivations and circumstances. It studies the conditions of freedom and responsibility underlying imputation of guilt and innocence.

The need for an ethical analysis of actions comprising clinical practice is demonstrated in daily news articles on euthanasia, transplantation, experimental trials. Serious efforts have been made to provide such an analysis. Jewish medical ethics is predominantly a doctrine of duties. Joseph Fletcher's pioneer work in medical ethics applies utilitarian theory of action to clinical acts. The present authors wish to use as an example the natural law theory of duties as it is found in Roman Catholic medical ethics. A volume on medical ethics in the Catholic tradition contains lengthy discussions of specific clinical actions such as euthanasia, abortion, transplantation, obstetrical techniques, and cosmetic surgery. Pope Pius XII had intense interest in questions of medical ethics, and his frequent statements, delivered before distinguished medical societies, lent authoritative tone to the theologians' efforts.[11]

The medical ethics of this tradition is, in a very proper sense, a doctrine of duties. Medical interventions and procedures are analyzed in light of an explicitly formulated ethical system of principles and argumentation which can be broadly described as natural law.

The first affirmative of the system is that God has dominion over His creation, the human body, while man is granted a derived dominion over his body, which he must exercise in view of the divinely appointed finality of his body and its functions. Because he is ultimately not his own, he has an obligation to preserve his life and health. Any mutilation of his body is an abuse of the derived dominion, unless that mutilation contributes to the good of the whole body. This affirmation, called the principle of totality, is the proximate governing principle of Catholic medical ethics.[12]

Other carefully defined principles allow the Catholic moral theologian to thread a precise path through the complexities of medical procedures. The principle of double effect can be invoked when an intervention involves the problem of finding moral justification for both the physical evil of mutilation, and some other evil such as the death of a fetus removed in a salpingectomy done for ectopic pregnancy. The distinction between ordinary and extraordinary means of sustaining life, elaborated within the context of the principles of divine dominion and totality, provide to physician and patient thoughtfully defined ethical grounds for making painful ultimate decisions about life and death.[13]

The theory of duty elaborated in Roman Catholic ethics describes an act in terms of: (1) the *object*, that is, the objective design of the act and its immediate consequences; (2) the *end*, that is, the intention of the agent; and (3) the *circumstances*, that is, time, place, office, and other relevant concrete conditions of the act. In this approach, all three elements of an act must be right before the act is considered objectively moral. Criteria for evaluating the rightness of the action and its elements are such principles as divine and derived dominion and, more directly, the principle of totality.

In this scheme, a surgical intervention in the case of an ectopic pregnancy, described in terms of its objective, might be called a salpingectomy. The circumstances are advanced erosion of the fallopian tube, the presence of a fetus, and the absence of any therapeutic possibilities other than radical resection. The surgeon intends the removal of the eroding tube and tolerates the inevitable death of the developing fetus. The act would be judged morally right, for in its object, in the intention of the surgeon, and in the given circumstances, it effects the restoration of the integrity of the patient. The abortion is neither intended nor is it the principle objective of the act. It is, in the technical language of this school, an "indirect" abortion.

The purpose of this description and evaluation of actions is to enable the agent to discern actions that are morally right from those that are morally wrong. Morally right actions must or may be performed. Morally wrong action must be avoided. Thus, this doctrine of duties contains a doctrine of obligation, grounded in the principle of divine and derived dominion, which distinguishes between obligatory, permissible, and forbidden actions. There is an absolute moral obligation to refrain from morally wrong acts and a conditional moral obligation to perform right acts. The purpose of the theories of duties is to guarantee the moral rectitude of medical intervention. Almost every medical procedure of diagnosis and therapy requires an invasion of the sphere of the patient's physical and psychological independence.

Two points are particularly noteworthy about this example of a theory of duties. First, the principle of totality is defined in terms of the integrity of the *physical* organism of an individual person. Efforts have been made, from time to time, to extend its range to *social* or *interpersonal* totality, but these have never been enthusiastically adopted. Thus, early discussions of homografts, such as renal transplants, tended to meet with disapproval because of the nonbeneficial mutilation of the donor. The suggestion that the bond of charity could thereby be strengthened between donor and recipient won little favor and the transplantation was finally justified on grounds more consonant with traditional doctrine of totality, namely that donation of one of paired organs did not absolutely impair functional integrity. Similarly, attempts to defend contraception by means other than periodic abstinence on the basis that hormonal alteration or tubal ligation would, ultimately, improve the psychological and physical well-being of a woman or benefit the total family situation were met with disfavor. The principle of totality remains tightly linked to physical integrity of single individuals, rather than their psychological or social integrity.[14]

This problem has been framed in terms of the traditional Roman Catholic use of the principle of totality. However, it is not a problem unique to that particular form of the theory of duties. Most efforts to formulate a theory of duties, in particular those influenced by Kantian ethics, have a tendency to thrust the single act or the isolated agent onto center stage and leave the interrelationships of acts and agents in the shadows.

Second, any theory of duties issues prescriptions, prohibitions, and permissions. The physician committed to this moral reasoning must refrain from prohibited interventions. Even though certain concessions are made for unwilling and compelled cooperation in immoral acts, the physician's moral duty is quite clear. Direct abortion, direct sterilization, positive euthanasia are clearly forbidden. Refusal to perform these actions assures the moral integrity of the physician's conscience. However, from the point of view of those who do not share the physician's conscience, his refusal to perform an act is perceived as denial of a benefit to the petitioner. While any single petitioner might seek that benefit elsewhere, could it be that the conscientiously acting physician, by accumulation of his decisions and by his efforts to effect public policy in favor of his conscience, might impede some public good? And what if all physicians were of identical mind on the issue and all patients of opposite mind?[15]

Both of these problems—the restriction of the principle of totality to the *physical* integrity of single persons and the possibility of disagreement between adherents of this theory of duty and the possible demands of a broader public—suggest that a theory of duties, while necessary, may not be sufficient for adequate ethics. To the extent that such theories concentrate on discrete acts and individual intentions, they neglect the ethical issues arising from the intersection of multiple actions in institutions and society. Thus, an adequate ethics calls for an explicit reflection on the morality of institutions and on the relationship, and possible clash, between social and individual values. Classical ethics has made such a reflection. It can be conveniently called a theory of the common good.

The ethical theories of virtue and of duty are complemented by a theory of the common good. A theory of the common good seeks to elucidate the nature of human communities. These are the institutional forms that human actions create and human virtues sustain, and that in their turn should become the objective conditions nurturing virtue and sustaining action. This theory should treat two principal questions: what the "common" good or goods might be; and the manner in which they should be distributed. The first question inquires about the goods and values that are necessary for individuals and for the society. In the present context, "health and health care" might be discussed as common goods. This is a crucial discussion for ethics of medical care. However, the second question, properly called the problem of social justice, will be the problem to which we shall attend in the remainder of this chapter.[16]

Before considering this problem, it is important to realize that the theory of the common good is not merely a separate third chapter of ethical concepts that should be glanced at from time to time whenever a "social question" arises. Properly conceived, the theory of the common good is a third dimension in which virtues and actions take on a depth and tone that they do not have in isolation. The very meaning of a virtue or an action depends upon its social or institutional setting. For example, lying and deception can be viewed and analyzed as a private interaction between two individuals, as in the recent drama *Sleuth*; but, when they are considered within the structures of public trust, authority, and responsibility that constitute an institution, for example government, quite different issues arise. In what sense, for example, does the problem of national defense security morally qualify an act of deception? And, analogously, would a national health security be sufficient warrant to deceive patients, or experimental subjects, about the nature of what was being done to them?

It must be clear that considerations of the common good do not ipso facto override considerations of individual rectitude of action. Rather, the purpose of the doctrine of the common good is to consider how conflicts may be avoided or reconciled; or, more important, how the institutional structure can be designed so as to avoid conflict, how to reconcile discord, and how to compensate unjust harm.

There is little or nothing that can be identified as a doctrine of the common good in contemporary ethics of medical care. There is, of course, a conviction on the part of most professionals that they do serve the common good in a significant way. Yet there is, further, a contention on the part of many professionals that the practice of medicine involves significant social injustices. The authors do not intend to argue either conviction or contention. Neither of them, however valid, constitutes a theory of the common good. Such a theory must consist of a comprehensive description of the exigencies of medical care and the institutional forms that presently serve these exigencies. It must propose criteria whereby these institutional forms can be analyzed and criticized, not only in terms of the exigencies of care, but in light of certain exigencies of human moral existence. These latter exigencies, when seen in the light of social institutions, have been most clearly expressed, by the great ethicists, in terms of a doctrine of justice.

Justice, while a virtue, or personal characteristic, of individuals, is above all the "virtue" of institutions.[17] An institution may be judged ethically "good" if it exhibits, in its organizational structure and in its procedures, the characteristics of justice. The establishment of a just society, for the great ethicists, required not merely the assembling of many just men, but the design of social institutions, of laws, of policies, of economics, in which the habits, inclinations, and intentions of just men could be realized in public policy and practice. It is curious that, while we often speak of just laws, just courts, just taxes, just contracts, we do not often speak of just medicine.

If, however, justice is pre-eminently the virtue of institutions, our failure to apply the criteria of justice to medicine may result from our failure to recognize that medicine has become, in fact, an *institution*. Medicine has, in recent years, evolved from a practice, a private technical interaction between two parties, through a profession, a socially coherent, publicly recognized group that defined the conditions under which those private transactions take place, to an institution.[18]

By an institution, we mean a complex interaction of professionals, paraprofessionals, and the public, on informational, economic, and occupational levels, in identifiable physical environments, whose coordinated decisions and actions have magnified public impact, and which is recognized culturally and legally as affecting the public welfare in a significant way. Law enforcement, the free market, religion, higher education, are institutions in this broad sense.

Just as the free market once consisted simply of a solo producer exchanging his product for consideration by a single buyer (and still, in essence, consists of that), so the medical transaction once was, and still essentially is, a solo physician diagnosing and treating a single patient. But that essential transaction has gradually been surrounded by the indispensable cooperation of other people, by accessory producers, by physical environments, by customary and legal prescriptions. The face-to-face decisions made in the private transaction have magnified public impact, since they now engage the attention of multiple other parties, nurses, druggists, insurance carriers, etc. The coordinated decisions and actions of the institutions have magnified public impact because accepted forms of diagnosis and treatment, of research, of prevention, engage the manufacture of products, the construction of buildings, and the enactment of laws.

Modern medicine, then, is an institution that incorporates a profession that practices a technique and an art. The practice remains, indeed, at the heart of the institution, but it cannot be adequately performed or understood outside of it. Doctrines of virtue and action supply ideals and norms and pragmatic directions for the profession and for the practitioner; a doctrine of the common good must be added to provide an ethics for the institution.

It must be emphasized again that a doctrine of the common good does not supplant the other two modes of ethical analysis. All three doctrines are required for an adequate ethics. The practice of medicine, once conceived as the relief of the suffering of one person by another properly qualified person, was adequately analyzed in ethical terms by the two doctrines of virtue and of duty. Today, however, the institutionalization of practice and profession calls for an institutional ethic. On the other hand, the possibility that misjudgments about the ethical exigencies of virtue and duty might be propagated throughout the institution still demands a careful ethical scrutiny of quality of individual character and rectitude of single actions.

Institutions are vehicles for the distribution of the benefits and burdens of social life, and it is the function of the principles of justice to determine fair and equitable assignment of rights and duties and fair and equitable distribution of benefits and burdens.[19]

An institution possesses an identity, an organization, and resources that enable activities performed by its members to have an extensivity and perpetuity that they otherwise could not have. By *extensivity*, we mean that activities can have effects on a broad contemporary population. By *perpetuity*, we mean that they can be prolonged in time by affecting future populations. It may be argued that medical actions always factually had effects that fulfilled these definitions of extensivity and perpetuity. However, the development of epidemiology and biostatistics has made the dimensions of this extensivity and perpetuity vividly evident in contemporary medicine.

Only the institutional form provides the exchange of information, the continuity and cooperation, the designation of qualified participants, and the utilization of physical and financial resources to support extensivity and perpetuity. A profession may have an identity based on possession of similar knowledge and techniques and may cooperate to share and assure possession of them, but a professional, as such, did not deliberately utilize information and resources to effect extensivity and perpetuity. Medicine has, in the last hundred years, in virtue of certain scientific and technical accomplishments, evolved from a profession with knowledge of limited effects in time and space to an institution with knowledge of extensive and perpetuated effects.

The most pressing ethical issues of modern medicine arise out of the potential for extensivity and perpetuity inherent in its new institutional status. A medical intervention was, at one time, perceived as a transaction between a physician and a patient. The benefits and the costs were, for the most part, thought to be quite strictly limited to that transaction. Today, benefits and costs are known to be distributed broadly, in many ways. Financial costs of medical research and education are borne by an extensive public. Costs of care are borne by insurance purchasers and tax payments. Resource allocation distributes benefits of research to certain afflicted populations at a cost to others. Certain treatment modalities impose burdens on persons other than those treated. The effects of certain medical interventions can be perpetuated into future generations; for example, the burden of heredity of certain genetic diseases such as diabetes and hemophilia. Formerly, *these patients* often did not live long enough to reproduce, and hence the defective gene was eliminated from the pool. Techniques for genetic diagnosis and control are directed toward modification of inheritable characteristics.

Where benefits and burdens can be so distributed, the problem of justice arises. Some who will benefit will not bear costs; some who will bear costs will not benefit. When this situation depends, not on chance or accident, but on planned and conscious decisions about the structure of the institution, it is necessary to ask, "What justifies the imposition of a burden, a cost, a risk, on any single individual?" Why should one individual benefit at the apparent cost to another? These are the questions at the heart of each of the serious ethical issues of medicine, as they are of those of justice.

The problem of access to medical care is the most obvious field for the application of the concept of justice. On its face, this appears to be a problem of distributive justice. A subset of this problem is the allocation of scarce resources, such as renal dialysis. However, many other problems that are not usually considered in terms of justice involve deliberate distribution of costs and benefits. Randomized clinical trials, particularly when one of the alternatives is a proven therapeutic agent, involves costs without compensating benefit to certain individuals. An increasing number of therapeutic modalities, such as drugs administered to pregnant mothers, lay burdens of risk on others than the beneficiaries. In the near future, nuclear-powered artificial hearts—and in the further, but real, future, DNA therapy through viral agents—will have this effect. The entire realm of genetic control, whether it utilizes elimination of births or elimination of defective genomes, raises the question of justice to future generations. Psychosurgery and psychoactive drug therapy, while they may be conceived as interventions beneficial to the individual, have the potential to impose stringent limitations on that individual's freedom from which others may benefit socially, politically, and economically. The classic problem of euthanasia is aggravated by the institutionally supported potential for prolonging dying at great cost, emotional and financial, to survivors.

Finally, the nagging, but ill-defined, problem of dehumanization of medical care may obtain clarity within the concepts of justice. The great jurisprudent Georgio del Vecchio wrote, "The ideal criteria of justice ... demand the equal and perfect recognition ... of the quality or personality in oneself as in all others for all possible interactions among several subjects."[20] Dehumanization is, at bottom, unequal and imperfect recognition of the quality of personality, an entity most difficult to quantitate under the criteria required for a just theory of the common good.

Many of the moral problems of medicine appear to be problems of justice. Many of the old problems of medicine, placed in the modern setting, seem to have been transmuted from problems of virtue or duty into problems of justice. Yet the theories of justice long familiar to ethics have not been fully mined for their relevance to the moral problems of medicine. The authors are not so naïve as to suppose that the ancient conflicts of individual versus institution and personal duty versus social good will be resolved by yet another invocation of the doctrine of justice. Still, to the extent that considerations of justice contribute to the design of institutions of medicine and to policies governing its practice, many of the moral problems may be either avoided or ameliorated.

The traditional definition of justice is "giving to each his due." The problem of justice is defining what is "due" to each. This is done, first, by recognizing that the "each" of the definition is both everyman, with a basic humanness shared by all, and this single person, different in ability, merit, and need from all others. Justice thus requires an impartiality resting on the fundamental similarity of all persons and an equity that allows for different treatment justified by different conditions of ability and merit. Effecting justice becomes the continual process of critical scrutiny of the reasons proposed for different treatment of persons. This scrutiny must measure particular considerations against universal characteristics, the claims of ability, merit, and need against the claims of equality of liberty, of consideration, and of treatment. So stated, the conundrum is not vastly different from the problem of reconciling the age-old precept to give to each according to his need with that of giving to each according to his merit.[21]

The requirements of a theory of justice are not satisfied by the proposition that an act or institution is ethically justified when it produces the "greater good for the greater number." This thesis, called *utilitarianism*, has been much disputed by ethicists, and its inherent defects revealed. Nonetheless, it appears to be the dominant ethic for many policy-makers in scientific medicine.[22] The problem of the lesser number, disadvantaged for the sake of the greater, remains unsolved.

In medicine, this problem can be particularly pressing, for traditionally medicine has favored the good of individuals, while the law has favored the common good. Today, the realization of extensivity and perpetuity of modern medicine places many medical interventions directly within the sphere of the common good. Whether the problems thus raised can be "justly" solved depends on how deeply modern medical practitioners and policy-makers reflect on the profound moral dilemmas and theses of the theory of justice. They must refuse to relax those dilemmas either by a facile appeal to the "inestimable social benefits of medicine," on the one hand, or the "inviolable individual rights of patient or practitioner" on the other. Neither assertion can stand alone; both must be comprehended within an adequate theory of justice. Above all, public policy relative to the shape of institutions, the flow of money and people through them, the regulation of their powers and vigilance over their performance, must be devised with the requirements of justice foremost in mind.

Several final points should be made about "just medicine." First, the cynical often say, "Ethics is no more than the simulation of good intentions." Doctrines of virtue, because virtue can be so easily simulated by scoundrels, are most susceptible to this pessimistic criticism. Doctrines of duty can take refuge in excuses and protestations of ignorance. But doctrines of justice are on different ground. Their concern is the fair and equitable structure and function of institutions. In this theory of ethics, we are concerned about the institutional forms that set up problems in certain ways and that restrict or expand the alternatives for their solution. We do not limit our attention to good intentions alone or to the outcome of single actions. We are concerned about the assignment of rights and duties, the design of offices and tasks, the currents of resources and support that can best eliminate problems of unfair distribution of burdens and benefits and can best enable virtuous character and right action.

Second, the advent of institutions heralds the appearance of laws. Medicine has always been governed, to a greater or lesser degree, by civil law. Medicine has seldom been happy under that governance. "Just medicine" raises the menacing threat of medical practice cribbed, cabined, and confined by statute and regulation. This need not necessarily be the case. Justice and law are not synonymous. A theory of justice is concerned basically with the design of institutions. Institutional design can be created and effected by innumerable agencies, other than the state. The profession, related professions and industries, interested and impartial groups, organized and unorganized consumers can, if allowed and enabled, assist in institutional design. However, to the extent that civil law and regulations are advisable, a doctrine of justice is indispensable. It alone can provide the vision of just and equitable distribution that the enacted law should—imperfectly, piecemeal, but steadily—seek to realize. Without a doctrine of just medicine, laws and regulations will be haphazard, aimless, and, for this reason, frustrating to profession and consumer alike.

In conclusion, then, the thesis of this chapter might be restated in terms of an ancient Roman definition of the entire field of ethics: *honeste vivere, nemini laedere, suum cuique tribuere*; live uprightly, hurt no one, give to each his due. The authors have attempted to state the conceptual foundations for an ethics of medical care under similar titles. It must consist, we maintain, of three essential theories of ethics applied to the unique enterprise of medicine and health care. The theory of virtue concerns those dispositions and qualities which define uprightness of life for those who practice medicine and engage in care. The theory of duties concerns criteria that enable the practitioner to recognize acts that ultimately harm those who seek his help. The theory of justice concerns the establishment of fair and equitable institutions for the practice of medicine and the provision of care. It is the authors' impression that in discussions of medical ethics these questions are often jumbled, that their theoretical bases are unrecognized, and that their intellectual history is unknown. We contend that fruitful progress might be made if future discussions acknowledge the distinction and the interrelation of these three theories of ethics and undertake their careful application to the difficult moral problems of modern medicine. This will make, we hope, for better medicine, for better ethics, and for a better ethics for medical care.

Notes to Chapter Two

1. *Lexicon of Medicine and Applied Sciences* (London: The Sydenham Society, 1881-89).

2. W. Frankena, *Ethics* (Englewood Cliffs: Prentice-Hall, 1963), pp. 1-10. G. Wallace and A. Walker (eds.), *The Definition of Morality* (London: Methuen, 1970).

3. *Opinions and Reports of the Judicial Council* (Chicago: American Medical Association, 1969). On the ethical nature of codes, cf. R. Veatch, "Medical Ethics: Professional or Universal?" *Harvard Theological Review*, 65 (1972), 531-59. On the history of the AMA code, cf. D. Konold, *A History of American Medical Ethics* (Madison: University of Wisconsin, 1962).

4. Our intention is to give an *ethical* analysis of codes. A sociological analysis can be found in E. Freidson, *The Profession of Medicine: A Study of the Sociology of Applied Knowledge* (New York: Dodd-Mead, 1970).

5. This echoes an early critique of the AMA code: "Were the great rule of Christian ethics present to the mind of the physician, 'do unto others as ye would that they would should do unto you,' there would be but little necessity

for societal codes." R. Duglison, "On the Present State of Medicine in the United States," *British and Foreign Medical Review* 3 (1837), 227.

6. C. Leake, *Percival's Medical Ethics* (Baltimore: Williams and Wilkins, 1927), 1-2, cf. Leake, "Theories of Ethics and Medical Practice," *Journal of American Medical Association* 208 (May 1969), 842-47. On the term "etiquette," cf. W.H.S. Jones, *The Doctor's Oath* (Cambridge: University Press, 1924) and "Ancient Medical Etiquette" *Hippocrates II* (Cambridge: University Press, 1923).

7. *Compleat Angler*, 1, 13, 1653. cf. L.S. King, *The Medical World of the Eighteenth Century* (Chicago: University of Chicago, 1958), 256.

8. G. Klubertanz, *Habits and Virtues* (New York: Appleton, Century, Crofts, 1965).

9. P. Ramsey, *Patient as Person* (New Haven: Yale University Press, 1970), Preface.

10. P. Lain Entralgo, *Doctor and Patient* (New York: McGraw, 1969).

11. Pius XII, *The Human Body* (Boston: St. Paul Press, 1960). cf. E. Healy, *Medical Ethics* (Chicago: Loyola Press, 1959); G. Kelly, *Medico-Moral Problems* (St. Louis: Catholic Hospital Association, 1958); J. Paquin, *Morale et Medecine* (Montreal: L'Immaculee-Conception, 1960).

12. Aquinas, *Summa Theologica* II-II, q. 65, a.1.

13. G. Kelly, "On the Duty of Using Artificial Means to Preserve Life," *Theological Studies* II (1950), 203-20; 12 (1951), 550-56.

14. M. Nolan, "Principle of Totality in Moral Theology," *Absolutes in Moral Theology*, ed. Charles Curran (Washington: Corpus, 1968). cf. Curran, *Medicine and Morals* (Washington: Corpus, 1970).

15. This problem is reflected in the debate over the *Code of the Catholic Hospital Association*, cf. "Catholic Hospital Ethics: Report of the Commission on Ethical Directions for Catholic Hospitals, *Linacre Quarterly* 39 (November 1972); J. Brennan, "Quicksands of Compromise," W. Reich, "Policy vs. Ethics," R. McCormick, "Not What the Catholic Hospitals Ordered," *Linacre Quarterly* 39 (February 1972).

16. Our use of the terms "common good" and "social justice" may be elucidated by the following: "Social justice [is] the equal treatment of all persons except as inequality is required by relevant, that is, just-making, considerations. . . . It takes equality of treatment to be a *prima facie* requirement of justice, but allows that it may on occasion be overruled by other principles of justice. . . . The differences in treatment are not justified simply by arguing that they are conducive to the general good life, but by arguing that they are required for the good lives of the individuals concerned. It is not as if one must first look to see how the general good is best subserved and only then can tell what treatment of individuals is just. Justice entails the presence of equal *prima facie* rights prior to any consideration of utility." W. Frankena, "The Concept of Social Justice," *Social Justice*, ed. R. Brandt (Englewood Cliffs: Prentice-Hall, 1962), 13, 15.

17. John Rawls, *A Theory of Justice* (Cambridge: Harvard University Press, 1971), Chapter 2.

18. D. Mechanic, *Medical Sociology* (Glencoe: Free Press, 1968), Chapters 10-11.

19. Rawls, p. 55.
20. G. delVecchio, *Justice* (Edinburgh: University Press, 1952), 116.
21. G. delVecchio; C. Perelman, *Justice* (New York: Random House, 1967); C. Friedrick and J. Chapman (eds.), *Nomos VI: Justice* (New York: Atherton Press, 1963).
22. "The dicta of that school [utilitarianism] ... are still used as part of the language of men of science." C. Singer, E.A. Underwood, *A Short History of Medicine* (New York: Oxford University Press, 1962), 208. For critique of utilitarianism see, among others, D. Lyons, *Forms and Limits of Utilitarianism* (Oxford: Clarendon Press, 1965).

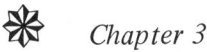 *Chapter 3*

Conceptual Foundations for an Ethics of Medical Care: A Response

Paul Ramsey

I must first indicate my extensive agreement with Jonsen and Hellegers concerning the need for general ethical analysis as the framework for discussing any problems in medical ethics, and with the clear and weighty things they have said on that subject.

For a reason our authors do not state, the overriding need is to enliven and articulate the genus "ethics" in which to locate medical ethics. If there are moral dilemmas in modern medicine, if—some would say—there is a moral crisis in the ethics of the medical profession, this is not because of recent triumphs in medical research or the great promise and grave risks stemming from medical technology. The fundamental reason is rather the continuing moral crisis in modern culture generally, which reverberates throughout all professions. It can no longer be assumed in the human community that we are agreed on moral action guides, the practice of virtue, the premises and principles of the highest, most humane, most bracing ethics, or what a moral agent owes to anyone who bears a human countenance.

In fact, serious ethical inquiry and discourse begin only when we discover we are in disagreement about what we ought to do. Then we are forced back upon our premises, and we must seek together in the human community and in the medical profession to find agreement at a deeper level. We must ask about what makes anything right. We need to find out if we can agree upon the right-making or wrong-making features of moral attitudes, actions, roles, or relations, before returning to the specific case where we first disagreed over what ought to be done. That is ethics proper.

In a period in which there is a moral consensus, ethics mainly gives backing to the consensus and few are needed for the important function of clarifying and strengthening that agreement. In an age, however, when ancient landmarks have been removed, and we are trying to do the unthinkable, namely, build a civilization without an agreed civil tradition and in the absence of a moral consensus, everyone needs to be an ethicist to the extent of his capacity for reflection and his desire to be and to know that he is a responsible person. In the present day, when nonutilitarian requirements in morality are eroded in society generally and can no longer be counted on silently to inform the physician's conscience, physicians and medical ethics generally must become more literate and establish explicit communication with the writings and reflections of ethicists. That conclusion I regret, since medical ethics worked better when moral consensus was intact and there was less need for ethical reflection and analysis.

I am not surprised, therefore, that our authors find codes of medical ethics to contain "faded tokens of their ancestry as ethics," or that they observe that "exhortations to virtue tend to dwindle, almost disappear, in more recent codes." To characterize those ancient codes, however, in their times as "the archeological ruins of a doctrine of medical virtue," seems to me to go far beyond the truth. I suggest that the physicians and medical societies who drew up codes in ages past pretty well knew the meaning of being honest, decent, courteous, vigilant, prompt, modest, sober, patient, of observing the Golden Rule and maintaining the most inflexible standards of personal honor; and—what is more important—they knew and were fairly well agreed on the kinds of actions and abstentions such virtues of the moral agent would lead to in the case of a physician. Few were the actions and abstentions that *needed* codifying. If exhortations to virtue tend to dwindle in the more recent codes, they (together with procedural regulations) tend also to get longer and longer. That necessity may reflect a decline and not an improvement in moral sensibility.

So moral character in the physician and its appropriate expression in action may have been largely presupposed in the earlier codes. To characterize those codes as "etiquette," or to condemn them for holding forth the ideal of the "gentleman physician," may not only be an exercise in futility. It may also be incorrect. Perhaps a gentleman and his behavior were simply silently understood—for example, that an ethical physician would not ordinarily have sexual intercourse with his female patients and then, when asked about it (in a recent survey), excuse that breach of the fiduciary nature of the relation of doctor to patient by saying he did it for "therapeutic" purposes.

In any case, behind admixtures of etiquette and ethics in the codes, we may be able to see more deeply into how moral sensibility and moral virtue are learned or acquired and transmitted. In the better moral ages of mankind, "manners" and "morals" have been joined by a cord not lightly to be broken. And when Aristotle exhorted his pupils to acquire virtues that were aptitudes to perform actions "to the right person," "in due proportion," "in the relative mean determined by reason," "at the right time," "with the right object," and "in the right manner," he customarily added: "or as the just man would do them" or "as the man of practical wisdom would determine."[1] Without Exemplars, no teaching of virtue. Moral education is unlikely except in the context of institutions that display rectitude. Nor is "just medicine" likely apart from a generally just society. How, then, can virtue be taught today?

Nevertheless, I am not altogether persuaded by J/H that exhortations to virtue constitute the heart of code ethics. Prima facie, is it not equally evident that an ethics of action or duties constitutes the heart of code ethics? Perhaps I ought instead to say that our authors have not demonstrated more than a provisional distinction between character and deeds, and that in this they faithfully record the nature of moral experience.

Virtues they define as "the goodness or badness of rather fixed states of persons who perform actions" or as "rationally intended, affectively rooted attitudes whereby persons seem consistently to incline toward certain sorts of behavior." If a theory of virtue is not vacuous, they write, it must provide some "practical guidance for action." With Aristotle, virtue is for them an aptitude for actions of a certain sort.

Of course, one can with Luther resolve all good works into some condition of the moral agent: good works do not make a good man, while a good man spontaneously (i.e. without much of a theory of action) does good works. Or, with a number of contemporary philosophers, one can try to resolve states of the soul of moral agents altogether into descriptions of sets of observable actions. Since J/H and the codes of medical ethics contain better moral philosophy than either of those extremes, I suggest that not only the moral character of the ethical physician (i.e. his "steady state" for acting in commendable ways) but also an ethics of right and wrong behavior are—indifferently—the moral background of code ethics, and the dual reason for calling them "ethics" at all.

In the belief that "medical ethics" is a species of "general ethics," Jonsen and Hellegers have placed before us an account of a theory of virtue, a theory of action, and a theory of the common good which they believe any adequate ethics must give attention to. I would describe their view as a threefold canopy of general ethics, suggesting by the word "threefold" that although its component parts can be distinguished they cannot be separated. They have disclosed the amplitude within general ethics, which means that the character of the moral agent alone, or the rectitude of his actions alone, or the common good alone, are insufficient. With that threefold amplitude of general ethics as model, they conclude that medical ethics cannot be built on narrower foundations; that "to live uprightly, to hurt no one, to give each his due" are irreducibly three distinct moral imperatives bearing upon the practice of medicine; that "Be an upright physician" alone, or "Do your medical duty" alone, or "Serve the common good" alone, cannot comprise the whole of medical ethics.

A practitioner of medicine might immediately object that J/H have provided a satellite photograph of "the main features of the topography of that ancient realm of the mind called ethics," but hardly a "roadmap" of that terrain. While articulating intellectual instruments for the analysis of morality, they have not come close enough to the old and new ethical issues in medical practice.

To an extent I agree with that objection, since I believe (as doubtless J/H do also) that ethics *as such* can come closer to decisional issues than was demonstrated in this chapter or could be demonstrated in a single chapter. Our authors have proposed where ethics must *begin* and what it consists in, not where it ends, nor have they described all the way to be traversed. At some point, ethical analysis can clarify the moral life *no further*, and prudent actors must stop deliberating and begin the business of doing (an entirely different enterprise). Our authors do not reach that point. They state, it is true, that ethics inquires "how one argues or should argue from norms and facts to decision"; but that final task, signaled, was not rigorously or comprehensively explored.

Instead we have the threefold canopy, a threefold conceptual foundation for an ethics of medical care. My task is to attend to those foundations, to ask whether the "folds" are straight.

In the main, our authors mean to exhibit a reciprocal three-in-oneness of general ethics: character, action, and the common good. I hear them saying that these three ingredients of ethics are coequal accounts each needing the others for completeness' sake; that they are interrelated and interacting aspects, none claiming primacy or sovereignty over the others. These are interpenetrating interpretations of the moral life. The absence or diminishing of any one of them would impoverish our apprehension of the full human good. Virtue, right action, social justice: these are polarities or three foci of the field of ethics, and so of medical ethics also.

Of course, at any time or place in the moral history of mankind, one can see a need for greater emphasis to be placed on one or another of these modalities, e.g. on personal moral character, or on the rectitude of actions, or on the common good. Such seems to be our authors' program when they tell us that "traditionally, medical ethics has dwelt mostly within two of those three theories [namely, virtue and duties]" and when they pronounce that "the nature of contemporary medicine demands that they be *complemented* by the third essential theory, the common good [italics added]." The prominence to be given to the common good comes as a corrective of a past deficiency. The contingent conditions of modern medicine call for the proposed redress. However, final justification of these three ingredients of medical ethics, and the weights assigned each, derives from general ethical theory itself.

What, we may ask, do the "folds" in the threefold theory of general ethics require as a critical corrective of medical practice? Were we not led to believe that an analysis of the constituent elements of general ethics themselves, and their interrelations, could help us delineate the shape of ethics in the medical context?

Before reaching that theoretical question, I must confess puzzlement as to our authors' meaning. After saying that a theory of the common good "complements" theories of personal moral virtue and theories of right action in traditional medical ethics, J/H affirm that "complement" does not mean merely added as "an appendix." I think I understand the difference between a "complement" and an "appendix." But what, then, are we to make of the assertion that a theory of the common good "can be the source of a new concept of the discipline [of medical ethics], which can affect profoundly the more traditional theories of virtue and duty"? If a "complement" is far more than a mere "appendix," still is it not too much to ask a "complement" to "affect profoundly" that which it supplements, to be "the source of a new concept of the discipline" of medical ethics which heretofore consisted of the virtues of the ethical physician and action-guides concerning his conduct?

What do our authors mean by a theory of the common good "affecting profoundly" the other components of medical ethics? And have they argued on theoretical grounds for the primacy of the common good over the other elements of morality? Have they reasoned within the conceptual foundations of general ethics to the conclusion that there should be a "profound" transformation of our understanding of physician virtue and/or of the right action and duties of physicians from the source for ethics in a theory of the common good?

It may be that when we bring the common good into view, personal "virtues and actions take on a depth and tone that they do not have in isolation," as J/H claim. For we can also affirm, in the alternative, that when true virtue and right action are given their full weight, the common good also takes on a quality and tone it does not have in isolation. But J/H surely err when they write that "the *very meaning* of a virtue or an action depends upon its societal or institutional setting [italics added]." Again, we can reverse that and say that the very meaning of the common good or a proper societal or institutional setting depends upon the kind of virtues or actions inculcated therein.

My plea, initially, whether it is an interpretation or a correction of the chapter, would be for parity and reciprocity among the threefold ingredients of ethics. J/H may mean this, since they promptly give illustrations that withdraw the proposition that the "very meaning" of personal virtues and actions depends upon their social setting.

Indeed, one could say that the very institutionalization, under the theory of the common good, of an error in analysis under the theory of virtues or of duties has the potential of propagating an evil with a multiplier effect. So it works the other way round: what one believes about moral character and about right action "affects profoundly" what one is allowed to say and do for the common good. Yet J/H still want to affirm that "the old problems of medicine, placed in a modern setting, seem to have been *transmuted* from moral problems of virtue or duty, into problems of justice [italics added]."

These various statements leave the present reader, candidly, somewhat confused. Clearly, J/H believe that the proper balance between the three theories of ethical analysis is the key to the development of an optional medical ethics. But what is that proper balance? Mutual parity? Or a balance in favor of the common good (which, however, in an optimal medical ethics, "does not supplant" the other two modes of analysis). Then does the common good only "complement," or "affect profoundly," or provide the "very meaning" of, or "transmute" into problems of justice the moral problems of personal virtue and actionable duties?

Such inexact and vascillating language betrays, if not conceptual uncertainty, at least a failure to give intellectual attention to the problem of the priority to be assigned to character analysis, to action analysis, and to analysis of the common good in making ethical appraisals.

This brings me to the first of several criticisms or complementary comments I wish to make of this chapter.

Jonsen/Hellegers have not directly and clearly addressed the problem of a lexical ordering, or some other value ranking, among the three modes of ethical analysis. The simple observation that our times call for greater stress on the common good raises no theoretical issues for ethics. Our authors, however, mean more than this. They have appealed to the contours and logic of general ethics to determine the specific shape medical ethics should take, and its modes of reasoning.

But within the amplitude or richness of general ethics, they fail to address clearly and rigorously the issue: Which of these moral claims has priority in case of conflict? Therefore, the shape of medical ethics and the weights to be assigned to its constitutive norms are left undetermined.

After all, even the assumption that ideals of good character, the requirements of right action, and the claims of the common good are in mutual parity is a kind of ordering that needs to be sustained by rational ethical argument. Departure from that likewise requires cogent warrant. A lexical order or any other weights to be given to theory of virtue, theory of action, and theory of the common good would seem to be a major task of general ethics. Whatever else it may be, medical ethics cannot claim to be a species of general ethics (and without such a claim it is not ethics at all) if it claims to incorporate norms for the physician as moral agent, norms governing his clinical action, and norms pertaining to justice in medical practice for the common good, but cannot rank these elements in medical practice in an order defensible within general ethics or defensible in terms of the examined morality of a wider human community. For all the amplitude of the ethical framework our authors have provided, they have not helped us either to order spheres of ethical reasoning or to assign primacy among the corresponding spheres of medical ethical justification.

At a crucial point *within* their consideration of a theory of the common good, our authors also avoid addressing the issue of determining a lexical or some other order among one's norms or principles. An "unseen hand" insures that mutual parity among moral virtue, right actions, and service of the common good will always endure, and these assessments never come into open conflict. So also in the matter of social justice; here again J/H rely on an "unseen hand" to avoid conflict. Enjoining medical practitioners and policy-makers to reflect on the profound dilemmas and theses of the theory of justice, our authors' assumption seems to be that such reflection will not lead to the need to establish a lexical (or some other ordering) among the elements in which justice consists, or any priority among its tests or claimants.

J/H write that as we reflect profoundly on a theory of justice we "must refuse to relax those dilemmas either by a facile appeal to the 'inestimable social benefits of medicine,' on the one hand, or the 'inviolable individual rights of patient or practitioner' on the other. Neither assertion can stand alone; both must be comprehended within an adequate theory of justice."

Granted. But *how* those moral appeals are to be comprehended may entail a decision within the ethical system itself (of which medical ethics is one species) as to which justification must first be satisfied before the other good or claim is taken up. (That is the meaning of lexical order.) Or it may require some other principle of adjudication or defendable weighing of the claims. What is or is not a "facile" appeal to overriding social benefits, or to inviolable individual rights, depends on foreseeing the possibility of conflict between justifications, and therefore the need for some priorities or principles for resolving such conflicts; first, within the canopy of general ethical theory, and second, in specifically medical ethics.

Several cases seem to me to represent potential or actual conflicts between "the inestimable social benefits of medicine" and "the inviolable individual rights of patients," which J/H assume too readily can be "comprehended within an adequate theory of justice" with no signaled need to decide which justification comes first.

1. Dr. Charles Ralph Buncher argues[2] that medical researchers ought not to stop their investigations when they have obtained "statistically significant" data. Nor should trials be suspended when "clinically significant" data are achieved. Instead, research should press on until "administratively significant" results are in. Administrators are responsible for all patients, not for those in the trial alone. The objective of research should be to persuade as many clinicians as possible, not only the rational clinical decision-makers. Research may need to be extended for a year or more beyond the time statistically and clinically significant results have been obtained—until more clinicians are convinced that *A* is the superior treatment. During that period, additional patients will be subjected to the less favorable treatment. Still, in the long run fewer patients will be exposed to the poorer treatment *B* if "administrative significance" is the objective. Dr. Buncher frames a hypothetical case in which the death rate for treatment *A* has already been discovered to be five per hundred, as compared to ten for treatment *B*. His rule of thumb is: "The finding should be declared

'administratively significant' only after the following imbalance is achieved: the likelihood that exposure of additional patients to the trial will persuade many physicians to adopt the better therapy is so small that it outweighs the risks to the patients continuing in the trials." To stop research earlier would be to fail to serve the common good. One of my correspondents compares that with making the hydrogen bomb in order to convince people who weren't persuaded by the atom bomb! Another suggested that "administratively significant" in Dr. Buncher's proposal could be better expressed by the words "rhetorically useful." Still, I let the case stand as Dr. Buncher worded it, since from ancient times rhetoric was regarded as also in the public interest. If the public interest or common good is overriding in ethics, I do not see how his conclusion can be avoided.

2. A document dated February 22, 1971 from the National Blood Resource Program entitled "Requests for Proposals RFP NHLI-71-18, Prenatal Diagnosis of Inherited Hematologic Diseases," sent to researchers *soliciting* their requests for research funds, stated in its preamble:

> The possibility exists that the prenatal diagnosis of homozygous sickle cell disease and hemophilia can be made from cells obtained at amniocentesis. These high morbidity diseases exert a demand disproportionate to their prevalence in the medical community and on the nation's blood supply and their prenatal diagnosis would be of great benefit to genetic counselors.

The stress clearly was on strengthening "a modern system which will assure adequate supplies of blood and blood components for the therapeutic needs of the American people and will utilize the national blood resource with maximum efficiency, economy, and safety." In this instance, that worthy objective was to be fostered, it seems, by getting rid of some of the sick who place inordinate demands on blood in their own therapy, for the sake of "the therapeutic needs of the American people."

3. What are we to say of the current practice of the use of sex chromatin tests to determine the sex of the fetus whose mother is a carrier of hemophilia or of Duchenne muscular dystrophy, followed by "genetic" abortion of *either* an afflicted *or* an unafflicted unborn? Consider the case of a normal male fetus given the treatment deemed appropriate for an afflicted fetus, had he been there. One fetus is interchanged for another nonexistent unborn. Such mistaken identification is rather like operating on the wrong patient—which no one would excuse by saying that the condition to be remedied (in someone else) was graver than the operation. Nor, in ordinary medical practice, if the wrong patient were caught in a mass screening, would the excuse be allowed that the mistake was statistically justified because the whole procedure accomplished the greatest good on the whole. That medical action and its medical outcome ought to be regarded as an ethically undefendable catastrophe even by those who defend the

general practice of "genetic" abortions. This should be our moral verdict, if for no other reason, in order to maintain a strong moral impulse for finding the means to overcome the necessity of doing what is now done.

4. The recently issued draft of regulations proposed by NIH entitled "Protection of Human Subjects: Policies and Procedures"[3] states that "research involving implantation of human ova which have been fertilized *in vitro* shall not be approved until ... the responsibilities of the *donor* and recipient 'parents' ... have been established [italics added]." It defines in vitro fertilization as "any fertilization of human ova which occurs outside the body of the female, either through admixture of *donor* sperm *and ova* or *by any other means* [italics added]." Thus, in the proposed regulations a quantum jump was made from the research to date, which may be described as attempts to treat oviduct blockage. Unless a husband is now to be called a "donor," the silent introduction of the word "donor," and in particular the addition of the words "and ova or by any other means," goes a long way toward changing the "moral species" of the action. That action might now be called research in "reproductive engineering." In any case, there lurks here a whole nest of issues, including the justice of marriage, requiring some ethical determination of the weights to be assigned to various competitive elements in a theory of common good. Not all claims can be regarded as equal and simply comprehended together.

5. The document "Protection of Human Subjects: Policies and Procedures" also substitutes the expression "supplementary judgment" for proxy or constructive "consent." "Supplementary judgment" is a clarifying expression when the issue was seeking the consent of *both* a parent and a child above the "age of discretion." The force of the new language, however, in regard to nontherapeutic research involving human subjects below seven years of age (instead of proxy consent or even *substituted* judgment) may be to further elide " the inviolability of individual rights" into "the inestimable benefits of research." That may be the way to go, but not as a result of a change of wording. That may be the way to go, but not before determining in ethical theory that the common good should have such weight over care for the infirm or incompetent person.

6. The majority report of the Artificial Heart Assessment Panel of the National Heart and Lung Institute[4] recommends that a nuclear-powered artificial heart not now (or soon) be implanted in human patients in view of the risks to spouses, children, associates, and more distantly, to the public and environment in general. (To say nothing of the recipients themselves, who risk leukemia and sterilization.) Research on the nuclear device should proceed in animals (including intense scrutiny of unborn generations of the progeny of the primary animal subjects). An electric-battery-powered heart was recommended instead.

The most extensive minority report—that of Clark C. Havighurst, Professor of Law, Duke University—argues to the contrary that while unknown and unborn persons may be protected by prohibiting the nuclear-powered device, such a policy would on balance more severely disadvantage recipients by placing them at higher risk from a less reliable or efficient device, subjecting them to the necessity of undergoing battery replacement operations, and noticeably lowering the quality of life sustained in them.

A careful reading of the majority statements and those opposed reveals, I believe, that the panel fell into dispute over which side was questionably using (or misusing) a social utilitarian calculus in reaching its decision!

Neither side, as I read the report, espoused an unqualified social utilitarianism. For the majority it seemed "crucial that the 'greater good' should not only flow to the 'greater number,' but that the greater number should emerge from the entire population with equal access to that good, and that the disadvantaged 'lesser number' not be excluded capriciously and that it be compensated in other ways" (p. 61). It was the unbalanced and uncompensated harm to nonbeneficiaries (in the presence of an alternate therapy for persons needing heart replacement) that led the majority of the panel to oppose giving priority to the nuclear device. While the majority called attention to the fact that much of its reasoning about advantages and disadvantages involved balancing "qualitatively different," "non-commensurable apples and oranges which cannot simply be added to or subtracted from one another" (p. 93), it still persisted in such speculations. For example, the majority thought that though it was true that women recipients would be less advantaged by an artificial heart because *women as a group* are slightly less prone to heart disease than men, still other women who are spouses of potential recipients would gain "improved expectation of deferred widowhood" (pp. 57-58).

I do not read Professor Havighurst to proceed from any other premise than the majority stated. He, too, believes that "making social choices solely on the basis of whether advantages or disadvantages predominate is ethically unsatisfying, for it involves a presumption that it is just for some to gain at the expense of others" (p. 232). He too believes that where there are winners and losers, the losers should somehow be compensated if possible. But this is not always possible to arrange.

Havighurst's substantive conclusion in the artificial heart implant case, however, follows from his identification of potential recipients of the "safer," less efficient device as "losers" (because the "better" nuclear device was forbidden them) as morally equivalent to those who may be the innocent, entirely nonbenefited "losers" if the optimal device is developed for heart patients. He equates *not* doing something for heart patients with *doing* damage to others, and so arrives at a balancing judgment regardless of who wins, who loses. "Since there are losers whichever way the decision goes," he writes, "private activities or public projects yielding net benefits should not be prohibited or given up just because there would be uncompensated losers."

In other words, Havighurst asks us to believe that greater harm would be affirmatively done by "a negative choice," i.e., by choosing to *do nothing*, for example, or by choosing not to develop some therapy, or by choosing an alternate one. So when compensation is impossible to arrange and "injustice therefore inevitable," Havighurst asks us to weigh *equally* the costs of *failure to develop* a therapy having fallout for others with the costs to the actual patients of developing the less efficient therapy. This explains his language, strange to ordinary ears, when he says that "it may still be unjust not to take action, since it would be to impose un-compensated costs (in the form of benefits denied) on the would-be beneficiaries."

Of course, if it is correct to speak of *injustice not done* and of *imposing* benefits denied, if it is correct to speak of *doing* "greater harm" by inaction, then in the case at issue one can make "each a possible gainer as well as a possible loser," and a pure utilitarianism may seem to be justified (p. 235). Therefore Havighurst ascends to outer space from which height a satellite photograph of medical policy decisions reveals no earthly "reason why the disadvantages ... should fall on would-be users of the nuclear device rather than potential recipients of radiation" (p. 241). So he can accuse the panel of using "different standards to weigh the patient's decision to expose society to risk on the one hand and the society's decision to expose the patient to risk of a poorer quality of life on the other" (p. 240).

But, of course, neither patient nor society have actually faced such a decision or made such choices. Society simply faces the choice between innovative therapies, both of which would benefit patients who now must die, or die prematurely. From that point of view, a technological and ethical assessment of avoidable and unavoidable costs to others would seem to be in order. Certainly it is possible to conclude from such an assessment (not a priori) that a patient's hypothetical preference for a higher quality of life that might flow from the rejected therapy at certain costs to others is "somehow immoral" (p. 240). That was what the assessment was all about!

Still, in this age of innovative therapies, one wonders what the conclusion of the panel majority would have been if the battery system did not exist as an alternative to the nuclear-powered system. Although the majority report began with a line of reasoning not unlike Havighurst's starting point, it notably rests some rather sweeping ethical verdicts upon contingencies, such as the availability of the battery alternative and the fact that it does not involve any known risk to the health and lives of other persons. "Accordingly," the panel concludes, "it is ethically unjustifiable, *regardless of the benefit-risk balance*, when (we are informed by experts) the battery-powered alternative is available, to subject the population at large to *any* significant degree of risk as a consequence of extending or improving the lives of particular recipients [italics added]" (p. 122). Suppose, we may ask, the battery system did involve significant but lesser risks to all concerned. Would the panel majority still have chosen risks that fall upon the potential recipient of the balancing benefits, and not on others close kin to him or randomly in the population? If those risks had been found acceptable but not the graver risks to others from the nuclear-powered device, would not such a conclusion require throwing into the balance the greater advantages of the latter to recipients? Then would not the panel have not only been engaged in quantifying the unquantifiable but also interchanging benefitees, like Havighurst, while reaching a different balancing judgment? Or suppose there were no alternative to the nuclear-powered totally implantable artificial heart, and its calculable adverse effects were still the same as detailed in this report, would the panel have had the courage to recommend that all research in nuclear technology of this sort be stopped? Or at least recommended that no such device be implanted in human beings until generations of "animal work" show genetic risks to be negligible, and efforts to decontaminate or control the radiation have succeeded?

Both sides in this disagreement charge the other with reversing the proper evaluation of an identifiable life in jeopardy more highly than "statistical lives" (cf. p. 241). The issue between them lies elsewhere, namely, over whether an unconveyed benefit counts the same as a harm done. And different viewpoints on that question, I suspect, are grounded in disagreement as to whether any patient has a *right* to medical progress, or whether medical progress is an optional goal.[5] The latter requires an ethical assessment of miracle cures, from which it may logically follow that we are forbidden to do or risk some sorts of harm to nonbenefitees for the sake of electable/nonelectable cures.

The foregoing cases represent some of the issues that must be addressed if ethical questions are to be not only asked but answered, anxieties not only aired but assuaged. And they must first be addressed by *ordering* our warrants in general ethics if medical ethics is to be more than special pleading.

Under the heading of "theory of action," Jonsen and Hellegers discuss the theory of natural law. That, indeed, is a worthy example of how, in general ethics, to talk reasonably about the justification for praising or blaming certain sorts of actions.

However, even if one were to conclude that the tradition of natural law has had its day and ceased to be, there are alternative theories of action in the writings of contemporary philosophers (indeed, there have been since Kant) that are quite credible candidates for the role "natural law" plays in J/H's chapter. From most of these less traditional, philosophical theories of action it is possible to derive some rather firm action guides, perhaps a number of unexceptionable action directives. It is important that an alternative theory of action of this order be made known to physicians and policy-makers for the following negative reason: It is commonly supposed that otherwise reasonable people hold to firm action guides only because of their adherence to natural law. If we could absent the relics of natural law, the furniture of our minds would consist solely of that footstool, situation ethics, or that loveseat, social utilitarianism, or both. Nothing could be further from the truth, as any even limited acquaintance with ethical writing today should make abundantly evident. We live, indeed, in an era of broken-down intellectual discourse, and no reader of Jonsen/Hellegers should conclude that natural law is the only theory of action that can supply anyone who exercises reason with some certainties about the morality of human actions, and therefore about physicians' actions.

One can simply begin in his ethical reflection with a moral agent or community of moral agents in interface with some cherished value. One can begin, in religious ethics, with *hesed*, or steadfast fidelity to the covenant of life, with life or with Christian love or compassion. Those standards in the Hebrew Bible and the Christian Scriptures root, of course, in conviction as to God's steadfast love for His created people; but the point here is that those ethical outlooks need not incorporate any articulation of "natural law." Or one can begin with "respect for life" or "respect for persons" (the outstanding philosophical proponents today of this standard expressly disavow what they understand "natural law" to mean). Or one can begin with the term "care" or "loyalty" as the requirement upon moral agents in their relation to anyone who bears a human countenance. I do not mean "care" in the sense of specific actions in a medical context, but "care" as a strong, ethical expression, the source of all particular obligations and one's court of final appeal for deciding the features of actions and practices that make what we do right or wrong in any context. That, then, would be a general ethics of actionable duties, the norm governing what anyone should do in his relations with others. Or finally, one might begin with "the preciousness of life" (unless that turns out to mean "price").

Let me take at this point "the preciousness of manuscripts" as a standard governing a scholar's conscience to show how from any of the foregoing nonnatural-law systems of general ethics can and indeed must be derived some firm, perhaps exceptionless, action guides. Anyone using manuscripts in the Beinecke Rare Book Library at Yale University is asked to read and sign, in order to indicate his understanding and acceptance of them, a set of "rules governing the use of manuscripts." Among other things, this codification of the principles of scholarly behavior states that "the use of any kind of pen is prohibited. Manuscripts may not be leaned on, written on, folded anew, traced, fastened with rubber bands, or handled in any way likely to damage them. Eating and smoking are prohibited in manuscript reading rooms." No mention is made of qualifications or exceptions allowed to anyone because he cherishes the preciousness of manuscripts only on the whole or in the long run, even though one can construct such justifiable sorts of exceptions in outlandish, unlikely examples. (Someone with a precious manuscript in hand and the whole building on fire may need to pop some pep pills or salt or vitamin pills to bolster his failing strength, and therefore might directly appeal beyond the rules to his need to "eat" in the manuscript room in order to act out successfully his true cherishing of that manuscript!) When recently I read this "code of scholarly ethics" and signed the card indicating I understood and meant to abide by those rules, I placed the card on top of a manuscript of Jonathan Edwards and signed with a pen, to the consternation of all the librarians! That was a lesson to me that there can be practically exceptionless rules stemming simply from the preciousness of manuscripts and an upright conscience in the moral agent relating to that value.

So when I read in the International Code of Medical Ethics, adopted by the Assembly of the World Medical Association, London, 1949, the following words: "As a stream cannot rise above its source, so a code cannot change a low-grade man into a high-grade doctor, but it can help a good man to be a better man and a more enlightened doctor. It can quicken and inform conscience, but not create one," I think the physicians who wrote that statement meant the informing of conscience as to the fitting actions. They presupposed "the preciousness of life" (or "the preciousness of manuscripts") and attitudes on the part of moral agents apt to cherish those things. At issue was only, or mainly, codes of conduct so that agents could be braced to act in accord with their best character and for the sake of the objects they valued most, or the loyalty their role requires.

Let us take "care" as standard in the strong sense explained above or "the preciousness of life"; and let us ask, What does care or the preciousness of life require of moral agents generally and of physicians in particular? That question breaks down into two sorts of questions productive of two sorts of answers.

1. One can say, first, that we are to tell what we should do in a particular dilemma by making sure we know the facts of that situation and the options it affords, and by then asking which specific action takes most care of human life—present lives and (in the case of research) future lives. In more or less discrete decisions in the face of more or less unique problematic cases we are to ask, What singular deed or design of ours is most likely to embody or convey care or respect for human life? We ask, Will this or that procedure care for the patient more? Or we ask, Will this or that research design be productive of the more significant benefit for the ongoing community of medical care?

This first form of our question is productive of balancing decisions to operate or not to operate in particular cases. It is also productive of the second Article of the Nuremberg Medical Code, which states that an experiment on human subjects "should be such as to yield fruitful results for the good of society, unprocurable by any other method or means of study, and not random and unnecessary in nature." These are essentially *prudential* decisions concerning what care requires, which only the physician or researchers are competent to make and which they decide case after case, from protocol to protocol.

2. The second form of the question, however, leads to answers of a different order. One can say in medical ethics that we are to tell what we ought to do, not only by asking which particular action or research design is most caring, but also by asking which *rules of practice*, what *principles* of action, what moral

institutions or "covenants of loyalty" (as I prefer to call them) would, if maintained or established in the regulations of the medical profession, prove generally most caring for the dignity of man in patients or research subjects. Some contemporary philosophers call answers to this question "rules of the game"; and I suggest that there are some universal rules of the game called "caring."

This sort of ethical reasoning from the ultimate norm "caring" or "the preciousness of life" is productive, for example, of the first Article of the Nuremberg Medical Code, which requires a free and informed consent in human experimentation. Now, the physician must also make prudential judgments in applying that principle in medical care and research. For this reason some physicians are under the impression that they are engaged in the same sort of activity when they judge a patient's or subject's consent to be an understanding, voluntary one as they are when they make balancing judgments to operate or not or in perfecting protocols.

In this I believe they are mistaken. In the latter case, the physician tries to respond aptly to a particular situation. In the former, he is asking the applicable meaning of a principle of medical ethics, a rule of professional practice. He is exploring the requirements of a governing "moral notion." He asks what he should to in order to *apply* a moral principle.

To repeat: the two forms of our original question are: What should we do in particular actions or designs in order, case by case, to extend the greatest care? and, What rules of practice render medical action most careful and respectful of the dignity of all concerned?

At this point we face again the question of priority of one over the other of these two sorts of ethical reasoning. I suggest that there are sound grounds for saying that rules of practice or regulative "moral notions" should be accorded priority over an ethics of doing the most good on the whole, if there are cases of irresolvable conflict between them.

To illustrate from another realm: the practice of promise-making and promise-keeping. If you promise a dying friend, no one else knowing, to take care of his two retarded children, why should you keep that promise if you come upon two other children who are very bright, equally destitute, your funds are limited, and there is no other recourse? Without here saying that promise-keeping is absolutely without exception binding upon us, I suggest that such a promise to one's dying friend ought to be kept even in face of the fact that one might do far more good on the whole by, instead, taking care of those other two children.

Dr. Henry K. Beecher made the same sort of priority judgment between the first and second articles of the Nuremberg Medical Code. If an experiment is moral it is moral in its inception; it does not become moral because it produces valuable data (or is wisely calculated to do so). Beecher goes on to criticize the language of the second provision because it opens the door to violations of the first, and much else besides. "The words 'for the good of society' must be viewed with distaste, even alarm. Undoubtedly all sound work has this as its ultimate aim, but such highflown expressions are not necessary and have been used within recent memory as cover for outrageous ends." Beecher repeats his negative verdict in his latest book: "The *bonum communum* was precisely the rationalization claimed by the Nazis"; "In Rule 2, the phrase 'for the good of society' is unsavory."[7]

That may go too far in downgrading the second article as also a manifestation of an ethics of care. Still, it needs to be acknowledged that there is a possible collision between these two requirements. One of the articles places an independent limit upon the use of the other; and fidelity to the being and well-being, and to the humanity, of everyone now engaged in helping to make medical progress takes priority. A major task in the ethical practice of medicine is to harmonize these requirements and to stay within the boundaries of permissible practice fixed by both together.

As an illustration of what goes on in normative medical ethics, it is most important for us to see that care leads to these two provisions through different modes of ethical reasoning. In the one case we are led to a *benefits* requirement by asking which particular actions or designs are productive of greater care for human life. In the other case, we are led to the *consent* requirement by asking which practice rule or principle of loyalty includes and exhibits care for all presently concerned.

Note also that if we assign priority to a benefits requirement (the second article), we are taken all the way to utilitarianism; and that, I will simply say, would be to try to revive a very sick horse. If that seems too extreme a statement, I can only cite the waning influence of utilitarianism among philosophers doing ethics today. If a crisis of medical ethics today is the threat that it will go overboard for utilitarianism, then such an eventuality would mean a most remarkable breakdown of communication without past parallel between two leading professions in our society, physicians and ethicists.

Let us now replay our model of an ethics of care in other illustrations. Here we come to some disputed conclusions, but ones that still show the crux to be our same two questions: What does care require in this particular situation? and What does care require as a general practice, in all like situations?

In hemodialysis, or like instances of placing a patient on a sparse medical resource whose absence would be fatal, decisions must be made as to who shall live, who die. If medical care asks only, what helps most in this particular situation? it unavoidably gets into judging competitively the comparative social worthiness of two patients who both need the only available kidney machine. However, if we ask, as we should also ask, What does care require as a rule of practice, expressive of loyalty and respect for all lives concerned in the issue? sound moral reasoning would, I suggest, incline us to adopt the controls of some form of lottery, or of a "first come, first served" arrangement, upon the vagaries of our private judgments about who most deserves to live. That alone would insure that, within the limits of possibility, care will be distributed equally to all who are in need, that we respect everyone who bears a human countenance. In the minimal form of equality of opportunity to live or to die when all cannot be saved, such a practice rule insures that everyone counts, and no one counts for more than any other (as would be the case if we applied criteria of comparative social worthiness).

Another illustration of a basic rule of medical practice is: Never directly take the life of a terminal patient, or intervene to hasten his death. Medical care as a moral institution can never mean that. This is a prohibition constitutive of the game of medical care, to be compared with rules of the game in football defining "offside" or forbidding more than eleven men in play. These proscriptions are without exception; they tell us the game we are playing, and lay down the basic roles of the players in relation to one another.

But in football there are other rules that are only advice to the players as to how they should play the game most of the time—Punt on fourth down, for example. Everyone knows there are exceptions to that rule. One should be prepared to violate it in appropriate situations. So also, there are summary directives to physicians within the institution of medical care that tell them how to play that game most of the time, but not always—for example, try and try again to cure your patient; struggle with him to save his life. Still, everyone should know that doctors ought not always do that. There comes a time when medical care no longer means continuing exquisite efforts to cure and to save life. To be sure, medical care always means to cherish and respect life, and that can never mean killing patients. But there comes a time when to cherish and respect life means to care, but *only* to care, for the dying. It means no longer to oppose death; instead, to accept its coming. It means not to prolong dying, but to comfort and to keep company with the dying, to make a human presence in that solitude, never deserting the dying patient, and insuring to him as much dignity as possible in his passage. In the words of the old revival hymn, medical care need not always mean trying to "rescue the perishing," but it does always mean to "care for the dying." So, unlike the prohibition of killing the innocent, the injunction to cure and save life is not a universal requirement of medical practice. How could it be, since cure is not always possible, and will finally become impossible in all cases? Care never ceases; yet care, never ceasing, has no duty to do the impossible, or the futile.

Thus, I argue that an ethics of care prolongs itself into a professional ethics consisting of several sorts of things: (1) rules constitutive of medical care, e.g the consent requirement, the prohibition of direct killing, and randomizing life-and-death decisions to insure equality of access to sparse resources, which are always binding; (2) directives to cure and save life which true care sometimes suspends and replaces by comfort and dignity for the dying; (3) balancing situational decisions, such as to operate or not to operate, or to use this or that research protocol.

Objection will be forthcoming to the more strenuous of these conclusions, to the view that professional medical ethics, like any other ethics, consists also of universally binding obligations. The objection will be that there are always "exceptions." But every ethicist knows that "exceptions" to rules of practice are themselves implied by the standard (the "care") in question; and also that "exceptions" themselves are "universals," only more specifically defined.

An "exception" indicates a *class* or *sort* of case having relevant moral features in common. The "exception" is a "moral notion," not a particular instance. The relevant moral features of cases are as universalizable as was the original rule before the exception was added. A chief exception to the need for consent—if such it is—still tells us, as a guide to action, that similar agents should do likewise in similar situations. *One* who is a physician, for example, not just *I* who am, should stop to help in emergencies, not just because that is a socially worthy individual over there by the side of the road, and even if he had no contract with me to be his physician. The moral judgment remains intact, even if all personal pronouns are removed (who I am or who he is—except for the relation of care). Even if suddenly there were no more crushed bodies along the highways, that would still in principle be the right thing to do. Even if never actually repeated again, what was done is essentially repeatable. In stopping to help without prior patient consent, the physician wills what he does to be a universal moral law governing medical practice. He prescribes for himself and all men a moral institution.

No man is good enough, or for that matter wise enough, to treat another without his understanding consent. Besides, medical care is a joint venture in which, ideally, patient and physician should both say, I cure. Therefore, the consent requirement is a universal rule of medical practice. Yet there is an evident sort of "exception" where consent seems not required, as in the case of highway accident victims. We might say that if a physician stops on the road to Jericho, instead of passing by on his way to read a research paper before a scientific gathering, or to visit his regular paying patients, he is self-selected as good enough to practice medicine without the needy man's expressed consent.

But the point is not whether or not that was subjectively an ethical physician, or not. The question is rather what makes us objectively certain that stopping was right to do. We could say that in these instances a physician practices medicine without consent—an exception to the rule. Instead we say—correctly, I believe—that the unconscious man "constructively" consented to procedures from which he may suffer harm if the physician bungles. Why do we imply that he did? The answer is by an application of the *reversibility* test, which shows that in the case of highway accident victims the requirement of consent is only being extended and applied. The physician exchanges places with the man by the side of the road, and thus sustains in himself the claims of the absolutely universalizable principle that human need calls for rescue, that a man in need "consents" to be helped.

Notice that the consent requirement is in no way weakened; its meaning might rather be said to be extended, explained, and applied.

To obtain another so-called "exception" to universal rules of medical practice, let us say—as I would argue—that one entailment of the consent requirement is that no one should give proxy consent for children or other incompetents to hazardous trials unless those are at least remotely in their behalf medically. (That "unless" is already an "exception," which again shows that exceptions to moral rules always define a *class* of actions, never unique situation.) Suppose we say, then, that a rule of medical practice is: "Never subject children to the unknown possible hazards of medical investigations having no possible relation to their own treatment." To that we must promptly add, "except in epidemic conditions." That exception simply explains, extends, and applies the rule. It takes account of the fact that the dangers from which the child needs protection need not be already resident beneath his own skin. He is already subject to predictable risks from exposure to crippling epidemic, for example, of polio. He can therefore be treated as one of a population and those risks be weighed against the risks, which are not negligible, of entering him into field trials of a vaccine. To do this *is* in his behalf medically, and therefore to put parental consent in place of the consent he cannot maturely give is quite valid. We only do what anyone, any parent, should do. This, again, illustrates the reversibility test and the universalizability test in deciding the ethical thing to do. The personal pronouns are removed, any idiosyncratic or situationally unique features are removed; yet the moral judgment remains intact. Such decisions are clearly not like deciding to operate or not to operate. In the latter case, one decides what care requires in a particular situation. In the former, one decides what actions fall under a rule of care and loyalty to the dignity of persons in need.

One cannot even do violence to the consent of another except within the consent requirement as a canon of medical practice (as but an instance of a wider ethics of respect for persons), any more than one can commit an "error" or draw a "walk" unless he is playing the game of baseball, which has some exceptionless rules. In the practice of medicine, too, there are constitutive principles. Otherwise, there are no infractions; and physicians are only technicians going about doing the most good on the whole, performing actions that can only be mistakes, never in any meaningful sense moral violations.

An important conclusion from the foregoing in criticism of the J/H paper is as follows: There are "rules of practice" and not only singular, particular duties to be derived from a proper theory of action. Of course, this is true also for natural law as a theory of action. It is strange that J/H do not take note of this fact when discussing the common good. Instead, too wide a gulf is set between the general justice of institutions and a physicians virtues and his actions in one-to-one relation to his patient's needs. Forgotten is the fact that the physician has a moral *role* in relation to that patient, a role having universalizable features and not particular features only. Justice is first of all a virtue of the physician's role, and of professional practice vis-à-vis patients. That justice is therefore quite compatible with the justice that is "above all the virtue of institutions."

I understand J/H to say that medicine as a "practice" means only one-to-one physician-to-patient relations, having few if any generalizable features. They define a "practice" as "a private . . . interaction between two parties." Only an ethics of institutional forms seems *not* to "limit our attention to good intentions alone or to the outcome of single actions." So they say, "Modern medicine, then, is an institution that incorporates a profession that practices a technique and an art. The practice remains, indeed, at the heart of the institution, but . . . a doctrine of the common good must be added to provide an ethics for the institution." There can be no objection to that statement, except to say that it bridges a gulf that ought not to have been perceived to be so wide. For with the backing and appraisals of a proper theory of *action*, a physician's practice of his technique and art already entails "rules of practice." These are as close to institutionalization under a theory of the common good as a physician's habitual aptitudes of character are to a theory governing the appraisal of his clinical actions.

Granted, that in appraising the relief of the suffering of one person by another properly qualified person, one does not perceive that situation or evaluate it primarily in terms of the action's external major effects in extensivity and perpetuity upon those not presently suffering or even not yet born. But in that quite personal situation of one qualified practitioner in relation to one suffering human being, we should also abstract all personal pronouns, letting what "care" requires remain intact. Then also we should treat similar cases similarly and universalize the right action to other, like cases. There is already a "design of offices and tasks," roles and relations, in a theory of blameworthy and praiseworthy individual action. Universalizable principles governing the practice of medicine do not arise alone when considerations of the common good come into view. There should be "just medicine" before the question of a just society is ever raised, or else later on there is not likely to be "just medicine."

Doubtless, it is the purpose of a theory of the common good to discover how to avoid moral conflicts; one of its chief tasks is to try to reconcile competing moral claims. But when J/H add to that the task of discovering "how to compensate *unjust* harm [italics added]," they reach and pass the point where most ethicists have already been forced to assign weights, priorities, and some order among ethical justifications. It is one thing to devise schemes for compensating for *acceptable* and *accepted* risks of injury and for any actual harm to "normal volunteers"—*no injustice done.* It is quite another thing to speak of compensating "unjust harm." Rather, one should say that harm ought not to have done it in the first place. A theory of right action claims priority over a theory of the common good, unless the "very meaning" of the latter is dependent upon the former. It may be that "the problem of the lesser number, disadvantages for the sake of the greater, remains unsolved" because it is unsolvable without a clear choice in case of conflict between some individual harms and some social benefits. Again, the smooth elision among all moral claims threatens to come apart when J/H speak of costs without compensating benefits to certain individuals in randomized clinical trials, "particularly when one of the alternatives is a proven therapeutic agent." Some would view the withholding of a proven remedy from a control group to be an instance of "unjust harm" that no medical research benefits could justify, even when redressed by extrinsic benefits to those less well treated.

Thus, Jonsen and Hellegers have not clarified the relation between the justice of moral actions and the justice that is definitive of the common good.

Notes to Chapter Three

1. Compare Aristotle: *Nicomachean Ethics*, 1107a, 1109a.

2. Charles Ralph Buncher, Sc.D., "Administratively Significant," *New England Journal of Medicine*, Vol. 289, No. 3 (July 19, 1973), pp. 155-57.

3. *Federal Register*, Vol. 38, No. 221, Pt. II (November 16, 1973), pp. 31738-48.

4. *The Totally Implantable Artificial Heart.* DHEW Publication No. (NIH) (June 1973), 74-191.

5. Hans Jonas, "Philosophical Reflections on Human Experimentation," *Daedalus*, Vol. 98, No. 2 (Spring 1969), 245; reprinted Hans Jonas, *Philosophical Essays* (Englewood Cliffs, N.J.: Prentice-Hall, 1974), p. 131. Also see Paul Ramsey, *The Patient as Person: Explorations in Medical Ethics* (New Haven: Yale University Press, 1970), pp. 107-109.

6. Henry K. Beecher, "Experimentation in Man," *Journal of the American Medical Association*, Vol. 169, No. 5 (January 31, 1959), 468.

7. Henry K. Beecher, *Research and the Individual* (Boston: Little, Brown & Co., 1970), pp. 77, 232.

※ *Chapter 4*

Self-Reliance and the Collective Good: Medicine in China

Victor W. Sidel and Ruth Sidel

The Chinese health care system illustrates a blend—which appears, in many ways, to be unique to China—of responsibility on the part of the individual to protect his own health and that of his neighbors, and of societal responsibility to organize and channel health care activity for local, regional, and nationwide well-being. Health care activity represents a complex mix of decisions made by individuals themselves, although within a common ideological and cultural framework, and decisions made at a series of organized societal levels. At the most local of these levels, where in a decentralized society such as China's many of the most important decisions are made, individual and societal decision-making are so tightly intertwined as to be almost indistinguishable.

The issue of the role of the individual in Chinese society is a complex one that can be understood only within the Chinese context and not within a Western one. Individualism never occupied the central position in China that it has in the West for the past several hundred years. In prerevolutionary China, the individual was seen as part of a group, part of his family, his clan, his village. His responsibilities to his living relatives and to his ancestors were clearly delineated and keenly felt.

Interviewed after a lecture in New York in 1974, the Chinese anthropologist Francis L.K. Hsu made some relevant observations that were quoted in *The New Yorker*: "From the Chinese point of view," said Dr. Hsu, "freedom is not the first concern. The importance of personal freedom is a Western premise—it has been from the time of the Greeks. On that premise, people always work for individual aggrandizement, individual sensuality, individual satisfaction. The

Chinese have never felt that way. In the old days, the Chinese were supposed to submit themselves to the family and to the kinship group; nowadays they are supposed to submit themselves to a larger group—a political group. In either case, they consider individualism to be selfishness."

But the comparison with the past has also been stated another way: "In the past the Chinese swept only in front of his door post; now he sweeps the whole street." Thus, while in postliberation China the individual is no more the centerpin around which all else turns than in the past, his devotion to the collective seems to have broadened and deepened. Not only is there the old devotion to the family or kinship group but now the devotion extends to the group with which the individual works, to those in his neighborhood or commune, and to the people of the country as a whole—even to non-Han "minority peoples" who live in the areas near China's border.

This change has many roots and many facets. Among the roots, certainly, is a socialist revolution, which changed the control of power and of resources in the society. But what has emerged is a special kind of socialism, forged by Mao Tse-tung and his followers, which makes both self-reliance and the collective good into the highest virtues toward which man can strive.

To "serve the people," to work for the good of the society, seems to be the prevailing ethic, expressed in countless signs and posters and in the conversation of all with whom we spoke in China. In order to understand more fully the role of the individual within the context of this ethical framework, it is helpful to distinguish between individuality and individualism as they seem to be viewed in China. Individual talents are carefully nourished and developed. The excellent Ping-Pong player is given extra help and plays on a local or national team; the scientist receives further training and is provided with facilities for research; the dancer and musician have the opportunity to employ their skills; and the person who exhibits special qualities of "caring" is recruited for medical school or into other helping roles. But these individuals are encouraged to utilize their talents not for their own sake, not for the sake of individual development and fulfillment, but for the good of the larger society. Thus individuality is encouraged, particularly when it meets the needs of the larger society; individualism is not.

The health care system has attempted to utilize and promote a commitment both to self-reliance and to the welfare of the group. The focus on mass participation, mass education, "mobilizing the masses" to engage in sanitation work or in wiping out schistosomiasis, and intense efforts in immunization and birth control programs can all be seen as part of a broader societal view. Within the context of this larger view, issues of privacy, considered an integral part of medical care in the West, take on quite a different character. The number of children a family has, for example, is no longer a private decision; "planned birth" is viewed as a collective problem, one that affects the whole society as well as each family. Whether one's child is immunized against polio becomes the formal concern of the local community, whose stake in the immunization program is emphasized over its importance to the individual. While the Chinese often seem reluctant to deal with traditionally private matters, particularly sexual matters, in a public manner, they nevertheless have developed mechanisms such as small group discussions and the intensive use of paraprofessionals which appear to deal with these issues effectively. They seem able to bridge the gap between the preservation of the family—which has been strengthened and protected in post-Liberation China—and devotion to a broader set of social responsibilities.

How the Chinese have managed to bridge the apparent gap between encouragement of "self-reliance"—which is also a widely esteemed virtue in modern China—and devotion to common societal goals is demonstrated in numerous examples in the health care system of people encouraged to take individual responsibility for the health of themselves, their family members, and neighbors, but within the context of broader social responsibilities.

URBAN HEALTH CARE

While rural health care provides some of the best examples of the intertwining of individual and societal decision-making and responsibility, we will concentrate in this chapter on the urban scene, a milieu much more recognizable to readers in the United States than are the peasants, villages, and communes of rural China. Cities are governed by revolutionary committees which are formal government bodies; city health services are coordinated by the local bureau of public health, which has responsibility not only for almost all service units and almost all health care personnel in the city, but also for the educational institutions of nonphysician health care personnel.

The next lower level of urban organization is the "district," which is also governed by a revolutionary committee. Hangchow, a city of 700,000 people, is divided into four districts; the city proper of Peking, with 4 million people, into nine districts; and the city proper of Shanghai, with 6 million, into ten districts. Districts are subdivided into "streets" or "neighborhoods," which are the lowest level of formal governmental organization in the city. The neighborhood is governed by a committee composed of representatives of the people in the area, cadres, and, in diminishing numbers since the end of the Cultural Revolution, members of the People's Liberation Army. The committee's responsibilities include the administration of local factories, primary schools, and kindergartens, a neighborhood hospital or health center, repair services, and a housing department, as well as the organization and supervision of "residents'" or "lane" committees.

The smallest unit in the urban areas is the "lane," with from 1000 to 8000 residents. Some lanes are further divided into "groups," for example, the residents of a single large apartment building, which are headed by a group or deputy group leader. The lane is governed by a committee chosen by, and from among, the "mass" living in the lane. The committee is, therefore, a "mass organization" rather than a formal governmental body, and thus does not usually have the three-in-one components of the revolutionary committees (ordinary people, cadres, army); the elderly play a key role in the organization and administration of these residents' committees. (Figure 4-1 is a schematic representation of the levels of urban organization.)

Each of the nine districts of Peking city proper, to use it as an example, has a population of about 400,000. Among the services provided at the district level are hospitals, sanitation facilities, middle schools (roughly equivalent to our junior and senior high schools), and "prevention stations" for illnesses such as tuberculosis and mental disorders. Within each district there are "neighborhoods" consisting of approximately 50,000 people. The West District of Peking has nine neighborhoods, of which the Fengsheng neighborhood, with a population of 53,000, is one. Within the Fengsheng neighborhood's jurisdiction are six factories, eight shops, ten primary schools, four kindergartens, and a neighborhood hospital.

Fengsheng is one of the older neighborhoods of Peking. It consists entirely of one-story dwellings rather than the four- or five-story apartment buildings found in newer neighborhoods. Courtyards, with several families living in each, are entered through doorways in the walls lining Fengsheng's 132 lanes. The people are grouped into twenty-five residents' committees, each of which encompasses about 2000 people. These committees usually provide a health station and other social services. Within each committee are "groups" of from 50 to 150 people, led by a group leader and a deputy group leader, who organize a number of services under what we might term social or welfare work.

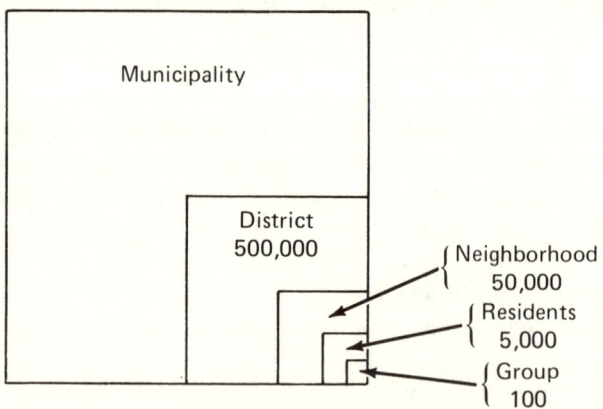

Figure 4-1. Organization of Cities in the PRC.

The health workers at the residents' committee level are local housewives called "Red Medical Workers." Three such workers serve the Wu Ting residents' committee, located in the western part of the Fengsheng neighborhood. Wu Ting has 400 families totaling approximately 1500 people. The chairman of the residents' committee, Chao Huan-ching, a seventy-year-old retired worker, serves as the director of the Wu Ting residents' committee health station, although he is not considered a health worker.

The major function of a residents' committee health station is preventive work, although it does treat some minor illnesses. The Wu Ting station is located in a single room off one of the courtyards, and its fairly typical equipment includes a bed for examination or treatment, a table with chairs for consultations, and a cabinet containing both Western-type and traditional Chinese medicines. On the walls are a picture of Mao Tse-tung, an acupuncture chart, and health propaganda posters.

Comrade Yan Hsio-hua, one of Wu Ting's Red Medical Workers, is thirty-eight years of age. After her marriage she worked briefly as a saleswoman, until she was nineteen, when her first child was born. Since then she has been home taking care of her children, now aged nineteen, fifteen, and eleven. Two years ago, responding to the call to "Serve the People" which grew out of the Great Proletarian Cultural Revolution, she volunteered for one month of training in the Fengsheng neighborhood hospital. During the training period she and her fellow housewives learned history-taking and simple physical examination techniques such as blood pressure determination. They were taught the uses of a number of Western and herb medicines, and techniques of acupuncture and of intramuscular and subcutaneous injection. Knowledge of preventive measures such as sanitation, immunization, and birth control procedures were an important part of the curriculum. But the most important thing Comrade Yang and her colleagues were taught, according to our hosts in China, was that there are no barriers to the acquisition of medical knowledge other than the person's own fears of not being able to learn. Once these fears are overcome, in part through sessions where life in the "bitter past" and the feelings of the students are shared and discussed, a lifetime of continued learning is anticipated. Comrade Yang continues to learn from the doctor at the neighborhood hospital who visits the residents' committee health station three times a week, from her own periodic visits to the hospital for instruction or to consult about a patient, and from the biweekly or monthly meetings of all the Red Medical Workers of the neighborhood.

Another Red Medical Worker, Chang Cheng-yu, is forty-three years of age. Her two children are now twenty-one and twelve years old. She has been a housewife all her married life and had never worked outside the home until she became a health worker. Both comrades Yang and Chang live in the residents' committee area within a few steps of the health station, which is staffed by them and their colleagues from 8:00 to 11:00 A.M., when they usually see from seven to ten patients, and from 3:00 to 5:30 P.M., when they see four or five more patients. If a resident feels ill when the station is closed, he or she may go directly to the home of one of the Red Medical Workers, although we were told that this rarely happens.

The Red Medical Workers are paid a modest sum for their work, about fifteen *yuan* a month, roughly one-third of a beginning factory worker's wages. The stipend comes in part from the small fees paid by patients, in part from the collective income of neighborhood factories and home industries. A patient's fee for a visit to the health station is never more than ten *fen* (about five American cents), and usually less. If the patient is a retired worker, he may present the health station bills to his former place of employment, where reimbursement is made in full. If the patient is a dependent of a factory worker or of one who has retired, the factory will reimburse half the health station charges. Currently employed workers are rarely seen in the health stations, because their primary medical care needs are taken care of at their place of work.

A large part of the Red Medical Workers' duties relate to sanitation work in the neighborhood; they are supervised by the Department of Public Health of the neighborhood hospital. In the summer there are campaigns against flies and mosquitoes and attempts to prevent the spread of gastrointestinal disorders. In the winter and spring the health workers are concerned mainly with the prevention of upper respiratory infections, for which they encourage morning exercises, washing the face with cold water, long walks, the use of traditional medicines, and the use of masks when a patient has a cold to prevent its spread. The public health department also supervises the Red Medical Workers in providing immunizations, which are usually given in the health stations.

The Red Medical Workers are also responsible for the provision of birth control information. They distribute oral contraceptives directly, often with no specific medical examination prior to initiation of treatment. Intrauterine contraceptive devices are available and insertion is performed by trained personnel in the neighborhood hospital. The Red Medical Workers make periodic visits to all women in the residents' committee area to encourage the use of contraception.

In addition to treating patients with minor illnesses the Red Medical Workers provide follow-up care after a patient has been treated in a hospital. For example, Red Medical Workers treat patients with arthritis, using a combination of acupuncture and herb medicines. They also check blood pressures and determine the dose of medication for patients with hypertension. The therapy has been started in the neighborhood or district hospital and the continuing dose of medication prescribed. The Red Medical Worker may herself change the type of traditional medicine given to a hypertensive patient, but can only vary the dose of Western medicine within certain limits. If a patient's blood pressure is found to be outside limits set by the hospital, the patient is sent back to the hospital for treatment and new instructions.

Self-Reliance & the Collective Good: Medicine in China 63

In another Peking neighborhood, adjacent to the Imperial Palace Museum, the Red Medical Workers discussed their responsibilities (see Figure 4-2). Through mass meetings and discussions with individual families, the Red Medical Workers in the twenty-three lane health stations of this neighborhood have educated the population of 49,300 about the importance of immunizations. The Red Medical Worker also informs parents when it is time for their children to receive immunizations. The lane health station is very near each family's home and therefore convenient to visit. If a family does not bring a child to the station for immunization at the appropriate time, however, the Red Medical Worker will sometimes bring the child to the station, or if necessary arrange for the immunization to be given in the home. A chart in one lane health station indicated that 95 to 100 percent of the children had been immunized against measles, diphtheria, poliomyelitis, pertussis, tetanus, encephalitis, meningitis, and tuberculosis. Other charts for this district indicated a marked decline in recent years in the incidence of measles, poliomyelitis, diphtheria, and pertussis. About 80 percent of the children had been vaccinated against smallpox. Since the last case of smallpox in China occurred in 1954, vaccination is not given if there is any contraindication. It is worth noting that in a society in which total, mass participation and distribution of the limited resources among all are important principles, individual exceptions can be made when there is good reason to do so. In technical terms, "herd immunity" tends to protect the

---

1. Hold high the great banner of Mao Tse-tung's thought. Stand up for proletarian politics. Study Chairman Mao's philosophical works creatively. Change our world outlook. Practice and apply it in every day's work.
2. Strengthen revolutionary discipline. Do not be late to work, do not go home early, do not be "thrice divorced": divorced from the mass movement, divorced from physical labor, or divorced from the masses.
3. Stress the policy of prevention. Initiate the patriotic health movement centered around the prevention of disease. Every week there should be a small general cleaning and every two weeks a big general cleaning. Proceed to inspect and increase the management of infectious disease. Emphasize prevention and vaccination work. Reach the unity of prevention and treatment.
4. Work on family planning. Do propaganda work constantly. Know the local situation clearly.
5. Be self-reliant. Observe the principles of diligence and frugality. Try to treat the patient at home. Take good care of chronic diseases. Work for the prevention of disease and the treatment of disease at a local level. Move forward (ride the horse of) the three traditions: traditional doctors, traditional medicines, and traditional methods. Use yourself creatively (collect the herbs yourself, plant the herbs yourself, and use the herbs yourself).

Figure 4-2. Instructions Posted at a Lane Health Station in Peking: Working Responsibilities of Red Medical Workers.

minority who are unvaccinated, and they can be spared the risk of vaccination.

Health workers in the lanes and neighborhoods also play an important role in birth control campaigns. In the period preceding Liberation, China's annual crude birth rate was said to be about 43 per 1000 population. After a lengthy period of widely varying policies toward population control, vigorous campaigns were launched—particularly in the cities in the 1960s. Education is one of the most important aspects of the program. This is done through booklets and illustrated materials, and, even more important, through street committees, Red Medical Workers, and other person-to-person contacts. The emphasis is placed on the importance of family planning in building a new socialist society, rather than on the Malthusian concepts of overpopulation leading to poverty and famine. The captions on a birth control poster illustrate this emphasis very well. People were urged to practice birth control in order to: 1) study and apply Chairman Mao's thought in a lively way; 2) consolidate the proletarian dictatorship; 3) prepare against war, against national disaster, and for the people; 4) support world revolution; 5) cultivate successors to the proletarian revolution; and 6) grasp revolution, promote production, and carry on work.

According to Han Suyin, family planning in China is

> based upon the emancipation of the woman, her equality, her right to study and participate in all political decisions, and her heightened social consciousness. Planned parenthood and marriage are factors for the promotion of a socialist society, but they must be based on full equality of both partners, self-respect, and knowledge. It is therefore essential that the masses themselves carry out the programs.[1]

The Chinese marriage law of 1950 provides that women may marry at age eighteen and men at age twenty, but a vigorous and successful campaign has been waged to delay the age of marriage. In the cities the ideal age for marriage for men is now said to be twenty-six to twenty-nine, and for women twenty-four to twenty-six. Late marriage is of course itself a powerful method of population control. Many first babies are being delivered to mothers in their late twenties or early thirties. The optimal family size in the cities is now considered to be two to three children, and tubal or vas deferens ligation is often urged after the second or third child.

In the urban lanes, Red Medical Workers are responsible for the dissemination of birth control information. In Silvery Lane in Hangchow, health workers trained by Red Medical Workers from the street hospital go from door to door talking with the women about the number of children they want and the birth control methods they are using. By means of monthly visits to the home of each woman of "childbearing age," which is defined as the time of marriage to menopause, the Red Medical Workers keep careful track of the contraceptives used. A chart on the wall at the Silvery Lane health station outlines the birth

Self-Reliance & the Collective Good: Medicine in China 65

control methods used in the lane (see Figure 4-3). Abortions are free and easily available but are almost never requested by unmarried women; pregnancies among unmarried women are exceedingly rare and out-of-wedlock births essentially unheard of. The annual crude birth rate in Silvery Lane was reported to be at the most incredibly low level of 7.9 per 1000 population. When the health workers in Silvery Lane were asked about possible reluctance on the part of the women to talk about the birth control methods they use, one health worker replied that sometimes the younger, newly married women were "shy," but that once they understood the importance of planned birth to China, they cooperated willingly.

In Kung Chiang New Village, part of the Yang Pu District in the industrial northeast section of Shanghai, Red Medical Workers conducted family planning

	Number	Percent of Total
Total married women of childbearing age	369	100
Vasectomies	10	3
Tubal ligation	89	24
Total permanently sterilized	99	27
Oral contraceptives	65	17
Condom	69	19
IUD	22	6
Rhythm	7	2
Other	9	2
Total using contraceptives	172	46
Husband outside the city	21	6
"Has not been pregnant"	6	2
Breast feeding	16	4
Newly married	7	2
Chronically ill	13	3
Other	25	7
Total not using contraceptives	88	24
Pregnant	10	3

Abortions, January-September 1971: None
Birth Rate, January-September 1971: 5.9 per 1,000

Figure 4-3. Family Planning Chart in the Silvery Lane Health Station Hangchow, Serving 2700 People, September 1971.

education at the residents' committee level. All of these trained housewives, each with two or three children, had had tubal ligations, so they served as models for the women they visited monthly. They told us that while no one was "forced" to limit the family to two or three children, they put great stress on educating people on the importance—not necessarily to themselves, but rather to Shanghai and to China—of population control. As a result of these intensive neighborhood campaigns the crude birth rate for the city proper of Shanghai in 1971 and 1972 was reported to be approximately 7 per 1000.

MAOIST PRINCIPLES

Implicit in these activities on the local level are a number of Maoist principles that have been widely applied in different ways throughout life in China. Mao Tse-tung in his 1937 essay "On Practice" wrote:

> If you want to know the taste of a pear, you must change the pear by eating it yourself. If you want to know the structure and properties of the atom, you must make physical and chemical experiments to change the state of the atom. If you want to know the theory and methods of revolution, you must take part in revolution. All genuine knowledge originates in direct experience.[2]

This theme of knowing by doing runs through essentially all aspects of Chinese life today. A peasant learns the difficulties of determining agricultural priorities by taking part in decision-making. The urban doctor learns about the life of the peasants by moving to the countryside for a period of time and laboring with them. The child learns what it is like to be a peasant or a worker by growing vegetables or doing a job on consignment from a factory. And, according to this theory, the way to teach 800 million people the principles of health prevention and health care is to involve them in it.

The mobilization of the mass has been the primary technique by which the Chinese have accomplished their feats of engineering: the construction of their canals, bridges, large-scale irrigation projects, dikes, and dams. The mobilization of the mass has also been the key mechanism in their feats of human engineering. Han Suyin describes the process of education of the masses since 1949 as one that has included the "eradication of the feudal mind," and "getting the masses away from the anchored belief that natural calamities are 'fixed by heaven' and that therefore nothing can be done to remedy one's lot." She continues: "To bridge this gap between scientific modern man and feudal man, the prey of superstition, and to do it within the compass of one generation, is a formidable task."[3] One important technique used to accomplish this "formidable task" has been the activating of the mass. In health care this has meant the broadest involvement of people at every level of society in movements such as the Patriotic Health Campaign; the recruitment of selected groups of people such as barefoot doctors from the population they are to serve; and the mobilization of the individual to "fight against his own disease." Individual concern with health reflects the Chinese belief in *tzu-li keng-sheng*, or self-reliance, more accurately translated as "regeneration through one's own efforts"—a virtue as honored today as its converse, mutual help.

This was brought home to us most strikingly while we were observing a kindergarten class of six-year-olds. They were being taught the life story of Norman Bethune, a Canadian thoracic surgeon who provided medical services for Mao Tse-tung's Eighth Route Army in the war against Japan until his death in 1939 from septicemia, secondary to an infection he acquired while performing surgery. Dr. Bethune is a national hero in China, celebrated for his "selflessness," his internationalism, and his self-reliance—all principles that are taught to Chinese children. After the audiovisual presentation the children were asked what they would do if they came upon a sick person on the street. "I would get water for him," and "I would get medicine for him," were typical replies, all suggesting things the child himself could do for the sick man rather than going to get help from a doctor or other adult.

THE ROLE OF THE MASS

In the early 1950s, as an implementation of the basic principle "Health work should be combined with the mass movement," the Patriotic Health Campaign was launched. The primary goal of this mass movement was the elimination of mosquitoes, flies, rats, and sparrows and the people were mobilized to exterminate these pests under the guidance of health personnel. The Patriotic Health Campaign has been maintained, and has been expanded to include the sanitary aspects of food, water, and the environment.

While environmental sanitation is a constant activity, it is attacked with particular intensity around festival days and in preparation for the May 1 and October 1 celebrations. Everyone participates, from retired people to health activists, and the general population works under the leadership of medical personnel. Thursday morning is Shanghai's fixed time for cleaning: the people scour the streets and their homes; cadres who work in the government usually do manual labor one day a week, often on cleanup day. There is interdistrict inspection whereby a group of people from one district come in and inspect another area and criticize or exchange experiences. Criticism most often takes the form of "promoting the strong points of another district, encouraging that district." The slogan used around cleanup time is: "It's a glorious thing to speak about hygiene and you should be ashamed if you're very dirty." (One assumes this sounds somewhat different in Chinese.) The importance of the involvement of the masses in breaking with traditional habits and in changing the spirit of the people is stressed. Health workers in a neighborhood health station in Hangchow, which serves 28,000 people, have established three days a month as general cleanup days. The entire population is mobilized into two groups, and certain individuals in each group are responsible for wiping out the pests, eliminating their breeding places, disinfecting water, and keeping the neighborhood clean.

"Health propaganda," as the Chinese put it, plays a crucial role in the participation of the community in health problems. Great attention is paid to educating the populace on the importance of immunizations, the handling of infectious diseases, and the need for "planned birth." In a district general hospital in Peking, mass meetings and study groups take place in the twenty-three neighborhood health stations under its jurisdiction; the meetings are organized by the district health workers to educate the people in hygiene and in the prevention of infectious disease, which they are taught to report to the health center immediately. These meetings are conducted on a regular basis as well as at special times during the year. The health station itself is considered a "mass organization."

Orleans and Suttmeier have emphasized the importance in China of mobilizing the masses in dealing with the problem of pollution. They describe people organized in the cities to "remove refuse that had accumulated in a residential district;" they mention specifically, "the spring patriotic sanitation movement" of 1970 that was organized by local revolutionary committees to mobilize the people to pick up litter and garbage from residences, farms, and factories, to clean up local water supplies, to eliminate pests, to collect reusable wastes, and to advocate public health measures. They also describe the efforts of the Shanghai Municipal Revolutionary Committee in July 1968 to clean up the Whangpoo River and Soochow Creek. The authors quote the New China News Agency as stating that

> 90,000 persons were mobilized on the industrial and agricultural fronts in Shanghai to form muck-dredging and muck-transporting teams, waging a vehement people's war to dredge muck from the Suchow River [sic]. After 100 days of turbulent fighting, more than 403,600 tons of malodorous organic mire had been dug out.[4]

The classic example of the use of mass organization in health has, of course, been the campaign against schistosomiasis. According to Joshua Horn this campaign was based on the concept of the "mass line"—"the conviction that ordinary people possess great strength and wisdom and that when their initiative is given full play they can accomplish miracles."[5] Before the peasants were organized to fight against the snails, Horn states, they were thoroughly educated in the nature of schistosomiasis by means of lectures, films, posters, and radio talks. They were then mobilized twice a year, in March and in August, and, along with voluntary labor from the People's Liberation Army, students, teachers, and office workers, they drained the rivers and ditches, buried the banks of the rivers, and smoothed down the buried dirt. Horn points out that in the antischistosomiasis program the concept was not only to recruit the mass to do the work but to mobilize their enthusiasm and initiative so that they would fight the disease.[6]

This method of attacking the enemy is an adaptation by Mao of the successful methods used in wartime Yenan to fire the enthusiasm of the population against the Japanese. Mao has transferred this ideology into campaigns against such "enemies" as illiteracy, disease, famine, and flood. In this case the enemy is schistosomiasis, and the technique used is the well-known "paper tiger" theory first used by Mao in 1946 to describe the United States-Kuomintang alliance. It states that there is a dual nature to everything. While one's enemies are real and formidable and must be taken seriously, they are, at the same time, paper tigers that can be defeated by the will of the people. One has to view one's enemies from this dual point of view, Mao teaches, in order to plan correctly one's strategy and one's tactics.

The antischistosomiasis effort is particularly revealing, since it mobilized the population in several directions: to move against the snails, to cooperate in case finding and treatment, and to improve environmental sanitation. Yukiang County in Kiangsi Province, for example, had been plagued by schistosomiasis for more than 100 years. According to one report, 1 million square meters of land were infested with snails, and the "average" infection rate among the peasants was 21.4 percent.[7] After investigating the prevalence of the disease, an antischistosomiasis station was set up in the county in 1953. When the campaign started, the personnel of the station began publicizing its purpose, as well as health work in general, using

> broadcasting, wall newspapers, blackboards, exhibits of real and model objects, lantern-slide shows, and dramatic performances. Related scientific knowledge was also popularized. To help the peasants raise their political consciousness, break their superstitious belief in gods, devils, and fate, and to build up their confidence in conquering disease, meetings were organized for recalling sufferings in the old society and comparing them with the happiness in the new society. Through these activities the confidence of the broad mass in the certain triumph of their struggle against schistosomiasis was gradually built up and further strengthened.[8]

Once the population learned about schistosomiasis, a "people's war" was launched against the snails. From 1955 to 1957, 20,000 peasants in Yukiang County filled up old ditches and ponds, dug new ditches, and expanded the cultivation area by roughly ninety acres. Special methods had to be used in some areas. For example, three lotus ponds three feet deep, covering several acres, had a high density of snails that people had attempted to exterminate by removing the surface soil, by burning aquatic vegetation, and by other methods, but the snails had not been completely eliminated. Finally the ponds were drained, all grass and vegetation at the bottom were burned, and snail-free mud was piled on top and pounded so that the snails were suffocated. Seven square or rectangular fish ponds were then created out of the three former snail-breeding ponds.[9]

After this massive war on schistosomiasis, however, it was still necessary to check for the recurrence of snails, as well as on water control and waste disposal, so the people had to be educated in the treatment of human excreta, the provision of safe drinking water, and improved personal hygiene. Production teams under the leadership of health workers are responsible for these public health measures. Horn reports the need to instruct the population on the importance of regular feces examination. At one commune he was told that the peasants did not always take the testing seriously and tried to play jokes on the testers by substituting dog or ox dung. The testers met this problem by reminding the peasants of what life had been like in the "bitter past" when schistosomiasis was common; cooperation was soon restored.[10]

Health work in Heilungkiang Province in the northeast was cited in an article in *China's Medicine* in 1968.[11] In order to spread health education in the province, mass meetings were called in sixty cities and counties, leaflets and pamphlets on health were distributed, and students then began to engage in health education among the workers and peasants. It was estimated that in two counties 250,000 middle and primary school students were mobilized for this work. Needless to say, the students learned as much as they taught.

THE ROLE OF INDIGENOUS HEALTH PERSONNEL

Since the Cultural Revolution it has been common practice in both urban neighborhoods and the communes to recruit health personnel from among the indigenous population. The barefoot doctors in the countryside, the Red Medical Workers in the cities, the worker doctors in the factories, and the health workers in the cities and on the communes are members of the mass recruited to provide health care and to communicate what they have learned to their friends and neighbors. In Silvery Lane in Hangchow, a community of 702 families, 50 residents work in the health center in official capacities; in other words, one member out of every fourteen families in the lane is directly responsible for health care. The high percentage of residents in any given neighborhood who are active in health work are responsible for instructing the rest of the community in the need for immunizations, the use of birth control, and the importance of good sanitation.

The commune health workers receive neither extra pay nor time off from their regular jobs. They do their health work during their lunch periods or at the end of the day. In addition to treating minor illnesses and giving immunizations, these individuals are responsible for disinfecting the water and treating human feces (night soil), which is used as fertilizer. These health workers are trained by, and are under the supervision of, the barefoot doctors.

The elimination of venereal disease in China provides another example of both the mobilization and education of the people and the use of indigenous health personnel. As Felix Green describes it, people were organized around the slogan: "We don't want to take syphilis into Communism." In the early 1950s checklists of symptoms were posted in every store and every community center throughout the country, and anyone with any of the symptoms was urged to get a blood test and be treated. Neighborhood pressure was brought to bear on those who tended to ignore symptoms or who had a history of promiscuity. Where the concentration of the disease was great, specially trained individuals in the neighborhoods made door-to-door visits to give examinations and blood tests. Prostitutes were identified, and suitable alternative jobs were found for them—if necessary by moving equipment, such as sewing machines, into the brothels and turning them into factories. Thus, prostitution was outlawed. Neighborhood committees had, and continue to have, the authority to eliminate prostitution and promiscuity. The technical details of the conquest of venereal disease are described in Edgar Snow's biographical chapter on Dr. Ma Hai-teh,[12] and in Ma's own article on the subject in *China's Medicine* in 1966.[13]

THE ROLE OF THE PROFESSIONAL

Health personnel are not, for the most part, self-selected, but are selected by the group with whom they work, and to whom they will return after their period of training is over. This selection is based on three criteria: academic ability, political ideology, and physical fitness. Both during their training period and afterward, health professionals are exhorted to put the needs of the patient and the needs of society ahead of their own preferences. Health professionals, particularly physicians, have also been encouraged to develop more egalitarian relationships with other health workers and with patients in order to maximize the effectiveness of every individual. The Chinese see this democratization process as an on-going effort, one hardly accomplished in the brief period since Liberation and one not without strains and the inevitable contradictions that characterize the Chinese goals and realities.

A striking example of the effort to decrease "elitism" and to "re-educate" the professionals to the needs of those they serve is the rotation of all urban health personnel through positions in factories or, more often, in the rural areas. The professionals, forsaking the greater comfort and intellectual stimulation of the city, live with the peasants and share their food, style of life, and problems. They also, of course, help provide needed medical services and help train the indigenous medical workers. Although this effort reached its peak during the Cultural Revolution, it still continues in some form in most areas today.

The same kinds of post-Cultural Revolution principles are seen in urban professional roles. Doctor after doctor in medical schools, teaching hospitals, and research institutes told us of their efforts to reduce the social distinctions between themselves and their fellow workers and patients. Although the salaries of the senior doctors are still substantially higher than those of more recent medical graduates and of other health workers—a legacy of the motivation-through-salary differentials encouraged during the period of Soviet influence in the 1950s—they try to follow life styles that will not distinguish them from the others.

In professional roles as well, efforts are made to reduce invidious distinctions. One of the most startling for researchers was the suspension of the publication of all scientific journals during the Cultural Revolution in order to find ways to reduce use of the journals for the "fame and gain" of the authors of articles. Since the resumption of journal publication in 1973 many articles have been attributed to institutions rather than to individuals, although this policy is still being actively debated in an attempt to find the most effective way to assign "responsibility" rather than "fame" for a specific publication.

When those affected by these changes are asked about their feelings, they invariably report that as individuals they are the better for them and that health services are better because of the changes as well. The doctors with whom we spoke did not deny, for example, that life during a rotation in the rural areas is much harder than their urban lives, but instead of bemoaning this hardship, they emphasized what they had learned and how much better physicians they were for it. This is not to say that tensions—"contradictions" is the Chinese phrase—do not exist, but rather that they seem usually to be resolved from the point of view of "social" good rather than the "individual" good.

THE ROLE OF THE PATIENT

Yet another way in which the Chinese people are encouraged to be involved in health is through mobilization of the individual patient. In the psychiatric ward of the Peking Third Hospital the staff tries to "promote the active factors so that the patient can struggle against his own disease." The patient studies the works of Chairman Mao in order to understand his illness and to be able to fight against it. As the psychiatrists reported: "Through the patient's studies his ideology is much elevated. The patient can then investigate his disease and recognize his condition in order to prevent a relapse." The following description of his illness was given by a thirty-eight-year-old male patient in the psychiatric ward of the Peking Third Hospital:

> My main trouble is suspicion. I think my ceiling is going to fall down; when big character posters are up I think it is criticism of myself; and when somebody is gossiping I think they are talking about me. After I was admitted to this hospital I gradually recognized my illness. As Chairman Mao says, when we face a problem we have to face it thoroughly, not only from one side. When I am discharged from the hospital, the doctors have said that I should have some problem of investigation in my mind. When I am in touch with people they have suggested that I make conclusions in

my mind after investigation not before investigation, in order to see if what I suspect to be true is just subjective thinking or is objectively correct. By studying Chairman Mao we can treat and cure disease.

The Shanghai Mental Hospital has carried the idea of a patient's disease as his enemy a step further. They have "adopted the system used in the army" and have divided the staff of the hospital into four divisions. The patients on the wards have also been divided into groups, and they now comprise a "collective fighting group instead of a ward." One of the psychiatrists told us, "It is not enough to have the doctors' or nurses' initiative; we need the patients' initiative to work together against the disease." This view of the patient's relationship with his mental illness is a curious combination of marshaling individual responsibility while viewing the illness as an external enemy; a dual attitude that perhaps serves to maximize the patient's efforts to fight his illness, while leaving him less guilt-ridden if he fails.

Patients are not only expected to participate in their own care; they are also expected to help one another. The Shanghai Mental Hospital has a buddy system whereby the healthier patients who have been in the hospital longer help the newer, sicker patients to adjust to their surroundings and to understand their illness. Horn describes a patient whose burns covered eighty-nine percent of the surface of his body. At one point during treatment the patient's appetite started to diminish and, as days went on, he ate less and less. The dietician tried to tempt him with delicacies, and chefs in Shanghai restaurants produced special menus to encourage him to eat; but, most important, "his comrades urged him to eat as a political duty, as his contribution to the fight for his life that was being waged with such determination by so many."[14]

In an article entitled "How We Have Struggled against Unstable Diabetes Mellitus in the Light of Mao Tse-tung's Thought,"[15] three patients write of their difficulties in dealing with their diabetes over the years and of the new approach they took in managing their disease: they studied the "pathophysiology of diabetes," "became familiar with the regulation of insulin dosage," and applied the theory of the paper tiger, that is, "we despised him and we took him seriously." Thus, the article states, the patient's initiative to fight against their diabetes was mobilized and their disease stabilized.

In health, as in other aspects of the Chinese brand of socialism, there are no passive bystanders. One is expected to participate "whole-heartedly" in community public health measures, in the organization of medical care, and in the conduct of all aspects of one's personal life, including one's health. It is a country of mass and individual participation, of mass and individual responsibility. John G. Gurley, an economist, has described China's current view of the role of the people in the following way:

To gain knowledge, people must be awakened from their half slumber, encouraged to mobilize themselves and to take conscious action to elevate and liberate themselves. When they actively participate in decision making, when they take an interest in state affairs, when they dare to do new things, when they become good at presenting facts and reasoning things out, when they criticize and test and experiment scientifically, having discarded myths and superstitions, when they are aroused—then the socialist initiative latent in the masses [will] burst out with volcanic force.[16]

SUMMARY

To the Western observer, much of this activity may produce an image of coercion, of "forcing" individuals to act "for their own good" or "for the good of society" as it is defined by local and national leadership groups. In the Chinese context, it appears quite different. Where the society rather than the individual is viewed as the basic unit ("If the Chinese people are not like cement, they shall be like sand"), the actions of any individual are always seen as irrevocably tied to the well-being of the larger group. Thus if a mother does not bring her child in for measles immunization, this is seen not only as a potential danger to his health, but as a danger to the health of those around him, and the mother is exhorted—using the strong relationships of neighborhood and the techniques of "education" and "persuasion"—to act in what is seen as the public interest. If for some reason it is difficult for the family to bring the child in, it is seen as the responsibility of the health establishment to provide that child with the immunization. Therefore, if the child is not immunized, it is also seen as a failure of the health establishment. The responsibility is viewed as a shared one between the family and the health system.

Perhaps even more dramatic are the individual-society relationships around birth control. There appear to be group discussions concerning the goals for the neighborhood and how many children each woman should have. This is then translated into decisions on which women should have babies over the next year and which should not. If the group collectively decides that a woman should have children in a specific year and she by accident or design becomes pregnant, the pressures on her to have an abortion—despite her "right of free choice"— must be very great indeed. Was she "forced" to give up her individual preference for the societal good? In a literal sense, no, but in a very real moral sense, yes.[17]

But there are perhaps even more important issues. For the poor of China prior to 1949, there were few of the individual freedoms that the West finds so important. Now, in the 1970s, while some freedoms still appear to be limited, the vast majority of the population appear to be free from starvation, free from homelessness, free from semifeudalism, free from disease. Furthermore, everyone seems to be sharing equally in the limited resources that their society has to offer. In many ways the "rights" of the individual—to life, to justice, and to fulfillment in work—have indeed been strengthened even as the societal "control" over the individual has in many ways been broadened and deepened.

In sum, the resolution of the issues of individual versus societal rights and responsibilities in China are far from clear, differ in some ways from one locality to another, and are continually changing. What is clear and relatively unchanging is that the Chinese, with their far different cultural past and politico-economic present, are attempting to deal with these issues in ways far different and far more "societal" in their orientation than are other countries. It seems clear from the changes of the past two decades that these techniques are working in China; whether they will continue to work as standards of living rise and expectations and problems change, and to what extent they are applicable to other societies with vastly different cultural, political, and economic conditions are critical questions whose answers are much less clear.

Notes to Chapter Four

1. Han Suyin, "Family Planning in China," in *Population and Family Planning in the People's Republic of China*, ed. by Phyllis T. Piotrow (New York: Victor-Bostrom Fund and Population Crisis Committee, 1971), pp. 16-21.

2. Mao Tse-tung, "On Practice," *Four Essays on Philosophy* (Peking: Foreign Languages Press, 1966), p. 8.

3. Han Suyin, "Reflections on Social Change," *Bulletin of the Atomic Scientists* 22 [6] (1966), 80-83.

4. Leo A. Orleans and Richard P. Suttmeier, "The Mao Ethic and Environmental Quality," *Science* 170 (1970), 1173-76.

5. Joshua S. Horn, *Away with All Pests: An English Surgeon in People's China* (New York: Monthly Review Press, 1971), p. 96.

6. Ibid., p. 97.

7. "A Great Victory of Mao Tse-tung's Thought in the Battle against Schistosomiasis," *China's Medicine* 10 (October 1968), 588-602.

8. Ibid., p. 593.

9. Ibid., pp. 598-99.

10. Horn, p. 99.

11. "Experiences in Health Work and Disease Prevention in Heilungkiang Province in the Past Year," *China's Medicine* 3 (March 1968), 148-53.

12. Edgar Snow, *Red China Today* (New York: Vintage Books, 1970), pp. 261-69.

13. George Hatem, "With Mao Tse-tung's Thought as the Compass for Action in the Control of Venereal Disease in China," *China's Medicine* 1 (October 1966), 52-67.

14. Horn, p. 108.

15. Chang Tze-han, Yang Teh-ching, and Tu Jui-fen, "How We Have Struggled against Unstable Diabetes Mellitus in the Light of Mao Tse-tung's Thought," *China's Medicine* 7 (July 1968), 400-407.

16. John G. Gurley, "Capitalist and Maoist Economic Development," in *America's Asia*, ed. by Edward Freedman and Mark Selden, Vintage (New York: Random House, 1971), p. 336.

17. Han Suyin, "Family Planning in China," *New York Times*, September 1, 1973.

Section B:
Justice and Health Care Delivery

PREAMBLE

If we concede that we must face social questions in delivering health care—either because ethics in general requires that we examine social impacts or simply because some health care planning decisions require budget and other allocation decisions—then the most central issue is a theory of social justice. We use the term "justice" here not in the broad sense where it is almost synonymous with being "morally right." We are using it in a more narrow, distributional sense. The question is, "How can we fairly or 'justly' distribute our health resources so that everyone in the society gets his or her due?"

In the first chapter of this section Gene Outka presents the classic alternatives. In doing so he introduces the reader to problems with many of the standard formulations, and concludes that a formal principle, "similar treatment for similar cases," must be applied. He maintains that this leads to the conclusion that all persons should have equal access to health care. The authors of the next three chapters propose three different interpretations of a just health care delivery—all claiming that, at least in some cases, health care is not necessarily distributed most justly when distributed so that all have equal access. Joseph Fletcher gives us a classical utilitarian solution: health care should be distributed so it produces the greatest good for the greatest number. Computers will be necessary to make the calculations, but the method is essentially mathematical—calculate the goods and the harms. Ronald Green applies the theory of justice of John Rawls to health care. The Rawlsian interpretation of justice—based in part on the principle that goods should be distributed so that they serve to benefit the least well off—has emerged as a storm exciting the *philosophical world in mid-twentieth century. It presents a radical challenge to the classical utilitarianism dominating health policy planning. Robert Veatch argues that this is a vast improvement on the simpler utilitarian principles, but still fails to capture the fundamental claim of equality that ought to be an essential part of a concept of justice. He argues that even the Rawlsian theory of justice can give rise to a very unequal distribution of health care. An egalitarian interpretation, he claims, would produce the most just health care delivery system.*

Chapter 5

Social Justice and Equal Access to Health Care[a]

Gene Outka

Is it possible to understand and to justify morally a societal goal that increasing numbers of people, including Americans, accept as normative? The goal is: the assurance of comprehensive health services for every person irrespective of income or geographic location. Indeed, the goal now has almost the status of a platitude. Currently in the United States politicians in various camps give it at least verbal endorsement.[1] I do not propose to examine the possible sociological determinants in this emergent consensus. I hope to show that whatever these determinants are, one may offer a plausible case in defense of the goal on reasonable grounds. To demonstrate why appeals to the goal get so successfully under our skins, I shall have recourse to a set of conceptions of social justice. Some of the standard conceptions, found in a number of writings on justice, will do.[2] By reflecting on them it seems to me a prima facie case can be established, namely, that every person in the entire resident population should have equal access to health care delivery.

The case is prima facie only. I wish to set aside as far as possible a related question which comes readily enough to mind. In the world of "suboptimal alternatives," with the constraints, for example, that impinge on the government as it makes decisions about resource allocation, what is one to say? What criteria should be employed? Paul Ramsey, in *The Patient as Person* thinks that the large question of how to choose between medical and other societal priorities is "almost, if not altogether, incorrigible to moral reasoning."[3] Whether it is or not

---

[a]Much of the research for this paper was done during the fall term, 1972-73, when I was on leave in Washington, D.C. I am very grateful for the two appointments that made this leave possible: as Service Fellow, Office of Special Projects, Health Services and Mental Health Administration, Department of Health, Education, and Welfare; and as Visiting Scholar, Kennedy Center for Bioethics, Georgetown University.

is a matter that must be ignored for the present. One may simply observe in passing that choices are unavoidable nonetheless, as Ramsey acknowledges, even where the government allows them to be made by default, so that in some instances they are determined largely by which private pressure groups prove to be dominant. In any event, there is virtue in taking up one complicated question at a time, and we need to get the thrust of the case for equal access before us. It is enough to observe now that Americans attach an obviously high priority to organized health care. National health expenditures for the fiscal year 1972 were $83.4 billion.[4] Even if such an enormous sum is not entirely adequate, we may still ask: How are we to justify spending whatever we do in accordance as far as possible with the goal of equal access? The answer I propose involves distinguishing various conceptions of social justice and trying to show which of these apply or fail to apply to health care considerations. Only toward the end of the chapter will some institutional implications be given more than passing attention, and then in a strictly programmatic way.

What stake does someone in religious ethics have in this discussion? If the issue is to how to justify morally the societal goal that seems so obvious to so many, whether or not they are religious believers, does the religious ethicist then simply participate qua citizen? Here I think we should be wary of simplifying formulae. Why for example should a Jew or a Christian not welcome wide support for a societal goal that he or she can affirm and reaffirm, or reflect only on instances where such support is not forthcoming? If a number of ethical schemes, both religious and humanist, converge in their acceptance of the goal of equal access to health care, so be it. Secularists can join forces with believers, at least at some levels or points, without implying that there must be unanimity on every moral issue. Yet it also seems too simple if one claims to wear only the citizen's hat when making the case in question. At least I should admit that a commitment to the basic normative principle that in Christian writings is often called *agape* may influence the account to follow in ways large and small.[5] For example, someone with such a commitment will quite naturally take a special interest in appeals to the generic characteristics all persons share rather than the idiosyncratic attainments that distinguish persons from one another, and in the playing down of desert considerations. As I shall try to show, such appeals are centrally relevant to the case for equal access. And they are nicely in line with the normative pressures agapeic considerations typically exert.

One issue of theoretical importance in religious ethics also emerges in connection with this last point. The approach in this chapter may throw a little indirect light on the traditional question, especially prominent in Christian ethics, of how love and justice are related. To distinguish different conceptions of social justice will put us in a better position, I think, to recognize that often it is ambiguous to ask about "*the* relation." There may be different relations to different conceptions. For the conceptions themselves may sometimes produce discordant indications, or turn out to be incommensurable, or reflect, when different ones are seized upon, rival moral points of view. I shall note several of these relations as we proceed.

Which then among the standard conceptions of social justice appear to be particularly relevant or irrelevant? Let us consider the following five:

1. To each according to his merit or desert.
2. To each according to his societal contribution.
3. To each according to his contribution in satisfying whatever is freely desired by others in the open marketplace of supply and demand.
4. To each according to his needs.
5. Similar treatment for similar cases.

In general I shall argue that the first three of these are less relevant because of certain distinctive features that health crises possess. I shall focus on crises here not because I think preventive care is unimportant (the opposite is true), but because the crisis situation shows most clearly the special significance we attach to medical treatment as an institutionalized activity or social practice, and the basic purpose we suppose it to have.

TO EACH ACCORDING TO HIS MERIT OR DESERT

Meritarian conceptions, above all perhaps, are grading ones: advantages are allocated in accordance with amounts of energy expended or kinds of results achieved. What is judged is particular conduct that distinguishes persons from one another and not only the fact that all the parties are human beings. Sometimes a competitive aspect looms large.

In certain contexts it is illuminating to distinguish between efforts and achievements. In the case of efforts one characteristically focuses on the individual: rewards are based on the pains one takes. Some have supposed, for example, that entry into the kingdom of heaven is linked more directly to energy displayed and fidelity shown than to successful results attained.

To assess achievements is to weigh actual performance and productive contributions. The academic prize is awarded to the student with the highest grade-point average, regardless of the amount of midnight oil he or she burned in preparing for the examinations. Sometimes we may exclaim, "it's just not fair," when person X writes a brilliant paper with little effort while we are forced to devote more time with less impressive results. But then our complaint may be directed against differences in innate ability and talent which no expenditure of effort altogether removes.

After the difference between effort and achievement, and related distinctions, have been acknowledged, what should be stressed is the general importance of meritarian or desert criteria in the thinking of most people about justice. These criteria may serve to illuminate a number of disputes about the justice of various practices and institutional arrangements in our society. It may help to explain, for instance, the resentment among the working class against the welfare system. However wrongheaded or self-deceptive the resentment often is, particularly when directed toward those who want to work but for various reasons beyond their control cannot, at its better moments it involves in effect an appeal to desert considerations. "Something for nothing" is repudiated as unjust; benefits should be proportional (or at least related) to costs; those who can make an effort should do so, whatever the degree of their training or significance of their contribution to society; and so on. So, too, persons deserve to have what they have labored for; unless they infringe on the works of others their efforts and achievements are justly theirs.

Occasionally the appeal to desert extends to a wholesale rejection of other considerations as grounds for just claims. The most conspicuous target is need. Consider this statement by Ayn Rand.

> A morality that holds *need* as a claim, holds emptiness—nonexistence—as its standard of value; it rewards an absence, a defect: weakness, inability, incompetence, suffering, disease, disaster, the lack, the fault, the flaw—the zero.
>
> Who provides the account to pay these claims? Those who are cursed for being non-zeros, each to the extent of his distance from that ideal. Since all values are the product of virtues, the degree of your virtue is used as the measure of your penalty; the degree of your faults is used as the measure of your gain. Your code declares that the rational man must sacrifice himself to the irrational, the independent man to parasites, the honest man to the dishonest, the man of justice to the unjust, the productive man to thieving loafers, the man of integrity to compromising knaves, the man of self-esteem to sniveling neurotics. Do you wonder at the meanness of soul in those you see around you? The man who achieves these virtues will not accept your moral code; the man who accepts your moral code will not achieve these virtues.[6]

I have noted elsewhere[7] that *agape*, while it characteristically plays down, need not formally disallow attention to considerations falling under merit or desert; for in the case of merit as well as need it may be possible, the quotation above notwithstanding, to reason solely from egalitarian premises. A major reason such attention is warranted concerns what was called there the differential exercise of an equal liberty. That is, one may fittingly revere another's moral capacities and thus the efforts he makes as well as the ends he seeks. Such reverence may lead one to weigh expenditure of energy and specific achievements. I would simply hold now (1) that the idea of justice is not exhaustively characterized by the notion of desert, even if one agrees that the latter plays an important role; and (2) that the notion of desert is especially ill suited to play an important role in the determination of policies that should govern a system of health care.

Why is it so ill suited? Here we encounter some of the distinctive features that health crises possess. Health crises seem nonmeritarian because they occur so often for reasons beyond our control or power to predict. They frequently fall without discrimination on the (according-to-merit) just and unjust, i.e., the virtuous and the wicked, the industrious and the slothful alike.

While we may believe that virtues and vices cannot depend upon natural contingencies, we are bound to admit, it seems, that many health crises do. It makes sense therefore to say that we are equal in being randomly susceptible to these crises. Even those who ascribe a prominent role to desert acknowledge that justice has also properly to do with pleas of "But I could not help it."[8] One seeks to distinguish such cases from those acknowledged to be praiseworthy or blameworthy. Then it seems unfair as well as unkind to discriminate among those who suffer health crises on the basis of their personal deserts. For it would be odd to maintain that a newborn child deserves his hemophilia or the tumor afflicting her spine.

These considerations help to explain why the following rough distinction is often made. Bernard Williams, for example, in his discussion of "equality in unequal circumstances," identifies two different sorts of inequality, inequality of merit and inequality of need, and two corresponding goods, those earned by effort and those demanded by need.[9] Medical treatment in the event of illness is located under the umbrella of need. He concludes: "Leaving aside preventive medicine, the proper ground of distribution of medical care is ill health: this is a necessary truth."[10] An irrational state of affairs is held to obtain if those whose needs are the same are treated unequally, when needs are the ground of the treatment. One might put the point this way. When people are equal in the relevant respects—in this case when their needs are the same and occur in a context of random, undeserved susceptibility—that by itself is a good reason for treating them equally.[11]

In many societies, however, a second necessary condition for the receipt of medical treatment exists de facto: the possession of money. This is not the place to consider the general question of when inequalities in wealth may be regarded as just. It is enough to note that one can plausibly appeal to all of the conceptions of justice we are embarked in sorting out. A person may be thought to be entitled to a higher income when he works more, contributes more, risks more, and not simply when he needs more. We may think it fair that the industrious should have more money than the slothful and the surgeon more than the tobacconist. The difficulty comes in the misfit between the reasons for differential incomes and the reasons for receiving medical treatment. The former may include a pluralistic set of claims in which different notions of justice must be meshed. The latter are more monistically focused on needs, and the other notions not accorded a similar relevance. Yet money may nonetheless remain as a causally necessary condition for receiving medical treatment. It may be the power to secure what one needs. The senses in which health crises are distinctive may then be insufficiently determinative for the policies which govern the actual availability of treatment. The nearly automatic links between income, prestige, and the receipt of comparatively higher quality medical treatment should then be subjected to critical scrutiny. For unequal treatment of the rich ill and the poor ill is unjust if, again, needs rather than differential income constitute the ground of such treatment.

Suppose one agrees that it is important to recognize the misfit between the reasons for differential incomes and the reasons for receiving medical treatment, and that therefore income as such should not govern the actual availability of treatment. One may still ask whether the case so far relies excessively on "pure" instances where desert considerations are admittedly out of place. That there are such pure instances, tumors afflicting the spine, hemophilia, and so on, is not denied. Yet it is an exaggeration if we go on and regard all health crises as utterly unconnected with desert. Note for example that Williams leaves aside preventive medicine. And if in a cool hour we examine the statistics, we find that a vast number of deaths occur each year due to causes not always beyond our control, e.g., automobile accidents, drugs, alcohol, tobacco, obesity, and so on. In some final reckoning it seems that many persons (though crucially, not all) have an effect on, and arguably a responsibility for, their own medical needs. Consider the following bidders for emergency care: (1) a person with a heart attack who is seriously overweight; (2) a football hero who has suffered a concussion; (3) a man with lung cancer who has smoked cigarettes for forty years; (4) a sixty-year-old man who has always taken excellent care of himself and is suddenly stricken with leukemia; (5) a three-year-old girl who has swallowed poison left out carelessly by her parents; (6) a fourteen-year-old boy who has been beaten without provocation by a gang and suffers brain damage and recurrent attacks of uncontrollable terror; (7) a college student who has slashed his wrists (and not for the first time) from a psychological need for attention; (8) a woman raised in the ghetto who is found unconscious due to an overdose of heroin.

These cases help to show why the whole subject of medical treatment is so crucial and so perplexing. They attest to some melancholy elements in human experience. People suffer in varying ratios the effects of their natural and undeserved vulnerabilities, the irresponsibility and brutality of others, and their own desires and weaknesses. In some final reckoning, then, desert considerations seem not irrelevant to many health crises. The practical applicability of this admission, however, in the instance of health care delivery, appears limited. We may agree that it underscores the importance of preventive health care by stressing the influence we sometimes have over our medical needs. But if we try to foster such care by increasing the penalties for neglect, we normally confine ourselves to calculations about incentives. At the risk of being denounced in some quarters as censorious and puritannical, perhaps we should for example levy far higher taxes on alcohol and tobacco and pump the dollars directly into health care programs rather than (say) into highway building. Yet these steps would by no means lead necessarily to a demand that we correlate in some strict way a demonstrated effort to be temperate with the receipt of privileged medical treatment as a reward. Would it be feasible to allocate the additional tax monies to the man with leukemia before the overweight man suffering a heart attack on the ground of a difference in desert? At the point of emergency care at least, it seems impracticable for the doctor to discriminate between these cases, to make meritarian judgments at the point of catastrophe. And the number of persons who are in need of medical treatment for reasons utterly beyond their control remains a datum with tenacious relevance. There are those who suffer the ravages of a tornado, are handicapped by a genetic defect, beaten without provocation, etc. A commitment to the basic purpose of medical care and to the institutions for achieving it involves the recognition of this persistent state of affairs.

TO EACH ACCORDING TO HIS SOCIETAL CONTRIBUTION

This conception gives moral primacy to notions such as the public interest, the common good, the welfare of the community, or the greatest good of the greatest number. Here one judges the social consequences of particular conduct. The formula can be construed in at least two ways.[1,2] It may refer to the interest of the social group considered collectively, where the group has some independent life all its own. The group's welfare is the decisive criterion for determining what constitutes any member's proper share. Or the common good may refer only to an aggregation of distinct individuals and considered distributively.

Either version accords such a primacy to what is socially advantageous as to be unacceptable not only to defenders of need, but also, it would seem, of desert. For the criteria of effort and achievement are often conceived along rather individualistic lines. The pains an agent takes or the results he brings about deserve recompense, whether or not the public interest is directly served. No automatic harmony then is necessarily assumed between his just share as individually earned and his proper share from the vantage point of the common good. Moreover, the test of social advantage *simpliciter* obviously threatens the agapeic concern with some minimal consideration due each person which is never to be disregarded for the sake of long-range social benefits. No one should be considered as *merely* a means or instrument.

The relevance of the canon of social productiveness to health crises may accordingly also be challenged. Indeed, such crises may cut against it in that they occur more frequently to those whose comparative contribution to the general welfare is less, e.g., the aged, the disabled, children.

Consider for example Paul Ramsey's persuasive critique of social and economic criteria for the allocation of a single scarce medical resource. He begins by recounting the imponderables that faced the widely discussed "public committee" at the Swedish Hospital in Seattle when it deliberated in the early 1960s. The sparse resource in this case was the kidney machine. The committee was charged with the responsibility of selecting among patients suffering chronic renal failure those who were to receive dialysis. Its criteria were broadly social and economic. Considerations weighed included age, sex, marital status, number of dependents, income, net worth, educational background, occupation, past performance, and future potential. The application of such criteria proved to be exceedingly problematic. Should someone with six children always have priority over an artist or composer? Were those who arranged matters so that their families would not burden society to be penalized in effect for being provident? And so on. Two critics of the committee found "a disturbing picture of the bourgeoisie sparing the bourgeoisie," and observed that "the Pacific Northwest is no place for a Henry David Thoreau with bad kidneys."[13]

The mistake, Ramsey believes, is to introduce criteria of social worthiness in the first place. In those situations of choice where not all can be saved and yet all need not die, "the equal right of every human being to live, and not relative personal or social worth, should be the ruling principle."[14] The principle leads to a criterion of "random choice among equals" expressed by a lottery scheme or a practice of "first come, first served." Several reasons stand behind Ramsey's defense of the criterion of random choice. First, a religious belief in the equality of persons before God leads intelligibly to a refusal to choose between those who are dying in any way other than random patient selection. Otherwise their equal value as human beings is threatened. Second, a moral primacy is ascribed to survival over other (perhaps superior) interests persons may have, in that it is the condition of everything else." Life is a value incommensurate with all others, and so not negotiable by bartering one man's worth against another's."[15] Third, the entire enterprise of estimating a person's social worth is viewed with final skepticism." We have no way of knowing how really and truly to estimate a man's societal worth or his worth to others or to himself in unfocused social situations in the ordinary lives of men in their communities."[16] This statement, incidentally, appears to allow something other than randomness in *focused* social situations; when, say, a president or prime minister and the owner of the local bar rush for the last place in the bomb shelter, and the knowledge of the former can save many lives. In any event, I have been concerned with a restricted point to which Ramsey's discussion brings illustrative support. The canon of social productiveness is notoriously difficult to apply as a workable criterion for distributing medical services to those who need them.

One can go further. A system of health care delivery that treats people on the basis of the medical care required may often go against (at least narrowly conceived) calculations of societal advantage. For example, the health care needs of people tend to rise during that period of their lives, signaled by retirement, when their incomes and social productivity are declining. More generally:

Some 40 to 50 per cent of the American people—the aged, children, the dependent poor, and those with some significant chronic disability are in categories requiring relatively large amounts of medical care but with inadequate resources to purchase such care.[17]

If one agrees, for whatever reasons, with the agapeic judgment that each person should be regarded as irreducibly valuable, then one cannot succumb to a social productiveness criterion of human worth. Interests are to be equally considered even when people have ceased to be, or are not yet, or perhaps never will be, public assets.

TO EACH ACCORDING TO HIS CONTRIBUTION IN SATISFYING WHATEVER IS FREELY DESIRED BY OTHERS IN THE OPEN MARKETPLACE OF SUPPLY AND DEMAND

Here we have a test which, though similar to the preceding one, concentrates on what is desired de facto by certain segments of the community rather than the community as a whole, and on the relative scarcity of the service rendered. It is tantamount to the canon of supply and demand as espoused by various laissez-faire theoreticians.[18] Rewards should be given to those who by virtue of special skill, prescience, risk-taking, and the like discern what is desired and are able to take the requisite steps to bring satisfaction. A surgeon, it may be argued, contributes more than a nurse because of the greater training and skill required, burdens borne, and effective care provided, and should be compensated accordingly. So too, perhaps, a star quarterback on a pro football team should be remunerated even more highly because of the rare athletic prowess needed, hazards involved, and widespread demand to watch him play.

This formula does not then call for the weighing of the value of various contributions, and tends to conflate needs and wants under a notion of desires. It also assumes that a prominent part is assigned to consumer free choice. The consumer should be at liberty to express his preferences, and to select from a variety of competing goods and services. Those who resist many changes currently proposed in the organization and financing of health care delivery in the U.S.A.—such as national health insurance—often do so by appealing to some variant of this formula.

Yet it seems health crises are often of overriding importance when they occur. They appear therefore not satisfactorily accommodated to the context of a free marketplace where consumers may freely choose among alternative goods and services.

To clarify what is at stake in the above contention, let us examine an opposing case. Robert M. Sade, M.D., published an article in *The New England Journal of Medicine* entitled "Medical Care as a Right: A Refutation." He attacks programs of national health insurance in the name of a person's right to select one's own values, determine how they may be realized, and dispose of them if one chooses without coercion from other men. The values in question are construed as economic ones in the context of supply and demand. So we read:

> In a free society, man exercises his right to sustain his own life by producing economic values in the form of goods and services that he is, or should be, free to exchange with other men who are similarly free to trade with him or not. The economic values produced, however, are not given as gifts by nature, but exist only by virtue of the thought and effort of individual men. Goods and services are thus owned as a consequence of the right to sustain life by one's own physical and mental effort.[19]

Sade compares the situation of the physician to that of the baker. The one who produces a loaf of bread should as owner have the power to dispose of his own product. It is immoral simply to expropriate the bread without the baker's permission. Similarly, "medical care is neither a right nor a privilege: it is a service that is provided by doctors and others to people who wish to purchase it."[20] Any coercive regulation of professional practices by the society at large is held to be analogous to taking the bread from the baker without his consent. Such regulation violates the freedom of the physician over his own services and will lead inevitably to provider apathy.

The analogy surely misleads. To assume that doctors autonomously produce goods and services in a fashion closely akin to a baker is grossly oversimplified. The baker may himself rely on the agricultural produce of others, yet there is a crucial difference in the degree of dependence. Modern physicians depend on the achievements of medical technology and the entire scientific base underlying it, all of which is made possible by a host of persons whose salaries are often notably less. Moreover, the amount of taxpayer support for medical research and education is too enormous to make any such unqualified case for provider autonomy plausible.

However conceptually clouded Sade's article may be, its stress on a free exchange of goods and services reflects one historically influential rationale for much American medical practice. And he applies it not only to physicians but also to patients or "consumers."

> The question is whether the decision of how to allocate the consumer's dollar should belong to the consumer or to the state. It has already been shown that the choice of how a doctor's services should be rendered belongs only to the doctor: in the same way the choice of whether to buy a doctor's service rather than some other commodity or service belongs to the consumer as a logical consequence of the right to his own life.[21]

This account is misguided, I think, because it ignores the overriding importance that is so often attached to health crises. When lumps appear on someone's neck, it usually makes little sense to talk of choosing whether to buy a doctor's service rather than a color television set. References to just tradeoffs suddenly seem out of place. No compensation suffices, since the penalties may differ so much.

There is even a further restriction on consumer choice. One's knowledge in these circumstances is comparatively so limited. The physician makes most of the decisions: about diagnosis, treatment, hospitalization, number of return visits, and so on. In brief:

> The consumer knows very little about the medical services he is buying— probably less than about any other service he purchases. . . . While [he] can still play a role in policing the market, that role is much more limited in the field of health care than in almost any other area of private economic activity.[22]

For much of the way, then, an appeal to supply and demand and consumer choice is not quite fitting. It neglects the issue of the value of various contributions. And it fails to allow for the recognition that medical treatments may be overridingly desired. In contexts of catastrophe, at any rate, when life itself is threatened, most persons (other than those who are apathetic or seek to escape from the terrifying prospects) cannot take medical care to be merely one option among others.

TO EACH ACCORDING TO HIS NEEDS

The concept of needs is sometimes taken to apply to an entire range of interests that concern a person's "psychophysical existence."[23] On this wide usage, to attribute a need to someone is to say that the person lacks what is thought to conduce to his or her "welfare"—understood in both a physiological sense (e.g., for food, drink, shelter, and health) and a psychological one (e.g., for continuous human affection and support).

Yet even in the case of such a wide usage, what the person lacks is typically assumed to be basic. Attention is restricted to recurrent considerations rather than to every possible individual whim or frivolous pursuit. So one is not surprised to meet with the contention that a preferable rendering of this formula would be: "to each according to his essential needs."[24] This contention seems to me well taken. It implies, for one thing, that basic needs are distinguishable from felt needs or wants. For the latter may encompass expressions of personal preference unrelated to considerations of survival or subsistence, and sometimes artificially generated by circumstances of rising affluence in the society at large.

Essential needs are also typically assumed to be given rather than acquired. They are not constituted by any action for which the person is responsible by virtue of his or her distinctively greater effort. It is almost as if the designation "innocent" may be linked illuminatingly to need, as retribution, punishment, and so on, are to desert, and in complex ways, to freedom. Thus essential needs are likewise distinguishable from deserts. Where needs are unequal, one thinks of them as fortuitously distributed; as part, perhaps, of a kind of "natural lottery."[25] So very often the advantages of health and the burdens of illness, for example, strike one as arbitrary effects of the lottery. It seems wrong to say that a newborn child deserves as a reward all of his faculties when he has done nothing in particular that distinguishes him from another newborn who comes into the world deprived of one or more of them. Similarly, though crudely, many religious believers do not look on natural events as personal deserts. They are not inclined to pronounce sentences such as, "That evil person with incurable cancer got what he deserved." They are disposed instead to search for some distinction between what they may call the conditions of finitude on the one hand and sin and moral evil on the other. If the distinction is "ultimately" invalid, in this life it seems inscrutably so. Here and now it may be usefully drawn. Inequalities in the need for medical treatment are taken, it appears, to reflect the conditions of finitude more than anything else.

One can even go on to argue that among our basic or essential needs, the case of medical treatment is conspicuous in the following sense. While food and shelter are not matters about which we are at liberty to please ourselves, they are at least predictable. We can plan, for instance, to store up food and fuel for the winter. It may be held that responsibility increases along with the power to predict. If so, then many health crises seem peculiarly random and uncontrollable. Cancer, given the present state of knowledge at any rate, is a contingent disaster, whereas hunger is a steady threat. Who will need serious medical care, and when, is then perhaps a classic example of uncertainty.

Finally, and more theoretically, it is often observed that a need conception of justice comes closest to charity or *agape*.[26] I think there are indeed crucial overlaps.[27] To cite several of them: the equal consideration *agape* enjoins has to do in the first instance with those generic endowments which people share, the characteristics of a person qua human existent. Needs, as we have seen, likewise concern those things essential to the life and welfare of men considered simply as men.[28] They are not based on particular conduct alone, on those idiosyncratic attainments that contribute to someone's being such-and-such a kind of person. Yet a certain sort of inequality is recognized, for needs differ in divergent circumstances and so treatments must if benefits are to be equalized. *Agape* too allows for a distinction between equal consideration and identical treatment. The aim of equalizing benefits is implied by the injunction to consider the interests of each party equally. This may require differential treatments of differing interests.

Overlaps such as these will doubtless strike some as so extensive that it may be asked whether *agape* and a need conception of justice are virtually equivalent.

I think not. One contrast was pointed out before. The differential treatment enjoined by *agape* is more complex and goes deeper. In the case of *agape*, attention may be appropriately given to varying *efforts* as well as to unequal *needs*. More generally one may say that agapeic considerations extend to all of the psychological nuances and contextual details of individual persons and their circumstances. Imaginative concern is enjoined for concrete human beings: for what someone is uniquely, for what he or she—as a matter of personal history and distinctive identity—wants, feels, thinks, celebrates, and endures. The attempt to establish and enhance mutual affection between individual persons is taken likewise to be fitting. Conceptions of social justice, including "to each according to his essential needs," tend to be more restrictive; they call attention to considerations that obtain for a number of persons, to impersonally specified criteria for assessing collective policies and practices. *Agape* involves more, even if one supposes never less.

Other differences could be noted. What is important now, however, is the recognition that, in matters of health care in particular, *agape* and a need conception of justice are conjoined in a number of relevant respects. At least this is so for those who think that, again, justice has properly to do with pleas of "But I could not help it." It seeks to distinguish such cases from those acknowledged to be praiseworthy or blameworthy. The formula "to each according to his needs" is one cogent way of identifying the moral relevance of these pleas. To ignore them may be thought to be unfair as well as unkind when they arise from the deprivation of some essential need. The move to confine the notion of justice wholly to desert considerations is thereby resisted as well. Hence we may say that sometimes "questions of social justice arise just because people are unequal in ways they can do very little to change and ... only by attending to these inequalities can one be said to be giving their interests equal consideration.[29]

SIMILAR TREATMENT FOR SIMILAR CASES

This conception is perhaps the most familiar of all. Certainly it is the most formal and inclusive one. It is frequently taken as an elementary appeal to consistency and linked to the universalizability test. One should not make an arbitrary exception on one's own behalf, but rather should apply impartially whatever standards one accepts. The conception can be fruitfully applied to health care questions and I shall assume its relevance. Yet as literally interpreted, it is necessary but not sufficient. For rightly or not, it is often held to be as compatible with no positive treatment whatever as with active promotion of other peoples' interests, as long as all are equally and impartially included. Its exponents sometimes assume such active promotion without demonstrating clearly how this is built into the conception itself. Moreover, it may obscure a distinction that we have seen agapists and others make: between equal consideration and identical treatment. Needs may differ and so treatments must, if benefits are to be equalized.

I have placed this conception at the end of the list partly because it moves us, despite its formality, toward practice. Let me suggest briefly how it does so. Suppose first of all one agrees with the case so far offered. Suppose, that is, it has been shown convincingly that a need conception of justice applies with greater relevance than the earlier three when one reflects about the basic purpose of medical care. To treat one class of people differently from another because of income or geographic location should therefore be ruled out, because such reasons are irrelevant. (The irrelevance is conceptual, rather than always, unfortunately, causal.) In short, all persons should have equal access, "as needed, without financial, geographic, or other barriers, to the whole spectrum of health services."[30]

Suppose however, second, that the goal of equal access collides on some occasions with the realities of finite medical resources and needs that prove to be insatiable. That such collisions occur in fact it would be idle to deny. And it is here that the practical bearing of the formula of similar treatment for similar cases should be noticed. Let us recall Williams's conclusion: "the proper ground of distribution of medical care is ill health: this is a necessary truth." While I agree with the essentials of his argument—for all the reasons above—I would prefer, for practical purposes, a slightly more modest formulation. Illness is the proper ground for the *receipt* of medical care. However, the *distribution* of medical care in less-than-optimal circumstances requires us to face the collisions. I would argue that in such circumstances the formula of similar treatment for similar cases may be construed so as to guide actual choices in the way most compatible with the goal of equal access. The formula's allowance of no positive treatment whatever may justify exclusion of entire classes of cases from a priority list. Yet it forbids doing so for irrelevant or arbitrary reasons. So (1) if we accept the case for equal access, but (2) if we simply cannot, physically cannot, treat all who are in need, it seems more just to discriminate by virtue of categories of illness than, for example, between the rich ill and poor ill. All persons with a certain rare, noncommunicable disease would not receive priority, let us say, where the costs were inordinate, the prospects for rehabilitation remote, and for the sake of equalized benefits to many more. Or with Ramsey we may urge a policy of random patient selection when one must decide between claimants for a medical treatment unavailable to all. Or we may acknowledge that any notion of "comprehensive benefits" to which persons should have equal access is subject to practical restrictions that will vary from society to society depending on resources at a given time. Even in a country as affluent as the United States there will surely always be items excluded, e.g., perhaps over-the-counter drugs, some teenage orthodontia, cosmetic surgery, and the like.[31] Here, too, the formula of similar treatment for similar cases may serve to modify the application of a need conception of justice in order to address the insatiability problem and limit frivolous use. In all of the foregoing instances of restriction, however, the relevant feature remains the illness, discomfort, etc. itself. The goal of equal access then retains its prima facie authoritativeness. It is imperfectly realized rather than disregarded.

These latter comments lead on to the question of institutional implications. I cannot aim here of course for the specificity rightly sought by policy-makers. My endeavor has been conceptual elucidation. While the ethicist needs to be apprised about the facts, he or she does not, qua ethicist, don the mantle of the policy-expert. In any case, only rarely does anyone do both things equally well. Yet cross-fertilization is extremely desirable. For experts should not be isolated from the wider assumptions their recommendations may reflect. I shall merely list some of the topics that would have to be discussed at length if we were to get clear about the implications. Examples will be limited to the current situation in the United States.

Anyone who accepts the case for equal access will naturally be concerned about de facto disparities in the availability of medical treatment. Let us consider two relevant indictments of current American practice. They appear in the writings not only of those who attack indiscriminately a system seen to be governed only by the appetite for profit and power, but also of those who denounce in less sweeping terms and espouse more cautiously reformist positions. The first shortcoming has to do with the maldistribution of supply. Per capita ratios of physicians to populations served vary, sometimes notoriously, between affluent suburbs and rural and inner city areas. This problem is exacerbated by the distressing data concerning the greater health needs of the poor. Chronic disease, frequency and duration of hospitalization, psychiatric disorders, infant death rates, etc.—these occur in significantly larger proportions to lower income members of American society.[32] A further complication is that "the distribution of health insurance coverage is badly skewed. Practically all the rich have insurance. But among the poor, about two-thirds have none. As a result, among people aged 25 to 64 who die, some 45 to 50 percent have neither hospital nor surgical coverage."[33] This last point connects with a second shortcoming frequently cited. Even those who are otherwise economically independent may be shattered by the high cost of a "catastrophic illness."[34]

Proposals for institutional reforms designed to overcome such disparities are bound to be taken seriously by any defender of equal access. What he or she will be disposed to press for, of course, is the removal of any double standard or "two-class" system of care. The viable procedures for bringing this about are not obvious, and comparisons with certain other societies (for relevant alternative models) are drawn now with perhaps less confidence.[35] One set of commonly discussed proposals includes (1) incentive subsidies to physicians, hospitals, and medical centers to provide services in regions of poverty (to overcome in part the unwillingness—to which no unique culpability need be ascribed—of many providers and their spouses to work and live in grim surroundings); (2) licensure controls to avoid comparatively excessive concentrations of physicians in regions of affluence; (3) a period (say, two years) in an underserved area as a requirement for licensing; (4) redistribution facilities that allow for population shifts.

A second set of proposals is linked with health insurance itself. While I cannot venture into the intricacies of medical economics or comment on the various bills for national health insurance presently inundating Congress, it may be instructive to take brief note of one proposal in which, once more, the defender of equal access is bound to take an interest (even if he or she finally rejects it on certain practical grounds). The precise details of the proposal are unimportant for our purposes.[36] Consider this crude sketch. Each citizen is (in effect) issued a card by the government. Whenever "legitimate" medical expenses (however determined for a given society) exceed, say, 10 percent of his or her annual taxable income, the card may be presented so that additional costs incurred will be paid for out of general tax revenues. The reasons urged on behalf of this sort of arrangement include the following. In the case of medical care there is warrant for proportionately equalizing what is spent from anyone's total taxable income. This warrant reflects the conditions, discussed earlier, of the natural lottery. Insofar as the advantages of health and the burdens of illness are random and undeserved, we may find it in our common interest to share risks. A fixed percentage of income attests to the misfit, also mentioned previously, between the reasons for differential total income and the reasons for receiving medical treatment. If money remains a causally necessary condition for receiving medical treatment, then a way must be found to place it in the hands of those who need it. The card is one such means. It is designed effectively to equalize purchasing power. In this way it seems to accord nicely with the goal of equal access. On the other side, the requirement of initial out-of-pocket expenses—sufficiently large in comparison to average family expenditures on health care—is designed to discourage frivolous use and foster awareness that medical care is a benefit not to be simply taken as a matter of course. It also safeguards against an excessively large tax burden while providing universal protection against the often disastrous costs of serious illnesses. Whether 10 percent is too great a chunk for the very poor to pay, and whether by itself the proposal will feed price inflation and neglect of preventive medicine, are questions that would have to be answered.

Another kind of possible institutional reform will also greatly interest the defender of equal access. This has to do with the "design of health care systems" or "care settings." The prevalent setting in American society has always been "fee for service." It is left up to each person to obtain the requisite care and to pay for it as he or she goes along. Because costs for medical treatment have accelerated at such an alarming rate, and because the sheer diffusion of energy and effort so characteristic of American medical practice leaves more and more people dissatisfied, alternatives to fee for service have been considered of late with unprecedented seriousness. The alternative care setting most widely discussed is prepaid practice, and specifically the "health maintenance organization" (HMO). Here one finds "an organized system of care which accepts the responsibility to provide or otherwise assure comprehensive care to a defined population for a fixed periodic payment per person or per family."[37] The best-known HMO is the Kaiser-Permanente Medical Care Program.[38] Does the HMO serve to realize the goal of equal access more fully? One line of argument in its favor is this. It is plausible to think that equal access will be fostered by the more economical care setting. HMOs are held to be less costly per capita in at least two respects: hospitalization rates are much below the national average; and, less often noted, physician manpower is as well. To be sure, one should be sensitive to the corruptions in each type of setting. While fee for service has resulted in a suspiciously high number of surgeries (twice as many per capita in the United States as in Great Britain), the HMO physician may more frequently permit the patient's needs to be overridden by the organization's pressure to economize. It may also be more difficult in an HMO setting to provide for close personal relations between a particular physician and a particular patient (something commended, of course, on all sides). After such corruptions are allowed for, the data seem encouraging to such an extent that a defender of equal access will certainly support the repeal of any law that limits the development of prepaid practice, to approve of "front-aid" subsidies for HMOs to increase their number overall and achieve a more equitable distribution throughout the country, and so on. At a minimum, each care setting should be available in every region. If we assume a common freedom to choose between them, each may help to guard against the peculiar temptations to which the other is exposed.

To assess in any serious way proposals for institutional reform such as the above is beyond the scope of this chapter. We would eventually be led, for example, into the question of whether it is consistent for the rich to pay more than the poor for the same treatment when, again, needs rather than income constitute the ground of the treatment,[39] and from there into the tangled subject of the "ethics of redistribution" in general.[40] Other complex issues deserve to be considered as well, e.g., the criteria for allocation of limited resources,[41] and how conceptions of justice apply to the providers of health care.[42]

Those committed to self-conscious moral and religious reflection about subjects in medicine have concentrated, perhaps unduly, on issues about care of individual patients (as death approaches, for instance). These issues plainly warrant the most careful consideration. One would like to see in addition, however, more attention paid to social questions in medical ethics. To attend to them is not necessarily to leave behind all of the matters that reach deeply into the human condition. Any detailed case for institutional reforms, for example, will be enriched if the proponent asks soberly whether certain conflicts and certain perplexities allow for more than partial improvements and provisional resolutions. Can public and private interests ever be made fully to coincide by legislative and administrative means? Will the commitment of a physician to an individual patient and the commitment of the legislator to the "common good" ever be harmonized in every case? Our anxiety may be too intractable. Our fear of illness and of dying may be so pronounced and immediate that we will seize the nearly automatic connections between privilege, wealth, and power if we can. We will do everything possible to have our kidney machines even if the charts make it clear that many more would benefit from mandatory immunization at a fraction of the cost. And our capacity for taking in rival points of view may be too limited. Once we have witnessed tangible suffering, we cannot just return with ease to public policies aimed at statistical patients. Those who believe that justice is the pre-eminent virtue of institutions and that a convincing case can be made on behalf of justice for equal access to health care would do well to ponder such conflicts and perplexities. Our reforms might then seem, to ourselves and to others, less abstract and jargon-filled in formulation and less sanguine and piecemeal in substance. They would reflect a greater awareness of what we have to confront.

Notes to Chapter Five

1. Edward M. Kennedy, *In Critical Condition: The Crisis in America's Health Care* (New York: Simon and Schuster, 1972), pp. 234-52; Richard M. Nixon, "President's Message on Health Care System," Document No. 92-261 (March 2, 1972), House of Representatives, Washington, D.C., 1.

2. Hugo A. Bedau, "Radical Egalitarianism," pp. 168-80 in *Justice and Equality*, ed. by Hugo A. Bedau (Englewood Cliffs, N.J.: Prentice-Hall, 1971); John Hospers, *Human Conduct* (New York: Harcourt, Brace, 1961), 416-68; J.R. Lucas, "Justice," *Philosophy* 47, No. 181 (July 1972), 229-48; Ch. Perelman, *The Idea of Justice and the Problem of Argument*, trans. by John Petrie (London: Routledge and Kegan Paul, 1963); Nicholas Rescher, *Distributive Justice* (Indianapolis: Bobbs-Merrill, 1966); Gregory Vlastos, "Justice and Equality," pp. 31-72 in *Social Justice*, ed. by Richard B. Brandt (Englewood Cliffs, N.J.: Prentice-Hall, 1962).

3. Paul Ramsey, *The Patient as Person: Exploration in Medical Ethics* (New Haven: Yale University Press, 1970), p. 240.

4. Nancy Hicks, "Nation's Doctors Move to Police Medical Care," *New York Times* (Sunday, October 28, 1973), 52.

5. Gene Outka, *Agape: An Ethical Analysis* (New Haven: Yale University Press, 1972).

6. Ayn Rand, *Atlas Shrugged* (New York: Signet, 1957), 958.

7. Outka, 89-90, 165-67.

8. Lucas, 321.

9. Bernard A.O. Williams, "The Idea of Equality," pp. 116-37 in *Justice and*

Equality, ed. by Hugo A. Bedau (Englewood Cliffs, N.J.: Prentice-Hall, 1971), pp. 126-37.

10. Ibid., 127.

11. See also Thomas Nagel, "Equal Treatment and Compensatory Discrimination," *Philosophy and Public Affairs* 2, No. 4, 348-63 (Summer 1973), 354.

12. Rescher, pp. 79-80.

13. Quoted in Ramsey, p. 248.

14. Ramsey, p. 256.

15. Ibid.

16. Ibid.

17. Anne R. Somers, *Health Care in Transition: Directions for the Future* (Chicago: Hospital Research and Educational Trust, 1971), p. 20.

18. Cf. Rescher, pp. 80-81.

19. Robert M. Sade, "Medical Care as a Right: a Refutation," *The New England Journal of Medicine* 285, 1288-92 (December 1971), 1289.

20. Ibid.

21. Ibid., p. 1291.

22. Charles L. Schultze, Edward R. Fried, Alice M. Rivlin, and Nancy H. Teeters, *Setting National Priorities: The 1973 Budget* (Washington, D.C.: The Brookings Institution, 1972), pp. 214-15.

23. Outka, pp. 264-65.

24. Perelman, p. 22.

25. See John Rawls, *A Theory of Justice* (Cambridge: Harvard University Press, 1971), e.g. 104.

26. E.g. Perelman, p. 23.

27. See Outka, pp. 91-92, 309-12.

28. See also Honoré, 1968.

29. Benn, Stanley I., "Egalitarianism and the Equal Consideration of Interests," pp. 152-67 in *Justice and Equality*, ed. by Hugo A. Bedau (Englewood Cliffs, N.J.: Prentice-Hall, 1971), p. 164.

30. Anne R. Somers and Herman M. Somers, "The Organization and Financing of Health Care: Issues and Directions for the Future," *American Journal of Orthopsychiatry* 42, 119-36 (January 1972), 122.

31. Anne R. Somers and Herman M. Somers, "Major Issues in National Health Insurance," *Milbank Memorial Fund Quarterly* 50, No. 2, Part 1, 177-210 (April 1972), 182.

32. William N. Hubbard, "Health Knowledge," pp. 93-120 in *The Health of Americans*, ed. by Boisfeuillet Jones (Englewood Cliffs, N.J.: Prentice-Hall, 1970).

33. Somers, p. 46.

34. See some eloquent examples in Kennedy.

35. See Odin Anderson, *Health Care: Can There Be Equity? The United States, Sweden and England* (New York, Wiley, 1973).

36. For one much-discussed version, see Martin S. Feldstein, "A New Approach to National Health Insurance," *The Public Interest* 23, (Spring 1971), 93-105.

37. Anne R. Somers, *The Kaiser-Permanente Medical Care Program* (New York: The Commonwealth Fund, 1971), p. v.

38. See also Sidney R. Garfield, "Prevention of Dissipation of Health Services Resources," *American Journal of Public Health* 61 (1971), 1499-1506.

39. Andrew Ward, "The Idea of Equality Reconsidered," *Philosophy* 48 (January 1973), 85-90.

40. See, e.g., Stanley I. Benn and Richard S. Peters, *The Principles of Political Thought* (New York: Free Press, 1965), 155-78; Bertrand de Jouvenel, *The Ethics of Redistribution* (Cambridge: Cambridge University Press, 1952).

41. The issue of priorities is at least threefold: (1) between improved medical care and other social needs, e.g., to restrain auto accidents and pollution; (2) between different sorts of medical treatment for different illnesses, e.g., prevention vs. crisis intervention and exotic treatments; (3) between persons of whom all need a single scarce resource and not all can have it, e.g., Ramsey's discussion of how to decide among those who are to receive dialysis. Moreover, (1) can be subdivided between (a) improved medical care and other social needs that affect health directly, e.g., drug addiction, auto accidents, and pollution; (b) improved medical care and other social needs that serve the overall aim of community-survival, e.g., a common defense. In the case of (2) one would like to see far more careful discussion of some general criteria that might be employed, e.g., numbers affected, degree of contagion, prospects for rehabilitation, and so on.

42. What sorts of appeals to justice might be cogently made to warrant, for instance, the differentially high income physicians receive? Here are three possibilities: (1) the greater skill and responsibility involved should be rewarded proportionately, i.e., one should attend to considerations of *desert*; (2) there should be *compensation* for the money invested for education and facilities in order to restore circumstances of approximate equality (this argument, while a common one in medical circles, would need to consider that medical education is received in part at public expense and that the modern physician is the highest paid professional in the country); (3) the difference should benefit the least advantaged more than an alternative arrangement where disparities are less. We prefer a society where the medical profession flourishes and everyone has a longer life expectancy to one where everyone is poverty-stricken with a shorter life expectancy ("splendidly equalized destitution"). Yet how are we to ascertain the minimum degree of differential income required for the least advantaged members of the society to be better off?

Discussions of "justice and the interests of providers" are, I think, badly needed. Physicians in the United States have suffered a decline in prestige for various reasons, e.g., the way many have used Medicare to support and increase their own incomes. Yet one should endeavor to assess their interests fairly. A concern for professional autonomy is clearly important, though one may ask whether adequate attention has been paid to the distinction between the imposition of cost controls from outside and interference with professional medical judgments. One may affirm the former, it seems, and still reject—energetically—the latter.

Chapter 6

Ethics and Health Care Delivery: Computers and Distributive Justice

Joseph Fletcher

Because of the subjective and personal nature of human values, teaching ethics, biomedical or any other kind, is inescapably a venture in controversy. Ludwig Wittgenstein said of the value factors in ethical reasoning, "This is a terrible business—just terrible. You can at best stammer when you talk of it."[1]

Nevertheless, values are the necessary parameters of moral judgments. Literally speaking, they are the quality standards or measures we set alongside a moral act to judge its rightness or wrongness. Or they are, in mathematical language, the independent variables we use in any set of ethical equations.

At first this may sound too strangely mathematical to be appropriate to ethical discourse, not fitting for the study of the moral qualities of good and evil. I confess that my own training in philosophical and theological ethics was deeply planted in the humanities, with the consequence that I like many others of my breed feel uncomfortable and incompetent whenever questions of distribution and the requisite quantifiers are raised. All the same, the main purpose of this chapter is to contend that any serious ethical analysis of health care delivery plunges us headlong and unavoidably into what I can only call "ethical arithmetic."

The mere phrase "ethical arithmetic" revives memories of the way seventeenth-century economists like Petty and North spoke of "political arithmetic." Any social inquiry, including ethics, has to calculate quantities.

Controversy or disputation can be either good or bad, depending on whether its payoff comes down to more light or more heat. T.P. O'Connor once said, "If only the Catholics and Protestants in Ireland were all good pagans we could get along like Christians." In situations like that there is too much heat, too little light. However, even though we hope that light and understanding will follow from the abrasions of ethical discourse, it is still true that the best model for ethical discourse is incandescent light. Incandescence, from sunlight down to the filament in an electric light bulb, comes from heat. The heat always needs minimizing and controlling, but it can never be entirely dispensed with.

For our purposes the best definition of health is the World Health Organization's. It is far more analytic and comprehensive than the individualist and one-to-one definition with which clinical medicine has functioned historically, until the twentieth century; yet no other definition will ever again be acceptable to enlightened citizens (medicine's "consumers") or to public policy-makers. WHO defines health as *a complex of physical, mental, and social well-being*: all three. Over against this, as Dr. John Knowles of the Rockefeller Foundation has charged, "The medical ostrich has buried its head in the sands of biological science and turned its backside to the major social issues of medical care today."[2]

In ethical language this means, it seems to me, that medical centers ought to be converted into health centers. Truly to understand the biomedical enterprise in terms of human well-being instead of in terms of physical health is a fairly radical proposal, even in the 1970s, because it broadens and deepens the obligations (a key ethical term) of health care to include treatment not only of mental disorders but of social causation too. I am talking here about honesty in diagnosis.

WHO's definition was certainly anticipated a long time ago in the bureaucratic rhetoric of medical reports and public health literature; but even so, it could be argued that the only branch of medicine to date actually to take mental and social well-being into account, as well as physical health, is cosmetic surgery!

In actual fact, physicians have tried steadily and stubbornly to cut or keep the practice of medicine loose from psychology and psychiatry, and from public health management. Psychiatry or psychiatric medicine is still only a cousin in conventional medical sentiments, and certainly not a "kissin' cousin" yet. From the medical citadel public health workers are looked at as only very distant relatives, not in the cousin class at all. As for sociologists, they are as scarce as ethicists in medical schools.

On any realistic view there is a nearly complete divorce of scientific and clinical medicine from the social and economic disciplines. This is the case educationally, institutionally, and ideologically. For example, schools of public health were separated a long time ago from medical education.

Biomedical thinking, it seems, is in more flux right now than ever before, and this may mean that the well-being concept of medicine has a good chance of prevailing. This flux or creative disorder in medical rethinking is due to three major factors in health care change: (1) the expansion (not to say "explosion") of medical knowledge through science; (2) the institution of social welfare programs—including various forms of prepaid medical care; and (3) the development of our present forms of medical education.

Looking back at the Greek experience, we find three models of health care. One was the Cult of the Dogmatists, the medical teachings of Pythagoras and Empedocles, based on metaphysical rather than pragmatic principles. This was what Hippocrates broke away from, in favor of etiology and natural causation and in revolt against the priests and Neoplatonists. The second was what they called the Cult of Aesculapius, a strictly one-to-one, patient-physician affair aimed at getting the particular individual physically well. The Aesculapian is still the real model of medicine ideologically, not only in the A.M.A. but in medical schools also. The third one was what the Greeks called the Cult of Hygeia, the cult of the daughter of Aesculapius, which was a social or public health model of prevention as well as therapy.

The term hygiene means "good for health." In the hygienic model prevention of disease is the *summum bonum*, rather than treatment, and the problem of human well-being is understood and approached socially rather than privately or individually.

It is this hygienic model of the biomedical disciplines and of health care that is presupposed in this chapter. It is the public health or public interest way of looking at the ethics of health care and its delivery to patients—patients who are seen not as paying customers privately contracted, but as consumers with a common concern and a collective need.

DISTRIBUTIVE JUSTICE

Even at the clinical level there are many ways in which delivery of health care in modern times poses new moral questions. I cannot undertake to deal with many of them here, but we might just take note of a few. For example, have husbands a valid moral claim ("right") to be present at the birth of their babies? The Montana Supreme Court recently ruled that they do not.[3] Yet Dad's presence at delivery is held by many, as in the Lamaze or psychoprophylactic method of childbirth, to be essential to providing good obstetrical health care. Again, there are any number of ethical questions raised about various items in the Patient's Bill of Rights lately promulgated by the American Hospital Association. Such issues are all a part of the "consumerist" perspective on medicine, being spelled out more or less militantly in terms of consumer protection and patients' rights.

Hormone therapy, especially for minors, raises questions of right and wrong when, as is frequently a consequence of the treatment, the patient experiences an increase of sexual vigor almost compulsive in its magnitude. And speaking of minors, what of the delivery of health care in the form of birth control (contraception, sterilization, and abortion) to minors, bypassing parental consent, which is now the practice under "mature minor" statutes in some states? As one last example of the morality of health care delivery at the clinical level, how are we to formulate the ethics of surrogate therapy—the provision of psychiatrically supervised sex practice with therapeutic partners for patients with impotence, frigidity, inexperience, phobias, and so forth.

Such clinical problems of judgment and decision-making, arresting as they are on their own level, do not quite enter the focus of this discussion. The social issues of health care delivery take shape more pointedly at the systems or programmatic level. Being neither a medical sociologist nor a public administrator I lack the competence to do much more than indicate them, yet it is here that essentially *social nature* of health care becomes manifest, and it is this social character or dimension that lies at the heart of this chapter.

It is precisely here, in the social dimension of medicine, that we run into the question of distributive justice, and distributive justice is the core or key question for biomedical ethics. Distributive justice is the biggest or most all-embracing ethical problem. Ultimately, the reputation of biomedical ethics is at stake in whether it deals with it or not, and in how it deals with it.

Since Aristotle we have distinguished between three orders of justice: commutative, legal, and distributive. It is still a meaningful typology. Commutative justice deals with what is due between people, as in professional ethics (e.g., medical), trade ethics or market morality, the ethics of sex, family, and human reproduction; all problems of obligation in one-to-one and group relations. Legal justice has to do with what we as individuals owe to the community and to the state, in terms of jurisprudence, civil and criminal law, taxation, and the like. Distributive justice is concerned with what society and the state owe to individuals, as in public services and public utilities, protection of the environment, and—our special concern here—health care.

At this point, I enter an area in which I not only have had little or no training or experience but where I find myself drawn to a conclusion that makes me decidedly uncomfortable. My conditioning in the grand tradition has instilled in me a "feeling" that values are one thing and numbers (digits or dollars) are something else. But all ethics should be based, as the scientific ethic is, on honesty; like Martin Luther, I'll go where my understanding takes me. "I can do no other." Like Wittgenstein on values, I approach the *allocation* of values with Kierkegaard's "fear and trembling."

It seems that the heart of the problem of distributive justice is how we are to allocate our resources; for example, as between rural and urban patients; or between preventive and curative care; or between care by physicians and care by auxiliary and paramedical personnel; or between high-cost specialties and low-cost care. What the Chinese have done under the banner of "barefoot medicine" using lay trainees is a specter haunting the old guard who want to hold the line for arcane medicine. HMOs have run into massive resistance by the medical establishment. But given a serious commitment to exploring these options, what reallocations of roles and funds would distributive justice require?

Two of the most fiercely fought issues in the U.S. lately have had to do with health insurance proposals and peer review or monitoring of the quality of medical practice. PSROs (Professional Standards Review Organizations) were a matter of civil law by 1972 but bitterly opposed none the less for two more years, by doctors who do not want their performance checked out. (The House of Delegates of the A.M.A. meeting June 26, 1974 in Chicago finally voted, 185 to 57, to support the PSRO law.) Yet it is obvious that monitoring is needed; one doctor in Massachusetts was found to be doing eighty disc operations per year—as many as are done by all the surgeons at Massachusetts General Hospital combined.

The screams of outrage against PSROs from the A.M.A. have an ironical sound, since the A.M.A. first began as a peer review organization 125 years ago, to expose diploma mills, quacks, and financial highbinders. Peer review is, of course, what goes on anyway in any teaching hospital or university medical center.

Almost certainly the preponderant ethical issue about the delivery of medical care lies in rival proposals for national health insurance. One is the Kennedy-Mills bill (NHI), in many ways modeled on the Swedish-English systems—a federally underwritten social welfare program advocated with a rhetoric somewhat less than candid. It would eliminate private profit-making insurance companies. The Nixon-Weinberger proposal, a Comprehensive Health Insurance Plan (CHIP) is a national scheme allowing private individual election or employer insurance plans, with federal backup. The A.M.A. has an alternative of its own called Medicredit, aimed at keeping medicine in the traditional fee-for-service, private-practice model through the manipulation of tax credits in the individual patient's tax returns. The Ways and Means Committee's eclectic plan merges features in many of these schemes, keeps private insurance companies in the picture, and aims at a ceiling of $1000 on any covered person's annual medical expense.

The salient fact in all of this is the public's anger at the ruinous cost of medical care. Medicine is in trouble and its self-image in immediate jeopardy because it has been priced out of the marketplace. From 1960 to 1974 the cost of living rose by 52.2 percent while physicians' fees rose 57.7 percent and daily hospital charges went up from $56 to $144—up 155 percent.

Now, having painted this picture, what about it? Not being an economist, a statistician, or a political scientist, I cannot speak to the question which of these plans and options and distributions is most fair, most just. Justice cannot work without numbers; that much is obvious. It seems to me that the task of the just man and of the legislature is precisely to choose whatever course appears to maximize the good (in this case health care), or—as I would prefer to say—whatever would realize the greatest good of the greatest number.

Yet the question still remains, how is this ethical imperative to be put into effect? How are we to get the numbers for our value choices? It is on this point that I want to put my emphasis. Let me start by saying that many of our historical modes of ethical thought are utterly *out*moded.

The scope and arena of ethical choice or preference has widened enormously since the days when being one's brother's keeper and loving one's neighbor was a direct matter between you and a handful of people personally known to you, in what anthropologists call a "primary community." The pastoral-agrarian and village society of the Bible no longer exists in our Atlantic civilization. We cannot continue simply to turn to the teachings of Moses or Jesus for direct ethical guidance.

Things are just not that simple any more. Ethics is perforce "social ethics" now; it is no longer, or at least less and less, what we might call interpersonal morality. The world is so tied together, due to the interdependence of technology and rapid transport, and to the density of urban culture steadily aggravated by irrational reproduction, that even the words "neighbor" and "stranger" are nearly archaic. We are caught up in a tight web of radical interconnectivity.

TELESCOPES, NOT ONLY MICROSCOPES

What is needed is a moral telescope to see our moral problems through, not a moral microscope only. This is an age of macroethical more than microethical analysis. In medicine we have to deal with many patients who coexist, for instance, not just with patients one at a time. Hans Jonas says, "In the course of treatment the physician is obligated to the patient and no one else."[4] That, alas, is the classical ethic at its most myopic. It looks at the problem of medical care through a rear-view mirror.

The ancient one-to-one medical ethic is too simple, and it therefore falsifies ethical problems. A moral calculus of some kind is required if we are to cope justly with the imperative of health care delivery. Along with the one-to-one ethic we can set aside other classical norms as outmoded and therefore actually unethical—for example, such vestigial bits of medical piety as "first come, first served," "*non nocere*, do no harm," and the "inviolability of medical secrets."

Any very sophisticated discussion of the problem of social justice and the delivery of health care is rich with such terms as priorities, relative claims, triage, value judgment, systems analysis, allocation of scarce resources, cost-benefit balance, tradeoff, games theory, decision-making, choice, options. This is what I take to be the contemporary and relevant language of ethics. As an ethical lexicon it predicates quantifiers, numbers, and weights. Ethical judgments need to be able to quantify qualities or to variate values.

Daniel Callahan was on target quoting Kenneth Boulding's definition, "A moral, or ethical, proposition is a statement about a rank order of preferences among alternatives, which is intended to apply to more than one person."[5] Whether the weights we assign to different values and interests in our ethical "mix" are monetary or arithmetical, somehow we must learn to program computers with preference questions.

Robert Theobald told a symposium at Vanderbilt University in 1971, "If you pulled the plug on the computers this country would come to a grinding halt." I have a feeling that Theobald is right. If so, this would mean that artificial intelligence is the only answer to the magnitude of human relations in a technological world of runaway material production and human reproduction.

We are all fairly familiar with tradeoff and cost-benefit judgment at the clinical level, and the notion of proportionate good—in so-called triage decisions. Selection committees face it in renal programs where patients outnumber the perfusion slot available on kidney machines. This can be difficult, of course; as when, for example, the choice is between a candidate with good prospects and a patient already in dialysis with a neurosurgical deficit, such as the loss of frontal lobes, or maybe one with hemorrhage of the GI tract.

But things get a lot more *statistical* when we look at an uptown New York hospital's ethical question about its relative obligations. Its hyperbaric chamber cost $750,000 to install, $600,000 per year to operate. In five years the total cost was $3,700,000—and only 900 patients were treated, at a cost of $4111.11 each. For the same amount of funds 20,000 outpatients could have been treated per year, or 100,000 altogether. Or a screening program could have been set up in East Harlem to detect lead poisoning and anemia in a million children, to keep their brains from being ruined. If you want to think about ethics and health care delivery, here is a good case, posing all the factors at stake—both numbers and competing values.

The numbers question gets lots harder when hundreds and thousands are involved, not just two or ten. There is the famous story about the medical corps problem in North Africa during the Second World War. They had a short supply of penicillin. It could be used to treat a few hundred badly wounded soldiers or it could be used in light dosages for several thousand who were out of action only because of venereal disease caught in brothels in the rest areas.

The American military's health care policy in front line stations is to give priority of treatment to those with slight conditions rather than overwhelmingly serious wounds. The U.S. government's civil defense policy in the event of nuclear war is the same—lightly injured first, badly injured last.

This is utilitarian ethics; the greatest good of the greatest number. But it would be a pity if our discussion got bogged down in a doctrinaire debate over the theoretical merits of utilitarianism. As a question on its own merits it would be an important subject, but in the present context I believe the main thing is the problem of distributive justice and whether or not we should maximize the recipients of health care and optimize the quality of the health care delivered. The utilitarians are in the picture inevitably, since from the start they set their sights and based their ethics on the public welfare and justice, as in Bentham's *Principles of Morals and Legislation*; they "politicized" ethics. But we can avoid a lot of energy loss by simply heeding Albert Jonsen's advice: "Ethics must learn to speak the language of public policy in order to function as easily in conference rooms and legislative halls as in the classroom."[6]

In Britain it was argued that the steroid contraceptive pill would cause embolisms due to the estrogen—which was true. But the health service persisted for the reason that fourteen such deaths per million users is preferable to 228 deaths per million nonusers—deaths, that is, resulting from pregnancy and childbirth. Since the mortality rate is seventeen times higher for pregnancies than for contraception, they acted for the greater good of the greater number.

This kind of mathematics only gathers and compares numbers, however. When we have to compare values as well as sums, which is the real problem of ethical arithmetic or mathematical morality, then things begin to get hazier and harder. Look, for example, at a problem of health care delivery faced by WHO and the government of Sri Lanka. The anopheles mosquito spreads fast in Ceylon, but by DDT spraying they cut malaria cases from 2.8 million in 1961 to only 110 in 1964 (three years' time). Appreciating that DDT does ecological damage, they then stopped spraying, in the belief that the pests were licked. The mosquitos returned at once; in 1968-69 malaria had again infected 2.5 million people.

Here is an ethical choice problem comprising both numbers and values. The numbers are easy, but how should we relate the values of ecologic balance as over against human mortality rates? It is my belief that this task of value ranking must itself be converted into numbers, dollars or abstract digits, or whatever, before we will be able to quantify the moral options we have to program into our computers' data banks. Without it we cannot optimize the widest benefit (the non-moral good) at stake in health care delivery, nor make the "optimific" calculations needed if the ideal we serve is human well-being for all.

QUANTIFYING QUALITIES (VALUES)

Here, then, is the heart of this chapter—that we must set out on a new task for ethics, an effort to innovate a mathematical morality or statistical ethics. Gordon Rattray Taylor put it neatly when he said we lack "a mathematics of mercy" with which to "calculate who, of thousands of sufferers, should receive the privilege of being saved by scarce facilities."[7] The ethics of delivering health care demands that we face the fact of the limits of growth and resources, the realities of a finite world. John Stuart Mill made this perfectly clear 150 years ago in his essay on the stationary state, and more recently it was brought home by the Club of Rome, in the English *Ecologist's* "Blueprint for Survival," and by the Meadows's *Limits of Growth*.

In 1961, there was a brief debate between Warren Weaver of the Rockefeller Foundation and Roger Shinn of the Union Seminary.[8] Weaver pointed out that the "five principle world religions of revelation" got their start too long ago to have much to say about our interdependent modern world. Our problem now is cost-benefit judgments about things like new expressways or highrise building construction when weighed against the predictable loss of life entailed. Accurate projective estimates by so-called actuaries are available and reliable. Tradeoff decisions of this kind go on all the time in medicine, transport, building, mining, everything.

Shinn argued, on the other hand, that "some aspects of ethics can never be reduced to statistics." As his example he took Jesus' nomadic-agrarian parable about the lost sheep and the shepherd who left ninety-nine sheep in the wilderness to hunt the one that was lost. Shinn's idea was that you cannot relativize the value of some things, such as a human life. But surely it would be unjust if leaving the flock actually risked losing ninety-nine for one. (Many exegetes say there was, in fact, no such risk.) He tried to furthur sharpen the issue by asking Ivan's question in Dostoievski's *Brothers Karamazov*: Would it be justifiable to make all men happy at the cost of torturing one little baby to death? If in this hypothetical case the world's unhappiness included the disease and deaths of countless people, then of course trading one for many would be hypothetically right—the preponderance of good over evil, of benefit over cost.

The ethical issue at stake is plain enough, uncomfortably so. Are the needs of the one or the few subordinate to the many? Which prevails in actual conflicts, the common or the private interest? Let it be carefully noted, by the way, that to be impersonal in the sense of counting noses is not by any means to be antipersonal. It is multipersonal. If some of us cannot see the trees for the forest, others cannot see the forest for the trees. The point is this: To sacrifice the one for the many is to sacrifice the one for many *ones*. The "greatest number" is not an abstraction; it is the sum of real, particular, and personal individuals.

Hegel, in his short essay on logic, reasoned that the headachy business of choosing between one good and another, or obversely between one evil and another, is true tragedy, whereas the simplistic collision of good and evil—black and white—is only melodrama, Sunday School ethics. It is hard for Shakespeare's Othello to decide between his love of Desdemona and Iago's testimony, or for Sophocles' Antigone to choose between her loyalty to her brother and her loyalty to King Creon. So it is with all competing value problems. All serious ethics, as in a socially just health care system, deals with tragedy, not with melodrama; with choices between competing values, not with obvious matters of good and evil, right or wrong.

In the ethics of health care delivery we must be utilitarians, at least in the sense of seeking the greatest good (health) for the greatest number possible. Or, as Kenneth Boulding puts it, without counting and cost-benefit analysis "all evaluation is random selection by wild hunches." He adds, "The fundamental principle that we should count all costs, whether easily countable or not, and evaluate all rewards, however hard they are to evaluate, is one which emerges squarely out of economics and which is at least a preliminary guideline in the formation of the moral judgment, in what might be called the 'economic ethic.' "[9]

Just as people like Paul Samuelson and Robert Dorfman have coined the term "econometrics" for mathematics and quantification methods applied to economic data, I suggest that "ethometrics" can be used for ethical analysis seeking distributive justice. It is a good label for applying statistical terms of amount and probability to macromoral problems, even down at the level of allocating funds as between developing an acceptable artificial heart and meeting the needs for patients in renal failure. To be ethical requires knowledge and careful calculation, because loving concern is the same as justice—it has to be distributed.[10]

All of this leaves many loose ends and unopened boxes. The overall questions are, presumably, whether ethometrics is (a) workable and (b) desirable. A great deal of thinking is called for, much of it new thinking, before we can catch sight of any consensual principles. Here are half a dozen worrisome questions:

1. Is it really necessary to weight values numerically, to quantify qualities? Why could we not just get the data numbers from the computers and then, with the factual data in hand, choose between the options thus measured according to our ranked but unquantified values? Some, like Toulmin, think the answer is Yes, we can. Some would even contend that "quantifying quality" is impossible, a contradiction in terms.

Jay Forrester at M.I.T. once told me that a middle course is called for: first to program a computer's bank with all the data of macroethical questions, then to assign relative numerical weights to the values involved (a basically ethical, nonmathematical step) and enter them into the computer too, and finally to ask "it" to compute which course will yield the greatest human benefit.

2. Will distributive justice if seriously pursued homogenize or mediocratize quality, reduce human valuations to a dead level, the least common denominator? In utilitarian theory there is a classic disagreement; should we seek total or aggregate happiness—five million totally happy people or ten million moderately happy people? Should we aim at the most for some, or the average (aggregate) for all? Distributive justice seems to favor the aggregate principle, but am I right about this, and how shall we regard the issue's bearing on ethometrics?

3. Is it the case, as ethicists of the school of emotive theory assert, that our values are inescapably subjective, in some degree personally arbitrary, even when shared widely with others? And even if they are, does this mean that a working consensus or common mind about what things are worthwhile, and in what order, is unreachable? If unreachable, what does this say about the claims of a democratic society? Does it and must it function without a common mind and common interests? Without consensus as its first premise how can a legislature or government justify itself?

4. Given a consensus about "the good" or human happiness, is the proper business of a legislature or law-making body anything but or besides the utilitarian task, i.e., seeking the greatest good for the greatest number?

5. Is there really a persuasive case to be made, as some have always contended, for refusing to select and choose among human beings' needs,

especially when human life is at stake? Or for resorting uncountingly to sortilège when face to face with tragic choices and distributions? To take the stance that some things, whatever that covers, may not be done no matter how much good would follow, is obviously deontological—opposed to the teleological ethics of calculating benefits and consequences. It appears that the tactics of absolute rules are incompatible with the tactics of value optimization. Is this contradiction real; if so, can deontologists get around it somehow?

6. Surely all values do not have to be politicized, in the sense of socially distributed. Which ones should, which should not? And of those which should be, should they be distributed on the democratic one-man-one-vote method, or what Garrett Hardin calls "mutual coercion mutually agreed upon"?[11] In democratic countries some values are usually excluded from the public dominion; tastes in music and the arts, for example. Furthermore, the logic of utilitarianism does not require the greatest good of the greatest number to be determined democratically, although almost all utilitarians in the West have been democratic for good reason.

An eminent bioethicist said to me recently, "It is time we began taking social medical ethics seriously." I agree, but it is going to take lots of work.

Notes to Chapter Six

1. Quoted in C.H. Waddington, *Science and Ethics* (London: Allen and Unwin, 1942), p. 7. A *viva voce* remark.

2. "The Unseen Ostrich in Our Teaching Hospitals," *Prism* 1 (November 1973), 13.

3. *Medical World News* 15 (June 14, 1974), 26J.

4. *Daedalus* 98 (Spring 1969), 238.

5. *The Tyranny of Survival* (New York: Macmillan, 1973), 184.

6. "The Totally Implantable Artificial Heart," *The Hastings Center Report* 3 (November 1973), 5, 1-4.

7. *The Biological Time Bomb* (New York: World, 1966), 211.

8. *Christianity and Crisis* 20 (January 23, 1961), 24, 210-15.

9. "Economics as a Moral Science," *The American Economic Review* 59 (March 1969), 7-8.

10. *Situation Ethics* (New York: Westminster, 1966), 87-99.

11. *Exploring New Ethics for Survival* (New York: Viking, 1972), 128-32.

Chapter 7

Health Care and Justice in Contract Theory Perspective

Ronald M. Green

No work in the field of social and political philosophy in recent years has been received with as much interest as John Rawls's *A Theory of Justice*.[1] Each passing month new articles in journals of philosophy and political theory appear either applauding or criticizing aspects of Rawls's social-contract view of justice. Whether it is the partisans or critics of Rawls's position who eventually prevail, it is safe to say that in the foreseeable future no responsible discussions of public policy, whether theoretical or applied, can afford to neglect Rawls's book.

In view of this, it is worth asking what are the implications of Rawls's view for health care policy. Certainly, questions concerning the supply and distribution of health care are central to contemporary discussions of social justice, and it is social justice that is the object of Rawls's inquiry. Despite this, the reader who searches *A Theory of Justice* for a discussion of health care will be puzzled and disappointed; not only does Rawls fail to devote any space to this topic in this lengthy book, but the index itself contains not a single reference to health, sickness, medicine, or medical care. It is true that there are some very brief references to these topics in the text, but these are mere afterthoughts to other discussions.[2]

Why, then, is this major work virtually silent on a matter that many persons believe to be at the forefront of questions of justice in our day? Several explanations might be offered. First, there is the fact that in this book Rawls is primarily interested in developing a theory for the distribution of those basic goods that are created by social cooperation and that are distributed by the social system. He calls these the "social primary goods," and they include

111

various civil rights and liberties, socially bestowed powers and opportunities, the material goods of wealth and income, and the important social good of self-respect. Rawls distinguishes these from the "natural primary goods" of intelligence, vigor, imagination, and good health whose distribution, he maintains, is only indirectly affected by the social structure, and he places the natural primary goods outside the scope of his concern (p. 62).

Is this move on his part valid? Not really, one is tempted to say. Critics of Rawls have repeatedly pointed out that for a natural primary good like intelligence, the distinction between what is directly and indirectly mediated by the social structure is artificial. In view of all we know about the effects of family circumstances on learning, for example, it does not seem right to say that intelligence is not in large measure distributed when income shares are decided. If this point has some force with respect to intelligence, it would seem to be even more pertinent where health is concerned. Modern medical technology, with its enormous preventative and therapeutic powers, renders almost archaic the notion that health depends on natural contingencies. Social decisions concerning medical care thus have a vital impact on everyone's health, even where health is construed only in the narrowest sense as freedom from physical disease.[3] Despite Rawls, then, health care ought to be considered a primary social good in his terms, and ought to be directly considered by a theory of justice.

A second reason Rawls may have neglected the issue of health care has to do with his extensive concern in his book with the problem of income distribution. It may be that he believes that the matter of medical care can be made a function of a just distribution of income. Indeed, this view may underlie his definition of health as a natural primary good only indirectly mediated by the social structure (p. 62). Thus, he might believe that once society has been set up so that everyone receives a just share of income, medical care can be arranged for privately out of that share with, perhaps, some special provisions made for those at the bottom of the income ladder. If this is Rawls's final view of the matter, however, it runs against the general tenor of his position. It is very doubtful that the rational agents whose choices define social principles in this theory would neglect to establish separate principles for medical care or would substantially leave its distribution to be determined by one's income share.

A final explanation for Rawls's neglect of health care is less involved than those I have mentioned, and it is the explanation I personally believe to be correct. This is simply that Rawls has not had the space in this book adequately to deal with this issue, and has preferred to pass it by, at least for the time being. *A Theory of Justice* is, after all, a very narrowly defined book. It may seem odd to say this of a volume six hundred pages long, but why should we assume that a topic as important as social justice can be handled in six hundred or even six thousand pages? As it is, the book omits treatment of a number of other vital issues of social justice. We should not be surprised, therefore, that Rawls neglects the issue of health care. It may be that his very silence on this issue reflects a deliberate decision to avoid discussion of an important but complicated problem.

Whatever the reasons for Rawls's unwillingness to engage this issue, it seems clear that a consideration of health care deserves an important place in the kind of theory of justice he advances. In the following discussion, therefore, I want to try to fill in this particular gap in contract theory by suggesting a "Rawlsian" or social-contract analysis of health care and social justice, accepting the basic lines of his theory and extending them beyond their present bounds.

The main ideas of the kind of social-contract theory worked out by Rawls may have been sketched out by writers in scholarly and popular journals so often by now as to preclude the need for a review of his position. But to help point up those aspects of the theory important for the matter of health care, I think it is useful to summarize the main features of his view. The theory as a whole has two different parts. First, Rawls offers a distinct and fairly novel procedure for arriving at the principles of social justice. Second, he advances several basic principles of justice that he believes a proper application of the procedure would produce.

The theory's choice procedure involves the thought experiment of an imaginary, hypothetical contract situation which Rawls calls "the original position" (chapter 3). The principles of social justice, according to Rawls, may be thought of as those that would be unanimously chosen in this original position by free, equal, mutually disinterested and rational persons (rational in the simple sense that they can select the best means to any desired end). Rawls further asks us to think of these contract parties as lacking any knowledge of the particularities that distinguish them from one another. They must be thought of as located, as he says, behind a "veil of ignorance" (pp. 136ff.). This prevents them from knowing their particular natural advantages or disadvantages (their intelligence level, for example, or their physical attributes), their respective places in any existing social order, or even the particular ends and values they actually wish to pursue, what Rawls calls their "plan of life." Finally, the veil of ignorance deprives them of the knowledge of those special features which distinguish their society from others, for example its pattern of income distribution or its relative stage of social and economic advance. They are permitted, however, to know true general facts about the human condition and natural and social laws.

The purpose of this elaborate fiction is to insure that strict impartiality rules in the choice of basic moral principles. The idea that moral rules are impartially chosen is not new to Rawls. Impartiality has been sought after by other moral devices such as the utilitarian idea that principles are selected by an impartial "sympathetic spectator" of the human condition.[4] But there are two reasons why the idea of the original position assists our moral reasoning. First, because it prevents the procedure designed to produce impartiality from completely effacing the important distinction between persons. Though they are stripped of the knowledge of their particularities, members of the original position can still defend their most vital human interests. This accords more with our conception of how moral principles should be produced, Rawls argues, than do some procedures associated with alternative theories, especially utilitarianism, whose "greatest happiness" principle focuses only on the social order as a whole. Second, the device of the original position assists our thinking by remarkably simplifying the moral choice process. It does this by converting moral choice into the simpler procedure of rational prudence. This means that to determine the principles of social justice, we need not engage in the complicated, opaque, and frequently unfruitful process of weighing one moral intuition against another or one common sense moral rule against other, possibly conflicting, rules. We need only ask, What principles would I as a rational agent in the original position find advantageous to myself? Because of the constraints that this situation imposes on our choice, the results of this prudential deliberation will be acceptable moral principles. Thus, while few of us are skilled in making complicated moral judgments, we are quite good at making individual rational choices, and contract theory seeks to exploit this fact.

From his discussion of the original position, Rawls moves on to the actual choice by contract parties of principles of social justice. These are understood to be enduring principles regulating the major political, social and economic arrangements of a society (pp. 7-11, 54, 64). A theory of justice must concern itself with this basic structure, Rawls argues, and not particular allocations of bundles of goods. This is so because the basic structure itself shapes all of our subsequent decisions and actions. Indeed, unless the priority Rawls gives to principles for the basic structure is kept in mind, his theory can be easily misunderstood. As he makes clear, principles suitable for individual allocations may not be suitable for the long-term functioning of a society's major institutions, and vice versa. Thus, while it is frequently rational to distribute goods on the basis of need (blood plasma on a battlefield), this same principle of distribution may prove inadequate as the sole basis for distributing income in a complex modern economy.

It may be thought that the veil of ignorance rules out the choice of social principles by the contract parties. How, after all, can they select principles advantageous to themselves when they do not know which ends are their own? Rawls responds to this difficulty with the concept of primary goods or values that are of instrumental use to virtually any plan of life. These include the natural and social primary goods mentioned earlier. Thus, the choice of principles of justice comes down to this: from the vantage point of the original position, each contractor selects those principles governing the basic structure that are likely to maximize his own share of the social primary goods, subject to the efforts of others to do the same and the obstacles presented by natural or social circumstances.

As might be suspected, Rawls's final principles are strongly egalitarian. Since the members of the original position are rendered fundamentally similar to one another, and since they are each interested in protecting and furthering their most vital interests, the outcome of the unanimous choice process are principles equally protecting the vital interests of everyone. To put this in a slightly more complicated way, the final principles represent a "maximin" choice by each contractor. Since each is zealously protective of his most important interests in this situation of uncertainty, he selects only those rules whose potential worst outcome for him in real life is as least damaging as possible (a maximum minimum; hence, "maximin").

Rawls concedes that a maximin procedure is not always the most rational one for choice under uncertainty. But it tends to become so, he maintains, when certain conditions obtain: when knowledge of the probabilities of various outcomes is limited, when the prospects of gain are not terribly enticing, and when the possibility of losing is intolerable (pp. 153-55). Now in Rawls's view, all of these conditions obtain for the choice in the original position of the basic and enduring principles of social justice. This is especially true, he argues, where the fundamental liberties of citizenship are concerned. These include the liberty to participate in the political process, liberty of speech and conscience, and the various liberties of person such as the freedom from arbitrary arrest and seizure (p. 61). These liberties are so important to many different life plans, Rawls maintains, that even a slight diminution or relative loss of them is a severe threat to the individual. Thus, within the original position, where the chances of winning or losing a greater share are unknown, a maximin choice becomes rational. In this case, a maximum minimum is secured by granting the most extensive equal share of these liberties to everyone.

Rawls's argument with respect to economic distribution is basically the same, but the outcome is less immediately egalitarian. The reason for this is that the contractors are presumed to know true basic facts about economic systems: they know, for example, that human beings naturally differ in their productive abilities and that economic systems can sometimes be made more efficient by employing various incentives (additional material goods or authority) to elicit the exercise of desired talents and abilities. By permitting unequal shares, therefore, the contract parties can insure a more productive society overall. But, of course, these parties are not primarily interested in society "overall." A higher level of total or average well-being does not interest them as it does the utilitarian with his "greatest happiness" principle. What each contractor wants to know is that his prospects in the worst possible representative position (say that of the unskilled worker or someone in the group with less than median income) are as high as possible. Ruled by this logic, the contractors might initially shrink away from permitting inequalities with the consequent loss of efficiency. But they need not do this, Rawls maintains. Instead, they can accept what he calls the "difference principle" (pp. 75-83, 100-108). This would permit inequalities in income, wealth, or authority only when these clearly work out, in a reasonable period of time, to the advantage of the least-favored representative groups and where the more privileged positions and offices are kept open on a fair basis to all. In other words, efficiency is both desirable and permissible but only when it advantages everyone, in the strictest sense of this term.

Rawls recognizes that inequalities can jeopardize those at the bottom of the income ladder. Though he refuses to define the hypothetical contractors as envious (because envy is an irrational and self-destructive propensity), he concedes that the important social primary good of self-respect can be affected by inequalities in income or authority (p. 546). Since they ordinarily lack many natural talents and abilities, those likely to end up at the bottom of the social order are already shaky in their self-respect: they lack a sense of the worth of their life plans and the confidence needed to fulfill them. Adding income differences to these differences in natural abilities only compounds the problem. But rather than scrap the difference principle and the efficiency it implies, Rawls believes that the contract parties can take various steps to preserve their self-respect. They can insist, for example, that equality of opportunity be implemented by various social measures so as to minimize the effect of class background on one's prospects for achievement. But the most important way contract parties can buttress their self-respect is to insist on the "lexical" priority over the difference principle of the principle guaranteeing the basic equal liberties of citizenship (pp. 243-50; 541-48). This means that these liberties would have to be insured before inequalities in income were allowed, and it also means that these liberties could not be traded off or made a function of income in any way. Apart from the difference principle, probably no aspect of Rawls's theory has been more controverted than this priority rule.[5] Nevertheless, the force of his view lies in the great importance the basic liberties have for rational agents. This priority is further strengthened by rational agents' unwillingness to permit the more problematically acceptable inequalities allowed by the difference principle to erode the self-respect of the least advantaged group.

Though I have certainly omitted many items needed both to understand fully or criticize Rawls's view, the intuitive sense of his position is clear enough, I hope, to permit its application now to the matter of health care. The immediate task is to follow the deliberations of members of the original position on this subject, or what is the same, to ask which principles I or any rational agent so placed would agree upon where health care is concerned.

Four very general questions would likely confront contract parties as they consider the matter of health care. First, there is the question of how important health services are to rational agents. Should they be considered a primary good (a value all rational agents would want, whatever their other values); and if so, how do they compare with other primary goods like liberty and income? Second, assuming health services to be a scarce good in most societies, how would rational agents want them to be distributed? Should equality prevail, for example, or should some privileged form of access be allowed? Third, there is the question of how extensive the health care services of a society should be, and what priorities a society should establish between health and other socially desirable objectives. This is not the general question of the relative place of health among the primary goods, but the more complicated one of how far a general priority should be carried out. Finally, there is the question of what mechanism, if any, it is rational to select for the implementation of a desired distribution. Should health care be distributed by the free market, by rationing, or by some other procedure? Obviously, these questions and their answers interpenetrate one another. But I shall try roughly to consider them in this same order.

On a very general level the first question permits a ready answer. Access to health care is not only a social primary good, in Rawls's sense of the term, but possibly one of the most important such goods. I have already indicated the central place Rawls believes contract parties would give to the civil liberties. But certainly the same can be said for health care. Even more apparently than governmental interference, disease and ill health interfere with our happiness and undermine our self-confidence and self-respect. Indeed, some who have disputed the priority that Rawls gives to the civil liberties have done so precisely because they believe that other values, especially physical well-being and security, are to be rationally preferred.[6] Fortunately, we do not have to enter this dispute, because conflicts between the civil liberties and health care are not so common as to force a relative evaluation of the two here. But there seems to be little question that in the priorities of rational agents health care stands near to the basic liberties themselves.

The very important place given health care in the prudential deliberations of contract parties has several important implications for the choice of a distributive principle. First, it appears to rule out any utilitarian distribution of this good whether to produce a highest total or highest average level of health care services. We can assume that rational agents in the original position are not primarily interested in aggregates of this sort, but would instead employ cautious maximin reasoning to secure the highest minimal level of health care for themselves and their loved ones.[7] Similarly, their reasoning would rule out any distribution on the basis of desert or merit, for the constraints of the original position rule out agreement on the meritorious qualities a person must possess to be worthy of preferential treatment in a matter as vital as this. As a result, we can expect the parties finally to opt for a principle of equal access to health care: each member of society, whatever his position or background, would be guaranteed an equal right to the most extensive health services the society allows.

This equal right would extend, presumably, only to equal access to health services. It would not signify an equal distribution of health care attention (for example, the same number of hours of medical care each year for everyone). The interests of the contract parties indicate the meaning of "equality" in its various employments. In this case, since the parties are primarily interested in securing services as they need them, equality extends only to access to the health care system. Within the system care would be distributed on the basis of need or in keeping with whatever other principles impartial rational agents consider appropriate.[8] The social-contract approach thus simplifies a problem that has bothered some writers at this point: how we are to make interpersonal comparisons of individual health care needs.[9] The difficulty is occasioned by the fact that, apart from objective differences in health, some persons experience a greater subjective need for health care than others. Should this be a basis for differing distributions of care? Contract theory bypasses this problem, both because it is not concerned with maximizing some social total of well-being (for which interpersonal comparisons are necessary), and because its focus is not on case to case allocations but on the basic structure of society. As far as this basic structure is concerned, the idea of equal access will suffice. To a large degree we can assume that the problem of differing subjective needs can be handled by professional judgments within the health care system.

An important further implication of contract reasoning at this point is that it would seem to rule out direct income-based distributions of health care. This follows from the value health care has in the plans of rational agents, and from their unwillingness to accept a less-than-equal share for any but the most important reasons. It is true that contract parties may sometimes accept a lesser share of a vital good in order better to secure this good in the future. Thus, during a just defensive war they forego some liberty through conscription in order to preserve their liberties (pp. 303, 380). And they might similarly be prepared to sacrifice some equal access to health care in order to secure such care more firmly in the future. (Permitting physicians to be innoculated first during a plague may be an example.) But they would not permit the tolerated inequalities in a less important good like income to affect their vital equal access to health care. That would allow the tail to wag the dog. Just as they insist on the priority of the basic liberties over the difference principle, in other words, contract parties could be expected to separate access to health care from income considerations. In this respect contract reasoning gives independent rational support to the assertion, common today, that health care is a basic right of all persons regardless of income.

The idea of equal access to health care has more ramifications and complexities than I can touch on here. Other questions come to mind. Should this right be affected, for example, by one's geographical location?[10] Should the health care "illiteracy" of certain classes and groups be allowed to compromise the exercise of their right of equal access?[11] In each case, I think, the cautious, self-protective reasoning of the contract parties behind the veil of ignorance furnishes a negative answer. Similar reasoning can also guide answers to the many specific questions that a right of equal access must raise.

The question of just how much of a society's productive energy and resources must go into health care poses a particularly difficult set of problems. In general, we have seen, rational agents would consider health care, like liberty, a more important good than income. But this general preference for health care must at some point be qualified, even more so than is the case with liberty. As many writers have noted, provision of the "best possible" health care is an unreachable goal whose pursuit can absorb all the resources of even the richest society. A right to health care, then, cannot be affirmed like other fundamental rights and liberties. It must eventually be defined in terms of its permissible claim on other resources, particularly those handled by the economic system. Very bluntly, the question is, How much should society spend on health?

It may be, as some have argued, that this question cannot be answered in any general sort of way, and that efforts to do so are "totalitarian."[1,2] Alternatively, it may be contended that this matter is best left to the discretion of legislators within particular societies and should not be handled in terms of general moral principles. But if either of these conclusions is morally acceptable then it would have to be shown that rational agents in the original position would choose either to neglect this issue themselves or leave their future health care prospects up to the whim of majority decision; and neither of these alternatives seems immediately acceptable. The members of the original position as the architects of the basic social system would certainly want to set some upper and lower limits on the availability of health services. They know, of course, that they cannot achieve utter precision in this endeavor, but they have a vital interest in the effort to do so. Furthermore, they are aware that they do not have to be absolutely rigid in their specifications. Since they are permitted to know that societies develop economically over time, they can make their health care principles flexible, as they do in the matter of savings (p. 287). This would allow an adaptation to altered circumstances even as it insured a measure of moral regulation.

Consider, for example, the lower stages of social and economic advance—those typically exhibited in our day by the underdeveloped societies. To neglect the issue of health care's priority at this stage is frequently to allow the health care industry to take a back seat to other social needs, especially economic development. Indeed, some would argue that this is the rational and moral thing to do. Since health care and many other activities require economic support, they ask, why not postpone consumption in this and other goods in order to allow the economy to develop? If many members of several generations suffer ill health, they argue, that will be more than offset by the rapid achievement of economic development and the better health of future generations.

Would contract parties accept this reasoning? It seems not. For one thing, the anti-utilitarian thrust of their thinking extends even to inter-generational issues and prevents, where possible, the sacrifice of any one generation's welfare for the sake of others (p. 286f.). Thus, while investment in health care during the early stages of economic growth may not be allowed to block economic development entirely, neither would such investment be prohibited or given low priority. Each generation, even the first, has an important interest in health. Indeed, there might be good reasons why contract parties would wish at these very early stages of development to give health a very high priority among social investments. We can understand this better if we keep in mind the fact that a savings process must always to some degree disadvantage the earliest generations. They can afford to save the least but must be asked proportionately to save the most, and they receive few immediate rewards for their sacrifices.[13] Health care may be a way of cutting this particular Gordian knot. For one thing, health investment certainly advantages the earliest generations, since even modest improvements in care at these earliest stages produce vast benefits. For another, at these stages health care can have an important effect on productivity by improving the numbers and quality of the labor force.[14] Finally, health care can be a key aspect of programs aimed at reducing the savings-consuming high birth rates of the less-developed societies. As a number of demographers have noted, the persistently high childhood mortality rates of the poorer nations continue to provide a major incentive for numerous offspring. Moreover, these incentives have remained relatively unaffected by mass public health measures. By generally lowering mortality rates, these measures have boosted population growth, but without really giving families any more security that all their children will survive. Despite rising population levels very many couples still aim to have large families. Lowering mortality on a family-to-family basis, therefore, by providing adequate personal health care, can, when supplemented by other measures, help to reduce population growth.[15] As such, health care would be a form of investment likely to receive significant attention from members of the original position.

How much attention? Enough, one might say, to insure that basic preventative and therapeutic services are rapidly brought within the reach of every member of society. Universal basic health care is the desirable goal at this stage. Less desirable, and perhaps actually to be prohibited, are expensive care of the highest quality and costly, esoteric medical research. At this stage such expenditures only distract from the goal of universal basic health care, as well as other health-related goals such as the development of food production and transportation. Among the less-developed societies, it is mainland China that has probably come closest in our day to implementing a program of this sort, even down to the priority placed within the health care system on patient care as against research.[16] This suggests that these priorities are as workable as they are desirable.

How would members of the original position choose to alter these priorities as a society developed economically? For one thing, it would seem rational as development proceeds to go beyond the provision of basic care to more intensive preventative programs, more sophisticated therapies, and more esoteric medical research. Maximin reasoning counsels protecting oneself as much as possible against ill health, whatever its cause. It goes without saying that improvements in quality at these higher stages cannot be made a grounds for departures from equality of access. That would represent an inversion of priorities.[17] At these stages, however, the problem of limitless expenditures poses itself anew. Given the sophisticated development of medical technology, there are virtually no limits to what can be spent to preserve individual life and health. To take a bizarre example, where costly research and therapies fail, cryogenic techniques might be used, whatever the cost, to keep the body intact for future revivication. Since each member of the original position seeks to protect his most vital interests, why should he not insist upon such expenditures as soon as the resources become available? And why not do this even if it absorbs all the income that could be devoted, above the level of bare necessities, to making life more satisfying and fruitful? As Arrow points out, a strict maximin solution to this problem could easily lead to the choice of medical procedures so costly as to reduce society to the subsistence level.[18]

Offhand, the logic of contract reasoning does not produce an unequivocal repudiation of such a priority. Indeed, the citizens of many industrialized countries whose economies are marked by abundant consumer goods and luxuries, but often less-than-extensive health services, may have adopted a policy they could not impartially or rationally advocate. Perhaps this is why when some are denied access to scarce dialysis machines, many decry the priorities that would place gadgets for the many over the lives of a few. Still, there are good reasons for not devoting all of the output of an economy above survival to health care. For one thing, economies are complicated mechanisms and developments in one area frequently produce benefits in another. Who would have believed, for example, that a device developed to produce cheaper telephones (the laser) would lead to a superior therapy for glaucoma? Thus, rational agents have good reasons on health care grounds alone to allow the modest development of many of the normal activities of an economy.

Added to this is the common sense consideration that health is thought to be a state of mental, physical and social well-being and not merely freedom from disease. As such, a healthy existence presumably includes various opportunities for the desired exercise of many human capacities and excellences. In contract terms, we can say that the members of the original position have very good reasons for not settling for a society whose members are free from physical disability but who otherwise live at a level of economic austerity. Thus it is rational for them here to qualify their maximin logic and sacrifice some health care to economic considerations. Just where they would draw the line is hard to say, but a reasonable test may be available. Since contract parties select principles in the original position that they would be prepared to live with in any representative social position, the test of any actual choice made concerning degrees of health care or research is whether those who fall ill would regret the social decisions that rendered the therapy for their condition unavailable. This test is not perhaps totally adequate. It breaks down where the very young are concerned, since they cannot be expected to have availed themselves of the opportunities opened up by the decisions that jeopardize them. But then, this may also mean that we should be cautious about decisions limiting young peoples' access to the most extensive health care services.

If it is true that social decisions limiting health care can sometimes be morally acceptable, this would seem to be the case only in a society whose basic structure otherwise conformed to the principles of social justice. No rational individual, after all, would agree to expose himself to grave health risks without at the same time requiring that the benefits produced by these risks be distributed in ways that he can accept. Though obvious, this awareness has sometimes been lacking in discussions of how scarce life-saving therapies should be allocated.[19] Claims of various contenders have been weighed by several common-sense rules without asking how the larger social context affects the moral acceptability of the final allocation. For example, where "social contribution" has been made a criterion for receiving scarce therapy, the questions of whether all candidates have had a fair, equal opportunity to make such a contribution, or whether all have really benefited from the contributions of others, have typically been ignored.[20] Here again, contract theory's prior attention to the society's basic structure reveals its moral importance.

The imprecision of any general effort to determine just how much of a society's resources should be devoted to health care leads to the final major question before contract parties: whether particular mechanisms for implementing health care policy might be agreed upon by members of the original position. Specifically, it might be asked whether there are not acceptable mechanisms of social choice that can help reduce reliance on a priori decisions by contract parties and that can allow real members of actual societies to establish their priorities in ways that all can accept. The principle possibility here is use of the free market mechanism, the advantage of the market being that it allows each individual or family to establish priorities between health care and other goods. Among the other advantages of this approach are facilitation of consumer choice in the "style" of health care delivery,[21] and the possible encouragement of both quality and efficiency in the health care system. In the past, it is true, consumer choice in this area has frequently worked against both quality and efficiency, and it may never be capable of promoting these objectives.[22] But a free market in medical care, in conjunction with such devices as health maintenance organizations financed on a per capita basis, have been thought by some to hold out encouraging prospects in this direction.[23]

The major objection to reliance on the free market is that it seems to reintroduce the income-based distribution of health care already repudiated by the contract parties. But this objection need not be decisive. Through the device of progressive rates on health care (or health insurance and its requisite copayments and deductibles), the goal of equal access can be preserved. Of course, in practice the stipulation and maintenance of just progressive rates may prove impossible, as it has in many other areas, and this would seriously undermine the acceptability of this method. Still, it is at least theoretically possible to proceed in this way.

Assuming truly progressive rates, the free market in health care would function as an instance of "pure procedural justice" on a parallel with Rawls's hope for the economic system as a whole (pp. 86f., 201). Once properly set up, in other words, the health care industry could operate in a morally acceptable way without the need for constant moral and political regulation. This is desirable in itself, but there are at least two respects (apart from the matter of setting rates) in which this mechanism could only be "quasi-pure" and would continue to require moral supervision through just political decisions. First, if what I have been saying about the rational importance of health care is correct, then a just society would be expected to have an extensive and well-trained corps of medical practitioners. It is the continuing responsibility of government to see that this is so. At the lower stages of economic development, this would probably require considerable direct governmental involvement in medical training and staffing. At higher stages, where the market mechanism could prevail, it would be the government's job to see that the supply of practitioners is not kept artificially low (or their wages artificially high) by monopolistic practices or by the political intervention of self-interested professional groups.[24] Presumably, in a just society a profession as socially important and as occupationally attractive as medicine would, even without especially high wages, attract competent personnel and be among the most heavily staffed. The government's job is to see that this is the case.

A second reason for assuming the continuing need for political intervention in this area has to do with the importance of collective decision where health is concerned. The matter of savings is an example. Left to themselves, members of any one generation might totally exhaust available resources on consumption, especially in an area as important as health care. Government's responsibility is to prevent this from happening, by establishing a just savings rate and deducting the funds for this prior to the distribution of income. But any savings decisions of this sort require judgments concerning which kinds of expenditures are morally permissible at a given stage, and these judgments must take into account moral principles stipulating permitted degrees of health care. Other instances where collective decision is needed could be cited. The point is that even the best-functioning health care system cannot totally eliminate the need for collective social choice. And whenever choice is made, if it is to be morally acceptable, it must conform to those broad principles established, in the first place, in the original position.

In attempting to sketch the outlines of the kind of health care policy I think would be generated by social-contract theory, I have had two important objectives: First, I have tried partly to fill what I believe to be a major gap in

Rawls's contract theory as it presently stands. Second, I have tried to show that the distinguishing aspects of this theory—the device of the original position, the identification of instances where maximin reasoning is appropriate, and the focus on the basic structure—all serve as sound and useful guides to our moral reasoning process. Many of the points I have made have already been emphasized by those using more traditional and intuitive moral approaches. But the aim of contract theory is partly to illuminate the more fundamental rational considerations that underlie our intuitive judgments. In tracing the reasoning of contract parties on this issue, I hope to have at least illustrated the usefulness of this method, and to have identified those basic points in rational deliberation about justice and health care where more focused future discussion and debate is in order.

Notes to Chapter Seven

1. Cambridge, Mass.: The Belknap Press of Harvard University Press, 1971. All further references to this book appear in parentheses in the text.

2. None of these brief mentions of health care appear in the index. They include the definition of health as a "natural primary good" (p. 62); the designation of innoculation procedures and health services as "public goods" in the special economic sense of that term (pp. 268, 270); and the brief, provocative, but unexpanded suggestion that the social minimum of a just society, those payments made to the least-favored groups, will include "special payments for sickness" (p. 275).

3. That mental health is a social primary good seems even clearer. For a criticism of Rawls's neglect of mental health see Vinit Haksar, "Autonomy, Justice and Contractarianism," *British Journal of Political Science*, III (1973), 496ff.

4. R.M. Hare notes this basic similarity between the original position and other procedures and concludes, wrongly I think, that this device makes no contribution to our moral reasoning. See his "Critical Study: Rawls's Theory of Justice—I," *Philosophical Quarterly*, XXIII (1973), 144-55.

5. For a good critical appraisal and qualified defense of this priority rule see Brian Barry, *The Liberal Theory of Justice* (Oxford: Clarendon Press, 1973), chapter 7.

6. See, for example, David Lyons and Michael Teitelman, "Symposium: *A Theory of Justice* by John Rawls," *Journal of Philosophy*, LXIX (1972), 535-57.

7. Assuming this minimal share to be above some low threshold where it acquires worth for rational agents. For a discussion of this threshold problem and maximin reasoning see Barry, chapter 9.

8. I mention need only as the foremost criterion of distribution within the system. Other common-sense rules may have their place. Thus, "desert" in some special, medically defined sense may properly affect in-system decisions or insurance rates (smokers possibly having to pay more). For a good discussion of this see Gene Outka, "Social Justice and Equal Access to Health Care," *Journal of Religious Ethics*, I (1974), 16f. The problem of allocating scarce therapy

poses problems that defy even common-sense analysis, however, and that require the more systematic approach that contract reasoning affords. For an application of contract reasoning to this issue, see James Childress, "Who Shall Live When Not All Can Live?" *Soundings*, LIII (1970), 350ff.

9. See, for example, Kenneth Arrow, "Some Ordinalist-Utilitarian Notes on Rawls's Theory of Justice," *Journal of Philosophy*, LXX (1973), 244.

10. The issue of health care and geographic location is treated at length by David Mechanic, "Problems in the Future Organization of Medical Practice," *Law and Contemporary Problems*, XXXV (1970), 239-45.

11. Low-income groups' failure to use medical services despite the elimination of financial barriers has been noted in Sweden. See Ronald Andersen et al., *Medical Care Use in Sweden and the United States* (Chicago: Center for Health Administration Studies, 1970), p. 133.

12. This seems to be the view of Paul Ramsey, *The Patient as Person: Exploration in Medical Ethics* (New Haven: Yale University Press, 1970), pp. 266-75.

13. Thus Alexander Herzen's observation that human development displays a kind of chronological unfairness. This is quoted by Isaiah Berlin in his introduction to Franco Venturi, *Roots of Revolution* (New York: Knopf, 1960), p. xx.

14. The great importance of health care and other forms of "human investment" in the development process has recently been noted by a number of development economists. For a review of these discussions, see Harvey Leibenstein, "The Impact of Population Growth on Economic Welfare—Nontraditional Elements," in National Academy of Sciences, *Rapid Population Growth* (Baltimore: Johns Hopkins Press, 1971), pp. 183ff.

15. See, for example, Howard Taylor, Jr. and Bernard Berelson, "Comprehensive Family Planning Services Based on Maternal/Child Health Services: A Feasibility Study for a World Program," *Studies in Family Planning*, II (February 1971), 21-54.

16. Ruth and Victor Sidel, "The Human Services in China," and Frank Riessman, "Postscript: The Politics of Human Service: China and the United States," *Social Policy*, II (1972), 25-34 and 35-39.

17. Here, perhaps, is the basis of a common criticism of the American health system. See, for example, Abraham Ribicoff, "The Healthiest Nation Myth," and John Knowles, "Where Doctors Fail," *Saturday Review*, LXXX (August 22, 1970), 18-20 and 21-23.

18. Arrow, 251.

19. Thus, the extensive discussion of this problem by Nicholas Rescher entirely omits to consider this issue. See his "The Allocation of Exotic Medical Lifesaving Therapy," *Ethics*, LXXIX (1969).

20. See for example the account of the deliberations of the Seattle Artificial Kidney Center's selection process in Ramsey, pp. 245ff.

21. Whether the medical system should preserve personal contact with a physician or whether clinically based care is to be preferred is not, I think, a matter of social justice so much as it is a part of one's social ideal. But the preservation of choice here is desirable. For a discussion of this matter see Michael Halberstam, "Liberal Thought, Radical Theory and Medical Practice," *New England Journal of Medicine*, CCLXXXIV (1971), 1180-84.

22. Kenneth Arrow points out that the consumer has the dual characteristic of being ignorant about medicine and loathing to take risks about his health. These characteristics make for poor consumer decision in this area. See his "Uncertainty and the Welfare Economics of Medical Care," *American Economic Review*, LIII (1963), 941. R.M. Titmuss argues that this problem has been exacerbated by the rapid disappearance of the general practitioner with his traditional role of patient-advocate. See his criticism of free market medicine in *Monopoly or Choice in Health Services?*, Occasional Paper Number 3 of the Institute of Economic Affairs (London, 1964).

23. Clark Havighurst, "Health Maintenance Organizations and the Market for Health Services," *Law and Contemporary Problems*, XXXV (1970), 716-95.

24. For a penetrating critique of the American Medical Association's activities in this area see Reuben Kessel, "The A.M.A. and the Supply of Physicians," *Law and Contemporary Problems*, XXXV (1970), 267-83.

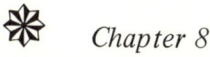 *Chapter 8*

What Is a "Just" Health Care Delivery?

Robert M. Veatch

Our problem begins when we realize that it would be obviously unjust for everyone to get an equal amount of health care services. This would be almost as unfair as the present distribution of health services. The problem becomes more complex if we realize that striving to maximize the usual indicators of the health of a people—average life expectancy, infant mortality rates, days of work lost because of illness—would possibly be even more unjust.

Many of the crucial contemporary questions in health policy planning are distributive. How do we allocate health care? Who gets the scarce intensive-care-unit beds or dialysis machines? Why should hemodialysis care be paid for by the federal government, but not cancer care? Who should pay for the coming national health insurance? And which diseases ought to be covered?

Traditional medical ethics is remarkably unhelpful in dealing with these problems. Physician ethics emerging out of the Hippocratic tradition tell us that the physician's duty is to do what he thinks will help his patient.[1] Taken seriously, this means that the physician has no duty to serve the health needs of the physicianless. In fact, put positively, he has a duty to ignore their needs. Furthermore, since this professional ethic focuses on the individual, isolated patient (in the singular), there is not even any guidance in deciding how a physician ought to allocate attention among his patients. What is desperately needed in order to make health policy is a theory of justice—a theory of distribution—for health care delivery. Beginning the construction of such a theory is my purpose.

128 Ethics and Health Policy

THEORIES OF JUSTICE IN HEALTH CARE

Let me begin the construction of a theory of justice for health care with the slogan "the right to health."[a] Converted to a principle of justice we might rephrase this slogan into the principle that (1) justice requires that everyone get the resources needed to be healthy. It is obvious, however, that healthiness is something society cannot deliver. It is strange, or at least impractical, for crucial public policy decisions to be based on a principle that is clearly impossible to fulfill or even approach. We might modify this to (2) justice requires that everyone get equal health care resources. The unusually healthy pose a problem, however. According to this principle either the sickly can get no more health care than the healthy would reasonably use, or the healthy should have extra health care forced upon them so that the sickly can consume an equal amount. The principle can be modified to (3) justice requires that everyone have access to an equal maximum amount of health care. This, however, means that the senile individual with metastatic cancer who has been relatively healthy throughout his life but now has completed most of his life's course has a greater claim on medical resources than the young, vigorous president of a nation who happens to have had a sickly youth. It also implies that the impoverished miner who, through economic circumstances and ignorance, has developed black lung disease has no more claim than someone who develops carcinoma of the lung through heavy smoking willfully and with knowledge that this choice would lead to increased risk of the disease.

Health Goods to be Distributed

The policy debate is made complex by the fact that there are two things varying simultaneously: the thing being distributed and the mode of distribution. We speak of distributing a long list of health related goods:

health
health care
opportunities for health
opportunities for health care
cost of paying for health care
burden for paying for health care
total goods including health

---

[a]Since the Greeks justice has always had two different meanings. Aristotle made the distinction sharply. He argues that, on the one hand, justice is complete virtue or excellence in relation to our fellow men (*Nichomachean Ethics*, Book V, Chapter I). He also recognizes, however, that justice can be used to mean a part of virtue. For Aristotle this narrower meaning referred to proper proportionality or fairness in distribution (Book V, Chapters II-III). On the one hand we say something is just when it is morally right; on the other, when it is morally right looking solely at the fairness of the distribution. This chapter will focus on justice in the latter, narrower sense.

votes for setting health policy
treatments for specific diseases

The list could go on. What makes the policy task tough is the fact that distributing one of these goods one way will be identical with distributing another one some other way. Distributing health equally will mean distributing treatments for specific diseases roughly in proportion to the presence of the disease. Distributing costs for health care equally will distribute the burden very unequally. Thus, any abstract argument about distribution principles in health care without pinning down precisely what is being distributed will be fruitless. However, I want first to catalogue the bases of distribution from which we may choose.

Ways in Which Health Goods May Be Distributed

What are the possible ways goods might be distributed? The list of candidates seems endless. Historically there have been advocates for distributing on the bases of ability, need, merit, previous injustices, and many others. In an effort to impose some system on the candidates I will identify ten of the most important ones. After mentioning two I will turn to three dichotomous variables that seem relevant to claims about just distribution. When crossed these give rise to eight candidates.

Flat equality. Some health-related goods seem justly distributed when every human gets the same amount. Votes on the community hospital advisory board would probably be an example. Some health insurance plans have a flat maximum of, say, $50,000 in benefits per policy.

In proportion to some objectively measured entity. Some goods are thought fairly allocated in direct proportion to something that can be objectively measured. Drug dosages are normally fairly allocated in proportion to body weight (but obese individuals may not have a full claim in the face of extreme drug shortage). Votes among stockholders in a privately owned hospital are normally presumed fairly distributed in proportion to the number of shares of stock owned.

In addition three dichotomous variables generate eight more claims for a fair distribution. First, we can distinguish more objective phenomena such as need and ability from more subjective claims such as desire or effort. Second, we can distinguish assets (virtues or talents) from liabilities (deprivations or harms). Ability and effort are assets, while need or desire are both deprivations. Third, we can classify claims on the basis of whether they make reference to the individual dimensions (such as effort or need) or to social dimensions (such as usefulness to society or previous social harm). It is clear that willingness to serve society (which is individual in its reference) is not the same as usefulness to society (which is socially referential). Thus there are at least eight additional bases of distribution:

Need. Health care and treatments for specific diseases might be justly distributed on this basis. Whether this is so I will leave to later argument.

Desire. The subjective correlate of need is desire. While few things are thought fairly distributed solely on the basis of desire, alternative medical treatments for a single disease might be. Likewise an individual's relative desire for health care and other nonhealth goods might be considered a just basis of governmental expenditure from an individual's share of the common resources. Pareto optimality depends among other things upon a sense that distributions based on desire are justified.

Usefulness. Usefulness to society is the social correlate of ability. A policy of preference in hemodialysis allocation to social leaders of heads of households would be built not on the individual ability of the patient, but the social value of that ability.

Willingness to Serve. Willingness to serve society is the subjective correlate of usefulness. We often feel compelled to praise or reward someone who tried to save a life or engage in a heroic military effort even though, through ineptness, he failed and was not "useful." (I recognize the qualification that the example of the inept one may itself be useful, and therefore shift the claim to real usefulness.)

Previous Social Harm. The objective, social deprivation of individuals and particularly social groups (such as blacks, chicanos, or women) through past social policies is a strong claim in health care delivery policy. Those who have been unjustifiably denied health care—particularly those who are now ill precisely *because* they have been denied previous health care—are claiming special priority for limited health resources. Whether these groups are fairly given priority over and above those equally ill but not sufferers of previous social harm forces a choice between this and the "needs" basis of a just distribution.

Feeling of previous social harm. This subjective, social deprivation basis of distribution completes the combinations of the variables. Feelings of past social harm, as opposed to real past social harm, seem to be of very limited value in accounting for perceptions of fair distribution in general and in the health area in particular. These last eight bases for distribution can be charted as in Figure 8-1.

In order to simplify the discussion, I shall focus on the distribution of only

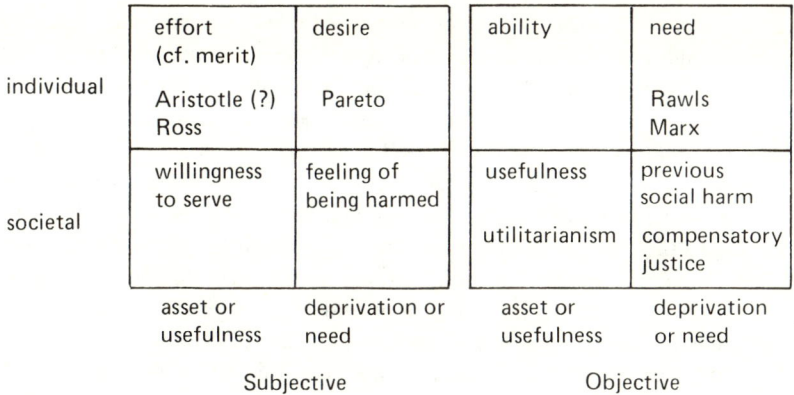

Figure 8-1. Bases of Distribution.

two things: opportunities for health care and the obligation to pay for health care (the obligation to provide funds for the national health insurance money pool). For this portion of the discussion I shall limit the bases of a just distribution to three major contemporary theories.

Major Theories of Distributing Health Care

All of these competing bases for distribution can, for purposes of policy analysis, be summarized in three major competing theories of justice. Each has been used to support some health care policy and implicitly some National Health Insurance proposals.

Utilitarian Theory of a Just Health Care Delivery. At first it seems reasonable to distribute health care so as to maximize the health of the society. The goal should be to improve the major social measures of health—infant mortality, average life expectancy, days of hospitalization, days of morbidity by disease—as much as possible. This is a health application of classical utilitarianism. According to the utilitarian position, the objective is to increase the net good in society to the greatest possible amount without regard to how that good is distributed except insofar as the distribution itself contributes to the total amount of good (through decreasing marginal utility or decreasing social unrest).

While health planning—as seen in the practices of cost-benefit analysis, PPBS, and the social indicators movement—seems based squarely on utilitarian, good-maximizing premises, I am convinced they are mistaken. The argument that utilitarian theory cannot account for our sense of justice is an old one. Suppose that in some hypothetical society the National Health Planning Council was considering ways of improving the health of the nation's citizens. Suppose also that the professional staff for the council had gathered data and made computer projections and had reached the conclusion that one particular plan would most improve the aggregate health indicators for the nation. It was the case in this society that one small group could be identified as having multiple chronic diseases consuming huge amounts of health resources. These individuals tended to be lower class, of low intelligence, and often brain damaged, so that health instruction had little usefulness. The proposed plan is to identify this group, amounting to 0.1 percent of the population, and ban them from the health care delivery system. The computers indicated that even though this would lower life expectancy for this particular group, it would in aggregate increase not only average life expectancy, but also all the other measures of health.

A second part of the plan would be the identification of the healthiest 10 percent of the population. This group would be encouraged to double their reproduction. Since their contribution to the health statistics would increase, all of the averages would improve.

The utilitarian theory of a just health care delivery would support the plan. In fact, since the sickest in the population would soon die off, morbidity (as opposed to mortality) would be directly improved.

Now utilitarian members of the National Health Planning Council may object. They may point out that the harm of death is critical and must be added to the calculation of goods and harms. Nonhealth harms also might have to be taken into account, such as social malaise or rebellion of the relatives of the sickest ones. It is not logical, however, that the feelings of social guilt would be one such harm, because one would not or should not feel guilty about doing what morality requires. Put more cautiously, the utilitarian should feel even more guilty if he fails to exclude the sickest, because he is consciously choosing to avoid producing the greatest good for the greatest number. One cannot appeal to nonconsequentialist feelings of justice, since those are ruled out by definition in the theory being advocated.

These additional harms would indeed increase the burden of the professional staff of the council—provided they conceded that nonhealth harms could be traded off against health goods. (That is a controversial concession to be taken up later.) New computer projections, however, might add in these nonhealth harms.[2] It is conceivable that even after these are added in, the banning of the one in a thousand still turns out to be utility maximizing.

It is the conclusion of nonutilitarians—and I would include myself—that such an outcome would not in itself be sufficient to justify the plan. Furthermore, even if it were the case that adding in enough social harms would always reveal that those policies we find morally objectionable were also not utility maximizing, it does not follow that they are morally wrong because they are not utility maximizing. It could be that they are not utility maximizing because they are wrong (and therefore generate guilt, which is a disutility).

I am convinced the plan of banning the sick is wrong because it is unjust. I am much more convinced that it is wrong than I am convinced of its disutility. In fact, since utility calculations in an area as complex as health care are so intricate, we should always be very uncertain of our judgments—much more uncertain than we actually are—if we based them on the utilitarian theory of a just health care delivery.

The Egalitarian Theory of a Just Health Care Delivery. I propose as an alternative to utilitarianism an egalitarian theory of a just health care delivery. An egalitarian theory of justice is fundamentally opposed to calculating goods—health or otherwise—in the aggregate. It is based on the premise that, at least insofar as health goes, every human being has an equal claim. Since it is health care we are trying to distribute we can formulate the principle as follows: (4) Everyone has a claim to the amount of health care needed to provide a level of health equal to other persons' health.

This sounds much like the first principle (that justice requires that everyone get the resources needed to be healthy). In this form, however, it recognized that healthiness as a goal can generate infinite demands so the egalitarian dimension is made more explicit: those whose health is worst are entitled to enough health care to get them as healthy as others. We would target our efforts on the sickest.

This sounds very similar to the principle articulated by Bernard Williams: "Leaving aside preventative medicine, the proper ground of distribution of medical care is ill health: this is a necessary truth."[3] It is also built on a similar understanding of equality. Williams, in his exposition of the concept of equality, recognized, as we must, that there are obvious physical, intellectual, and genetic differences among humans. There are also differences in ascribed and achieved roles. Beyond this, however, there are fundamental equalities. Common to our humanity is our ability to suffer and feel pain, our desire for affection, and related psychophysiological qualities. Humans may even be unequal in these; however, at least the question is open to empirical testing. Beyond these is what Williams calls "desire for self-respect." Drawing in part on the Kantian maxim that humans are to be treated each as an end and never as a means, Williams argues that each human is "owed the effort of understanding, and that on achieving it, each man is to be (as it were) abstracted from certain conspicuous structures of inequality in which we find him."[4] There is something essential about humans independent of their social, economic, and intellectual condition. This essential quality is sufficient to generate a claim of equality of treatment—at least in certain fundamental ways. This quality (which must be something closely related to Williams's notion of a claim of respect) produces a strong egalitarian claim that cannot be refuted by empirical arguments pointing to the differences among humans in other less essential ways.

The present form of principle (4) also sounds rather similar to Outka's. Beginning with the formal principle that justice requires similar treatment for similar cases, Outka maintains that this leads to the substantive principle that access to health care should be equal for people with similar categories of illness.[5] However, he recognizes a fundamental problem with the formula of this type. To return to our fourth formula, if everyone has a claim to the amount of health care needed to provide a level of health equal to other persons' health, the system will collapse as soon as the person most in need of health care is in need because he has a condition that cannot be treated. If health care is distributed strictly in proportion with ill health, as Williams at least considers "a necessary truth," a group of the incurably sick who are the most ill must end up with *all* the medical resources. This is certainly inefficient. Furthermore, if they do not benefit from the commitment of resources, it is hard to see why it is just that they get those resources. Outka apparently recognized that and thus allows for discrimination according to categories of illness. In doing so, however, his formula of treating similar categories of illness similarly could justify the National Health Planning Council's scheme to ban the 0.1 percent with serious multiple illnesses. Similar cases are treated similarly, but the priority for the neediest can be lost.

A modification might be to recognize that the neediest have a just claim only when something fruitful can come from the resource commitment. Thus: (5) Everyone has a claim to the amount of health care needed to provide a level of health equal, insofar as possible, to other person's health. This principle still will have to be both clarified and modified, but that is the principle in its stark form.

Another qualification is to shift from the duty to actually produce equal health (as far as possible) to a duty to provide an opportunity of equal health. One should not be required to improve his health (if, for instance, he prefers to abjure exercise or proper diet), and justice does not demand that we impose health care or that we provide repeated treatments because an individual does not take advantage of treatments rendered. Thus: (6) Justice requires everyone has a claim to health care needed to provide an opportunity for a level of health equal, as far as possible, to other persons' health.

Two other qualifications may be necessary in the egalitarian principle—one correcting for merit and another correcting for previous social wrong. Both of these qualifications are discussed later in this chapter.

The Rawlsian Maximin Theory of a Just Health Care Delivery. The third major theory of justice is receiving a great deal of attention in contemporary policy analysis because of the provocative and exciting work of John Rawls.[6] In brief summary Rawls concludes that two distributional principles are required:

1. Each person is to have an equal right to the most extensive total system of equal liberties compatible with a similar system of liberty for all.

2. Social and economic inequalities are to be arranged so that they are both: (a) to the greatest benefit of the least advantaged, consistent with the just

savings principle, and (b) attached to offices and positions open to all under conditions of fair equality of opportunity.[7]

It is often now presumed that this set of distributional principles is the major competitor to the utilitarian societal-good-maximizing principle, and that it properly captures the sense of moral commitment to the least well off that I have attributed to egalitarianism. But that is not the case. The maximin principle is a hybrid principle of moral right in a social distributional context, not a principle of justice that withstands Rawls's own tests.

In order to choose among the three principles of justice there must be a test of justification. There are a number of standard tests—techniques sometimes called "metaethical theories." We might ask what God would approve, what an ideal observer would approve as morally required, what accords with personal or societal feelings or institutions, or what accords with the natural law. Rawls's own method is not precisely the one I would normally support,[8] but it produces conclusions generally consistent with my own ideas.

Rawls asks us to imagine a society of persons formulating rules for social practices. These individuals are self-interested, rational, have access to relevant scientific facts including knowledge of human psychological traits. One clearly counterfactual condition is added, that these individuals have no specific knowledge of their own place in the society, his class, social status, "his fortune in the distribution of natural assets and abilities, his intelligence and strength and the life."[9] They are under a "veil of ignorance." Rawls now asks us to formulate a theory of justice using the original position method as a test. Would such a group indeed accept Rawls's two principles as principles of justice, as Rawls claims?

I am persuaded they would not uniformly adopt them as practices considered most just or fair.[10] Consider a hypothetical test case. Suppose that total amount of primary goods could be quantified for purposes of comparison. Those in the original position are presented with two alternatives (health policies or policies from other areas). One (policy A) would provide every member of the society with 10,000 units of the good, while the second (policy B) would provide everyone with 11,000, except that one percent would receive 100,000. Presumably the incentive to the elite would produce breakthroughs that would trickle down.

Since policy B clearly is more beneficial to the least well off, according to Rawlsian principles it is more just. I am not convinced that people in the original position under the veil of ignorance would find B more just. In fact I do not even find it plausible to conclude that B is always more right. Some (but not necessarily all) reasonable people might choose A. The smaller the marginal increase to the least well off in comparison to the increase in goods to the elite, the less plausible is the Rawlsian formula of justice. The egalitarian theory of justice is one that finds equality of distribution per se a just-making characteristic.

If equality of distribution per se is a just-making characteristic (perhaps one that has to be qualified by consideration of merit or previous social harm), then the maximin formula is not a pure principle of justice at all, but rather a synthesis of both just-making and other right-making characteristics (such as utility maximizing). Rawls specifically acknowledges that he is using the term "justice" in the narrower sense. Justice "is not to be confused with the principles defining the other virtues, for the basic structure, and social arrangements generally, may be efficient or inefficient, liberal or illiberal, and many other things, as well as just or unjust."[11]

Suppose in a health crisis resulting from a hurricane three people are in equal need of health care but the rescue team can treat only one. One of the injured is a physician who, if treated first and well, will be able to treat the others, but only to the point of partial restoration of their health (because of the time that passes). I find it plausible to conclude that it is prudent and right to give the health care to the physician first, and that even the other injured parties would agree to the priority for the physician; but I am not prepared to say that is just or fair. Furthermore, the waiving of the claim to equal treatment by the other injured parties seems to have more weight as a justification than would say the maximin argument offered by the physician. In other words, the waiving of the claim to equal distribution in favor of the maximin distribution is more justified if it comes from the least well off themselves rather than other members of the society. This claim that the least well off have more right to waive the equal right to health care than the more well off do cannot, I believe, be accounted for by Rawlsian theory.

If that is the case the maximin principle may (under certain partially indeterminant conditions) lead to the most right social policy; it would not, however, be the most just. I would argue that often the maximin would not lead to the most right policy—especially in cases where the least well off would prefer equality.

A health policy that focuses on a distribution that will maximize aggregate health indicators or aggregate economic indicators is most suspect. One that focuses on maximizing the health of the least well off is far superior, but it too is questioned. Justice requires health care sufficient to provide an opportunity for a level of health equal, as far as possible, to the health of others, and requires equality as the ordering principle for funding of health care.

REMAINING SPECIAL PROBLEMS

At several points in the development of the egalitarian principle of health care delivery I have had to postpone consideration of particularly vexing problems. I want now to take up: (1) the conflict between the generally least well off and the medically least well off; (2) claims based on merit; (3) claims of compensatory justice; (4) the question of which diseases have priority; and (5) the conflict between justice and rightness in a health care policy.

The Least Well Off: Generally and Medically

The principle that justice requires that everyone has a claim to the amount of health care needed to provide an opportunity for a level of health equal, as far as possible, to the health of other persons produces a priority for health care for the sickest insofar as health care can improve their health, qualified by individual freedom to reject that health care if it is not desired. This forces us to deal with the question why the medically least well off ought to be the focus of our distribution principle rather than the generally least well off. This basis of distribution means that the very wealthy, but sick, have a greater claim to a part of the national resources than the very poor person who happens to be healthy. The principles of Pareto optimality would require that the good be given out in as general a form as possible. In this case we might give funds to the generally least well off permitting them to buy housing or food rather than health care if that were their particular need. Since the wealthy but sick individual is not least well off, the funds would, in this example, not be spent for health care at all. According to this approach desire would be one basis on which health care is distributed.[1,2]

This is a critical challenge to the claim that justice requires that health care be distributed so as to provide an opportunity to equalize the health of the medically least well off. The question is, Why should the wealthy, even the sick wealthy, be included in a health care program at all?

Two answers seem appropriate. First, it could be argued that health is a prior requirement for receipt of any other goods. Rawls has argued that liberty is such a good. One cannot trade off liberty for other goods, because liberty by its very nature is required for enjoyment of the others. Health is, in some ways, like liberty. Certainly death-preventing medical care is like liberty in this respect. However, other forms of health care are not always prior in this way. I think it is meaningful to say that one is generally well off or well off on balance though sick, while it is not meaningful to say that with regard to either death or lack of liberty. Thus it appears that some kinds of health care could receive an absolute priority, taking them out of the general calculation of goods, but by itself is not an altogether convincing argument for separating all health care allocation from the general allocation of goods.

Another argument is a more pragmatic one. While I am not convinced that all with a particular illness, in principle, have an equal claim to health care at government expense without regard to their general financial means, I am convinced that adopting a practice of behaving as if they *did* have an equal claim will serve the interests of the generally least well off as well as the medically least well off, and may promote equality as well. The test case is deciding whether two individuals equally sick, one of whom is poor, the other wealthy, ought to be given equal access to health care under a national health insurance program, or whether their general state ought to be taken as relevant in deciding about health care allocation.

Two arguments support the decision to give the two equal health care independent of how well off they are generally. First, to support the policy of giving funds to the generally least well off one has to be convinced that distribution of a more generalized medium (money) would really be the policy adopted as an alternative. There is strong reason to believe that that is not the case. It is dangerous to assume that if a national health program is not adopted the funds saved will be allocated so as to be more beneficial to the generally least well off. The generally least well off should take what they can get, even if it also benefits those who are not generally least well off. This is, of course, not necessarily an argument from egalitarian justice as we have defined it. If, however, giving equal health care to the poor and the rich added to the welfare of each, it would at least reduce the ratio of their relative welfare and might, if one assumed decreasing marginal utility, decrease the absolute difference. It would not, of course, be the policy that would most radically decrease the difference; giving health care only to the poor would decrease it even more. That policy might suffer from the same practical consideration as giving the more generalized medium only to the poor: it might simply never be adopted. This argument for giving equal opportunity for health to the rich and the poor is not a very strong one from the point of view of egalitarian justice.

The second argument for including the medically least well off who generally are better off is stronger. There is reason to believe that having the more wealthy included in the same health system as the poor directly benefits the health care given to the poor. There are at least two ways the poor might benefit from including the wealthy. First, some goods are what might be called social or collective goods. They are not readily divisible. Some practices count as good if, and only if, a critical mass of people participate in the practice. The good of voting or of not walking on the grass accrues only if a critical mass join in the practice. Not everyone need participate, but a large number must. Those who do not will be "free riders." Society can tolerate a certain number of these free riders, but when the critical threshold is crossed, it is not simply the free riders who lose, it is everyone. Some elements of a national health care program may be social or collective goods of this type. Support for health research, for complex equipment, and for highly specialized skilled workers requires a large base of support. If the mass of the middle class were excluded it is quite possible there would not be sufficient support for the social good to result.

This is not the only, or even the primary, way that the poor will benefit by the participation of the relatively wealthy in a national health care program. If those in powerful places must participate in the same health care system as those least well off, the quality of that system may improve not because it adds a critical mass, but because it adds a group with sufficient power to make sure that the care is of high quality and that the patient is treated with respect and dignity. Inclusion of the wealthy might not improve their health at all; it might, in fact, decrease it. An inclusive system, then, might improve the health opportunity of the least well off (improve it even more than if only the poor were included), while it would not improve and might even diminish health opportunity for the better off. The interesting implication of these arguments centering on benefit to the poor if the more wealthy are included is that those well off might have an obligation to participate in the national health care system, whereas if the basis for their inclusion was the general priority of health over other goods, there might be a right to participate, but hardly an obligation.

All arguments considered, a strong case can be made for the general rule of treating the distribution of health care as a phenomenon independent from the more general distribution of goods. The wealthy sick as well as the poor sick should be treated as if they had an equal claim on health care, independent of their general condition. This, of course, may not mean that the burden of paying for the health care would necessarily be the same for the two groups.

Merit

One historically significant qualifier of the egalitarian principle of distribution is merit. Merit (or some modification of it) can, in principle, be a legitimate qualifier to the egalitarian principle that everyone should have an equal claim to health care sufficient to provide an opportunity to achieve a level of health equal, as far as possible, to other persons'. Consider two individuals (say identical twins) who have had equal genetic and environmental opportunities. Both open small grocery stores, but one works diligently, putting in a sixteen-hour day for twenty years, while the other is slothful, working short days and squandering his resources. It seems to me to be fair (or just) that the first brother has more accumulated goods at the end of the twenty years (even if the memories of experiences may possibly have been richer for the slothful brother).

In principle, justice requires taking into account effort or merit as a consideration of a fair or just distribution of health care. At the same time, I see the gravest danger in including effort or merit as a qualifier of a principle for just distribution of health care. ("Merit" is a confusing term because it seems to include not only the subjective component of effort, but also native abilities as well. "Diligence" or "effort" seems to me to generate the stronger claim.) It seems almost impossible to separate merit or effort from class privilege, inherited wealth and skills, and the social and value biases of those who would be doing the classifying. The error rate in ranking on the basis of effort or merit would seem to be extremely great. Furthermore, the enterprise of ranking individuals on the basis of merit or effort is itself potentially malicious and degrading. Qualifying the egalitarian distribution principle for merit or effort could be justified for some practices in some forms of social organization. However, we are talking about a national policy on the distribution of health care. The dangers appear so great that with one qualification, any such effort ought to be abandoned.

That one exception is the case of health need resulting from what is seen as a voluntary decision to take a health risk to engage in behavior that is not worthy of public subsidy, such as professional automobile racing, alcohol consumption, smoking, and recreational stunt flying. All are presumed to be voluntary behavior and are thus radically different from health needs as they are normally conceptualized. (If alcoholism were judged a nonvoluntary genetically or psychiatrically determined "disease" it would be excluded from the list.) Furthermore, all are generally not considered activities worthy of public subsidy. This separates them from professional fire fighting, which is voluntary behavior, but worthy of subsidy.

Even if these voluntary health-risky behaviors not worthy of public support are thought to generate a lower claim for just health care allocation, humaneness still requires including treatment for such conditions in a national health system. The source of funding for such care, however, might be radically different because of the nature of the medical condition. I have elsewhere supported the view that while all such conditions should be covered by national health insurance, the behaviors should be taxed, where possible, in an amount that would equal the projected costs of the medical treatment.[13]

Compensatory Justice

Another major problem with the general egalitarian principle that everyone has an equal claim to health care sufficient to provide an opportunity for a level of health equal, as far as possible, to the health of others is the claim of those who have suffered previous social wrongs that have previously deprived them of health care opportunities. The question is, Do we have a special obligation of justice to provide health care to those who are sick because of previous social wrongs over and above the obligation to distribute health care on the basis of equality for opportunities for health? Of course, those who have suffered significant social wrongs will often rank high solely on this criterion of need, but is there an additional claim for those whose need derives from previous social harms? In general there is. The duty to provide compensatory justice is a legitimate modifier of the general principle of egalitarian justice. I am not persuaded, however, that the compensatory justice qualifier ought to have significant bearing on the general egalitarian principle for purposes of health care distribution. The question is once again a pragmatic one. If we assume that health need alone will tend to identify those who have suffered previous social wrong, we must compare the justice resulting from the established preference for health care to the wronged group with the risks of singling that group out for an additional priority. I see a great danger in singling out any group for special health care on any basis other than ability to meet medical need. Creating a special class will once again create a two-class health system, with all of the risks involved. While compensatory justice is, in principle, an appropriate qualifier to the egalitarian principle of distribution, I am not convinced that it would add materially to the welfare of those who were previously wronged by society. I remain open for such evidence including expressions of opinions of the wronged groups and would readily incorporate a compensatory justice qualifier if such evidence were found. In this particular case, however, it seems prudent not to create a special health system with special priorities over and above the criteria related to health need.

Which Diseases Have Priority?

The thrust of the entire argument has been toward the position that priority go to the diseases or disease combinations that create the most hardship or suffering—to those which make one medically the least well off. The medically worst off have a complete claim of justice on health care resources in order to bring them, as far as possible, up to the level of health of others. This is strikingly different from the usual criteria of distribution in most of the national health insurance proposals, which for the most part focus heavily not on the nature of the diseases or medical conditions but on absolute limits on health care consumption in dollars or days or, in the case of catastrophic illness proposals, the size of the medical bill. These proposals will be examined in more detail in the next section.

The task of ranking diseases from worst to most benign is rather repulsive as well as gargantuan. Fortunately much of the ranking is unnecessary. We have the capacity to provide available health care necessary to improve the health, insofar as possible of the medically least well off. In fact we can probably work our way up the list of the worst diseases before the question of limits is even raised—if we approach the allocation of health care from this medical egalitarian perspective. Furthermore, we probably can agree on some medical conditions that impose (or ought to impose) so slight a burden that they should not be included in any national health program at this point in history. Alopecia (baldness), most cosmetic surgery, and personal attendance by a physician-traveling companion for general reasons of health safety are examples. The use of certain futuristic biomedical technologies for the satisfaction of medical tastes such as in vitro fertilization, prenatal sex selection, or electrical stimulation of the brain's "pleasure centers" might be others.

The real difficulties come in a fairly narrow range. We may not be sure whether patients claiming a need for hemodialysis, semiannual or annual physical examinations, nuclear-powered artificial hearts, dental prostheses, experimental treatments of the aging process, or psychoanalysis have the greatest medical need. If our task is to identify those most in need of health care we need not choose between penicillin for pneumonia and insulin for the diabetic. Certainly both qualify. Only when we get to the borders of our capacity to provide health care does the problem arise. Here the egalitarian claim is that, difficult though it may be, we must include those conditions which constitute the greatest assault on one's health—however that may be defined. The answer will clearly require an understanding of the human norms of healthiness, something requiring arduous philosophical reflection. This, however, is the appropriate task, rather than arbitrarily assigning dollar or day limits to the use of health care resources in a national program. To choose the latter is to distribute health in proportion to the luck of the natural and social lottery and according to our ability to buy health care in the private market.

Justice and Rightness in Health Care Delivery

The health care program that is most just is the one that will recognize a claim to health care necessary to provide an opportunity, as far as possible, to a level of health equal to others'. Before going on to look at national health insurance proposals in this light, I need to qualify the analysis with an explicit recognition that other ethical claims may require a modification of the claim of justice. The most obvious competing claims are those of efficiency. Coinsurance and deductibles included in many proposals seem to be incorporated as a means of reducing "unnecessary" use of health facilities. They may be efficient, but it is at the same time unjust. One disease that ranks very high as an assault to the normal health of a group of citizens may be within our capacity to treat, but only at a cost that would consume the health resources capable of treating a group hundreds of times as large, but less sick. Justice cannot be the only criterion for allocating health care, especially when the medically least well off prefer inequalities in order to promote their own medical welfare; efficiency and aggregate utility may have a legitimate place in the list of right-making characteristics. The dangers of appealing to such criteria as a means of overcoming the claims of justice are so serious, however, that such appeals must be minimized. This is a discussion of what makes health care *just*, not what makes it *right*.

JUSTICE IN NATIONAL HEALTH INSURANCE PROPOSALS INSURANCE PROPOSALS

Two different dimensions of the twenty-two proposals introduced into the 93rd Congress will be examined: how health care is distributed and how the costs of the funding pool are distributed.[14]

Health Care Distribution in National Health Proposals

Limits Based on Amount Paid. There are at least three basic kinds of limits on health care services possible in a national health policy. The first, health care in proportion to the amount one has paid into the system, has long been the distributional principle for private life insurance. A student of mine once advocated that national health insurance be limited to the healthy because it is unfair to add the sick to the same risk pool. Present Medicare has two levels of coverage, with those who pay an optional additional monthly premium getting a higher level of coverage. With these precedents, it is striking that, with one exception, none of the twenty-two proposals we have reviewed links benefits in any way with the amount one has paid. The one exception is the Nixon C.H.I.P. plan. It provides for optional better coverage at additional cost.

"Insurance" is really a misnomer for most of the health plans in the current dispute. Insurance is normally a device for sharing of risks where all entering the risk pool are a roughly similar risk (or those at greater risk are rated). If the objective is to distribute opportunities for health care so as to give every person an opportunity, as far as possible, to be as healthy as other people, limits on health care based on the amount one has paid in will be highly suspect. Presumably need for health care in order to be healthy is not very closely related to the amount one has paid into the insurance system, or to the ability to pay. It would seem preferable to include only one level of coverage in the basic national health program. If individuals want to buy insurance for coverage not included in that national health program, they might have that option, but it should be done through other channels based on actuarial pooling of risk.

Limits Based on Dollars or Days of Hospital Care. Of the twenty-two proposals introduced into the 93rd Congress fifteen place limits on the number of days or dollars of hospital care, normally without regard to how sick the patient is or how serious is his medical condition. Table 8-1 shows the day limits on hospital inpatient coverage, physician visits, nursing home care, and home health services listed in order of increasing hospital inpatient coverage. The Pell-Mondale proposal (S 2796) was the most restrictive. It limits utilization to twelve days per year for hospital inpatient care and ten days per year in a nursing home. However, it also includes a catastrophic coverage for cases when medical costs exceed 25 percent of annual gross income. The Railsback bill (HR 2618) provides thirty days per year of hospital inpatient care and eight visits per year for outpatient physician services. In addition there is a lifetime maximum limit of $50,000 on payments per person with a $2000 annual restoration. This, in effect, means that each person is entitled to one disaster per lifetime at government expense.

Proposals introduced by Dingell and by Staggers offer two months of hospital coverage. The Staggers proposal (the National Comprehensive Health Benefits Acts of 1973) also has limits of thirty days per benefit period for skilled nursing home facilities, and provides for a limit of fifty visits per year to a physician, one hundred visits per year for home health services, and one visit per year to a dentist. In addition other proposals have a basic limit of sixty days, but then switch to catastrophic coverage.

The Javits bill (S 915) would provide ninety days of inpatient hospital services per benefit period with a "lifetime reserve" of sixty additional days. In

Table 8-1. Day Limits of National Health Insurance Proposals, 93rd Congress

Chief Sponsors	Number	Hospital Inpatient Coverage	Physician Visits	Nursing Home	Home Health Services	Other
Pell-Mondale	S2796	12 days/yr	No limit	10 days/yr		Catastrophic coverage of medical costs which exceed 25% of annual gross income
Railsback 1. Family health insurance plan	HR2618	30 days/yr	8 visits/yr		Substitute 7 days for 1 day hospital in-patient care	Lifetime limit of $50,000 plus $2,000 annual restoration
2. Employer-employee plan		No limits	No limits			2-day deductible and 25% co-insurance
Dingell	HR33	60 days	No limit		No limit	Limit on unusually expensive drugs
Staggers	HR11345	60 days	50 visits/yr	60 days	100 visits/yr	30 days skilled nursing facility 1 dental exam/yr for children ages 7-12 drugs limited to specific conditions 1 pair eyeglasses/yr for children (to age 15) catastrophic coverage after noncovered expenses reach a specified limit
Javits	S915	90 days/benefit period		100 days/benefit period	100 days/benefit period	"lifetime reserve" of 60 additional days in hospital; 190 day lifetime limit in psychiatric hospitals

Burleson-McIntyre	HR5200 S1100	300 days/ illness*	No limit	180 days/ illness	270 days/ illness	
	*Note: Illnesses must be separated by 60 days to be considered different illnesses					
Fuqua						1 dental examination/year
Fulton-Broyhill-Hartice	HR2222 S444	300 days/ illness	No limit	180 days/ illness	270 days/ illness	
1. Basic		60 days	No limit	Can be substituted for hospital days on 2:1 basis	No limit	Dental care for children (through age 17)
2. Catastrophic coverage		No limit		Additional 30 days		
Ashbrook	HR288					
1. Basic coverage		60 days	No limit	Can be substituted for hospital days on 2:1 basis		
2. Catastrophic		No limit		Additional 30 days		
Ullman	HR1	90 days/ benefit period	10 visits/ yr	90 days	100 visits/ benefit period	30 days/benefit period skilled nursing facility; catastrophic coverage when noncovered limits reach a specified limit; 1 dental visit/yr for children 7-12; 1 set eyeglasses/yr for children to age 12
Mills-Schneebeli-Packwood	HR12684	No limit	No limit	100 days/ yr	100 visits/ yr	Dental care, eyeglasses and hearing aids for children under 13
Roy	HR13603	No limit	No limit	100 days/ yr	100 visits/ yr	Dental care, eyeglasses and hearing aids for children under 13

Table 8-1. (continued)

Chief Sponsors	Number	Hospital Inpatient Coverage	Physician Visits	Nursing Home	Home Health Services	Other
Griffiths-Kennedy	HR22, S3	No limit	No limit		No limit	120 days skilled nursing facilities per "spell of illness"
Mills-Kennedy	HR13870 S3286	No limit	No limit		100 visits/yr	100 days/yr post hospital extended care; eyeglasses, hearing aids and dental care for children under 13
Long-Ribicoff-Wagonner	HR14709 S2513					
1. Catastrophic plan		No limit	No limit		No limit	100 days skilled nursing facilities; 190 day lifetime limit in psychiatric hospitals
2. Medical assistance plan		60 days	No limit		No limit	No limit to skilled nursing facilities
Long-Stanton	HR8380 S1416					
1. Catastrophic plan		No limit	No limit		No limit	400 days skilled nursing facilities; 190 day limit in psychiatric hospitals
2. Medical assistance plan		60 days	No limit		No limit	No limits to skilled nursing facilities
Scott-Percy	S2756	No limit	No limit	No limit	No limit	Maximum of 60 days/yr with lifetime limit of 180 days in psychiatric hospital; dentists; for children under

Sponsor	Bill	Col1	Col2	Col3	Col4	Col5	Notes
Fannin	S3353	No limit	No limit				12, physical checkups; children under age 5; limit on drugs required for chronic illnesses
Lujan	HR15006	No limit	No limit	No limit			No dental care
Brock	S3670			No limit			No limit on extended care facility; Gives credit against personal income taxes if medical expenses exceed 15% annual gross income
Roe-Beall	HR1054 / S587	No limit	No limit	No limit			All services eligible as medical expense deductions under the income tax law covered after family medical expenses exceed a specific amount
Saylor	HR1916	No limit	No limit	No limit			Covers 90% of family health care costs after just $5,000 of expenses

addition there is a 190-day lifetime limit on stays in psychiatric hospitals. Limits for skilled nursing home facility services and home health visits are one hundred days per benefit period.

The Burleson-McIntyre bill (HR 5200, S 1100) which is supported by the Health Insurance Association of America, would introduce benefits gradually over a ten-year period, leading to a final plan that would provide three hundred days of hospital services per illness. (Illnesses must be separated by sixty days to be considered different illnesses.) There would also be a 180-day limit per illness on extended-care facilities, and 270 days for home health services. The Fuqua bill (HR 4349) would have benefits identical to the Burleson-McIntyre proposal.

The next group of proposals have no hospital inpatient care limits, but do place limits on other services. The Fulton-Broyhill-Hartke bill (S 444, HR 2222) is the Medicredit proposal sponsored by the American Medical Association. It has a limit of sixty days per year of hospital inpatient care, but added catastrophic benefits with unlimited additional hospital days. Nursing-home days can be substituted for hospital days on a 2 for 1 basis, but there is a limit of thirty additional days under the catastrophic illness coverage. The Ashbrook bill (HR 288) is similar, but excludes home health care and certain dental care services. Not surprisingly, the American Hospital Association's bill (introduced by Ullman as HR 1), provides generous hospital care. The limit is ninety days, but a catastrophic coverage plan pays hospital costs without limit once a specified limit is reached, which varies with family income and age. Both the Nixon administration's plan (the Comprehensive Health Insurance Act of 1974, HR 12684) and its major competitor supported by labor, the Griffiths-Kennedy "Health Security Act" (HR 22, S 3) provide no limit on hospital coverage. The administration proposal, however, places a limit of one hundred days per year on skilled nursing facilities and one hundred visits per year on home health services. The Griffiths-Kennedy plan places a limit of 120 days per "spell of illness" on skilled nursing facilities and forty-five consecutive days per spell of illness on psychiatric hospital inpatient care. The compromise Mills-Kennedy plan adopts the more conservative administration limits of one hundred days per year for skilled nursing facilities and one hundred visits per year for home health services.

The catastrophic coverage plans have no limits on hospital coverage (although they tend to have large deductibles, which will be discussed later). The Long-Ribicoff-Wagonner bill (S 2513, HR 14709) and the identical Long Stanton bill (S 1416, HR 8380), for instance, have no limits for general hospital coverage (after the first sixty days), but have a lifetime limit of 190 days for psychiatric hospitals. The Scott-Percy bill (S 2756) has a limit on psychiatric hospital care of sixty days per year and 180 days in a lifetime.

Finally there is a group of bills that place no limits at all. These include the proposals introduced by Fannin (S 3353), Lujan (HR 15006), Brock (S 3670), Roe-Beall (HR 1054, S 587), and Saylor (HR 1916). While the question of day and dollar limits is not addressed in these bills, quite possibly such limits would be included in the insurance policies or administrative regulations. The point of this survey is not to compare the merits of specific bills, for they will certainly be revised in future sessions of Congress; the point is to show that benefits can vary widely from very modest coverage (a few days a year with constricting lifetime limits) to practically limitless coverage.

From the point of view of a theory of justice the relevant question is, What principle of distribution stands behind these day and dollar limits? Apparently it is the notion that everyone is justly entitled to an equal maximum amount of health care per year. While at first that seems plausible, I have already discussed the obvious limitations. Upon reflection it seems difficult to defend the view that the sickest individuals are entitled to no more care than others in society, regardless of their need. If the goal is to produce greater equality of health, arbitrarily limiting the hospitalization coverage for the sickest probably will not achieve that goal.

Limits Excluding Medical Conditions. The third major method of limiting the benefits in a national health program is to exclude certain diseases or certain treatments. If the objective is to provide health care so that everyone has an opportunity to a level of health equal, as far as possible, to that of others, focusing on exclusions of marginal and trivial medical conditions would be extremely important. Nevertheless, very few of the current health insurance proposals discuss these limits. It seems most implausible that there will in fact be no limits. Someone at some point will eventually have to say No to requests for certain kinds of medical coverage. Thus, insurance proposals that ignore the question of limits are probably only postponing a critical element of a national health policy.

Among the bills we reviewed several kinds of exclusions were found. The Nixon Administration Comprehensive Health Insurance Program specifically excludes dental care, eyeglasses, and hearing aids except for children under thirteen. (Congressman Roy's proposal [HR 13603] follows the CHIP exclusions.) The Kennedy-Griffiths proposal (SR 22-23) excludes adult dental care, psychiatric care, nursing-home care, and some prescription drugs. The Long-Ribbicoff Proposal (S 2513) also excludes nursing-home care, dental care, and psychiatric care together with drugs. The proposal by Stanton and Long (HR 8380; S 1416) has the same exclusions. Even in these cases, however, the limits are described at a very high level of generality excluding such things as "dental care," "psychiatric care," "nursing home care." It seems that at least some dental and psychiatric and nursing home care might be required under our criteria of justice. At the same time many other kinds of care (hair transplants, in vitro fertilizations) may be excluded. Probably the decisions cannot be made using as gross a decision-making device as legislation. It would seem wise to establish a policy-making committee as part of any national health program to make these crucial value choices. It is important to realize that they are indeed value choices, deciding which medical conditions and medical treatment are sufficiently serious that they warrant public support. The alternative to a policy-making board will be case-by-case litigation in the courts.

Funding of National Health Insurance Proposals

The second point where a theory of justice is significant for national health proposals is in the funding. I have argued that health care should be distributed so as to give everyone an opportunity for a level of health equal, as far as possible, to the health of others, and that therefore general socioeconomic levels should not be relevant when it comes to providing the health care. Funding of health insurance is quite another matter, however. There are a number of ways of raising the money for the pool to pay for a national health care plan. Presumably the obligation to contribute funds to that pool should not be a function of how well off one is medically, but rather how well off one is more generally. General equality is the primary consideration of a just funding according to an egalitarian theory of justice. Thus it is critical to determine how progressive the funding is.

In rough terms we can divide the funding mechanisms into three groups: (1) those charging equal flat dollar amounts; (2) those charging amounts directly proportional to income; and (3) those where costs increase faster than income.

1. The least acceptable funding mechanism from the standpoint of egalitarian justice would be a system where everyone pays the same amount for his health coverage regardless of ability to pay. Several of the proposals sponsored by more conservative individuals and groups have this kind of a funding mechanism. (Here we are making the normal presumption that fringe benefits received from one's employer can be treated as equivalent to income to the employee. If compulsory employer contributions to a national health insurance funding pool resulted in the equivalent of real income increase to low income employees these comments would have to be modified.) The Nixon administration's CHIP Plan, the conservative Railsback Bill, the Chamber of Commerce's National Health Standards Act, and the Health Insurance Association's National Health Care Act would all charge flat dollar amounts—the most regressive of the funding mechanisms in the twenty-two proposals. Some of these also provide for special assistance for low-income groups, however. These provisions are mentioned below.

2. Funding mechanisms that require payment in direct proportion to income are limited to those that use a social-security type of payroll deduction. The Kennedy-Griffiths and the Javits Bills use a payroll deduction but have a cutoff point of $15,000. The Mills-Kennedy proposal has a cutoff of $20,000. Like the social-security deduction itself, this is in effect a relatively regressive taxation— first, because there is no graduation in the percentage as a function of income, and second, because after a cutoff point additional income creates no additional

responsibility to pay at all. An improvement from the standpoint of our theory of justice would be if a payroll tax is to be used to have no cutoff point, thus creating the same percentage of income contribution for the wealthy as for the poor. This of course would still not create as great a burden on the wealthy to pay for health care as it would for the poor. This gives rise to the more progressive proposals.

3. Funding of national health care out of general revenues is a method based on a more progressive tax. It distributes the burden the same way that the burden for raising general revenues is distributed. Some health insurance proposals, including some that are otherwise quite regressive, include provision for federal or state payment of premiums out of general revenues for the lowest income groups. The National Health Insurance Act and the Chamber of Commerce proposal are two examples. Others such as the Railsback proposal have a low-income provision with no fee for the lowest income groups and then a premium graduated according to income. The Lujan National Family Health Protection Act uses the progressive method of a 5 percent federal tax surcharge. This method of funding National Health Insurance takes advantage of the progressive income tax rate.

Deductibles and copayments provide another source of funding for the total health care program, and have a great relevance to the justice of the distribution of the funding burden. In general, a flat deductible or copayment will be the most regressive, placing the greatest burden on those with the lowest incomes. Flat-rate deductibles and copayments are thus very unacceptable according to egalitarian principles of justice. Some deductibles and copayments, however, have been graduated. The Roe and Beall National Catastrophic Illness Protection Act of 1973 would have had no deductible for low-income families, but the deductible would have increased rapidly to $15,500 for those with an adjusted gross income of $20,000. Thus it is possible to graduate the deductible and copayment dimensions of health care funding as well as the general contribution to the funding pool.

Unless a graduation is included, deductibles and copayments impose a unique burden on those least well off. The lower the amount of these features, the more just the proposals. The Kennedy-Griffiths proposal, for instance, had no deductibles and no copayments and no waiting periods for coverage. One of the real policy dilemmas is to harmonize the claims of justice with those of efficiency. Deductibles and copayments are introduced into the proposals in order to discourage frivolous overutilization of health resources. The challenge to Congress and to health policy planners is to come up with a scheme that would provide a disincentive for overutilization without being regressive. This would seem to call for a deductible or copayment feature that was pegged to an index of ability to pay. For instance, a deductible equal to a certain percentage (say 5 percent) of the income tax one paid the previous year would be graduated. It would approach an equalization of the burden and would still provide protection against overutilization.

152 *Ethics and Health Policy*

Some of the most progressive funding mechanisms have not even been proposed. Readjustments of the present income-tax tables increasing the percent tax at the high of the income scale would be one progressive funding source. One worth considering would be a payroll tax like social security, but one which began where social security leaves off—beginning presently with incomes of $14,100.

There are remarkable differences in the national health insurance proposals viewed from the perspective of egalitarian justice. While the most just health care program may not necessarily be the most *right*, any program that ignores the claims of justice will certainly be unacceptable. Only by exploring the claims of justice can the coming National Health Insurance debate be successfully completed.

Notes to Chapter Eight

1. See discussion of the paternalism of the Hippocratic ethic in Ludwig Edelstein, "The Hippocratic Oath," in his *Ancient Medicine* (Baltimore: Johns Hopkins Press, 1967), pp. 3-63, especially pp. 22-23.

2. See Chapter Six, "Ethics and Health Care: Computers and Distributive Justice," by Joseph Fletcher.

3. Bernard Williams, "The Idea of Equality," in *Justice and Equality*, ed. by Hugo Bedau (Englewood Cliffs, N.J.: Prentice-Hall, Inc., 1971), p. 127.

4. Ibid., p. 125.

5. Gene Outka, "Social Justice and Equal Access to Health Care," *Journal of Religious Ethics* 2 (No. 1, 1974), pp. 23-24.

6. John Rawls, *A Theory of Justice* (Cambridge, Mass.: Harvard University Press, 1971).

7. Rawls, p. 302.

8. Robert Veatch, "The Metaethical Foundation for an Ethic of the Life Sciences," *Hastings Center Studies* (No. 1, 1973), pp. 50-65.

9. Rawls, p. 137.

10. Others, some for different reasons, hold that Rawls's principles do not meet his own tests. See Robert Paul Wolff, "A Refutation of Rawls' Theorem on Justice," *Journal of Philosophy* 63 (1966), 179-90; Brian Barry, "On Social Justice," *The Oxford Review* (Trinity Term, 1962), 33-43; Robert Nozick, "Distributive Justice," *Philosophy and Public Affairs* 3 (No. 1, 1973), 45-126; Brian Barry, *The Liberal Theory of Justice* (New York: Oxford University Press, 1973).

11. Rawls, p. 9.

12. Several analysts have advocated market mechanisms and direct money transfers to the poor rather than social service programs. See Vincent Taylor, "How Much Is Good Health Worth?" *Policy Sciences* 1 (1970), 49-72; Martin S. Feldstein, "A New Approach to National Health Insurance," *The Public Interest* 23 (Spring 1971), pp. 93-105.

13. Robert M. Veatch, "Who Should Pay for Smokers' Medical Care?" *Hastings Center Report* 4 (November 1974), pp. 8-9.

14. Two government resource books have been used as the source of information on the bills, in addition to numerous other references, including the bills themselves. These are *National Health Insurance Proposals:* Provisions of the Bills Introduced in the 93rd Congress as of July 1974. U.S. Department of Health, Education and Welfare; Social Security Administration, Office of Research and Statistics DHEW Publication No. (SSA) 75-11920; and *National Health Insurance Resource Book*, April 11, 1974, prepared by the Staff of the Committee on Ways and Means for the Use of the Committee. U.S. Government Printing Office (Washington, D.C.; 1974).

Section C:
The Right to Health Care

PREAMBLE

"The right to health care" is a phrase that has become widely accepted in public debate about medical care delivery. The casual and often sweeping way in which it is used, however, had led some thinkers to further reflections on the notion. This use of "rights" language in connection with health and medical care raises new problems and new perspectives. Daniel Callahan places the appeal to a "right to health care" in the context of the ambiguous character of medical progress and the expanded concept of "health" current in our affluent and individualistic society. Unless society scales down its demands on medicine and accepts the practical and inherent limits of a right to health care, Callahan believes that appeals to such a right will reinforce unfulfillable expectations, increase the waste and maldistribution of resources, and endanger other rights.

Peter Steinfels agrees with many of the warnings in Callahan's presentation, but questions both the logic of some of his arguments and the fact that the public's concept of health and its demands on medicine have reached the runaway state Callahan describes. He argues that the potential dangers of guaranteeing medical care to all are largely due to faulty institutional arrangements, and that the pessimism about reform expressed by Callahan stems from a philosophical view of "liberal man" that ultimately undermines Callahan's concerns.

The open market is much more attractive to Peter Singer. He argues that the debate about justice in health care and the right to health care is misplaced. Rather than siding with either Callahan or Steinfels, he claims we should shift our attention to freedom and utility as the basic ethical claims in deciding how *health care should be distributed. The result is a greater attraction for marketplace modes of allocation.*

✳ *Chapter 9*

Biomedical Progress and the Limits of Human Health

Daniel Callahan

In thinking about the ideal of human progress and biomedical procedures, it is tempting to concentrate on the most dramatic possibilities: genetic engineering and positive eugenics, in vitro fertilization and extracorporeal gestation, sex selection, and the like. All these possibilities have been celebrated as potential occasions for human progress, primarily on the grounds that future people will be able to transcend the mischief and vagaries of nature by devising a human being who is brighter, more creative, more benign, and better adapted to modern life. An attractive vision. Yet even those most optimistic about human affairs can discern a few problems: What assurance would we have that the humans thus produced would actually be "better"? What does "better" mean? And who will decide what it means? In short, whether these radical biomedical developments would represent "progress" is highly problematic. Worse still, because of the inevitable time-lags, it will not be our generation that will have to live with any of the consequences. Our whole generation may be willing to bet that indeed it will represent progress, but it will be our children or their children who will either collect or pay up on the bet. We can *guess* whether it will represent progress, but they will be the only ones who will *know*. Looked at in that way, there is all the more reason to be wary of labeling something like genetic engineering as "progress."

More pertinent at the present historical moment are those far more subtle, less dramatic developments which are already upon us: safe and simple abortion on request, prenatal diagnosis (via amniocentesis) of genetic defects, new surgical techniques for treating deformed newborns, increasingly sophisticated methods for sustaining the life of the aged and injured, the use of a wide range of drugs

---

This chapter is included in a forthcoming book, edited by Florian Stuber and Michael Mooney © 1976; to be published by Columbia University Press. Reprinted here with permission of the author and publisher.

for increasingly focal effects on emotions and psychological predilections. The list could easily be extended. The importance of these developments, from a cultural and ethical point of view, lies less in their actual existence—they will help some people, harm others, and create terrible dilemmas for still others—than in their cumulative and total effect upon the way people begin thinking about themselves, their children, and other human beings.

If one can speak of an historical dialectic between technology and culture, it would probably amount to this: the advance of technology requires a set of affirmative cultural attitudes in the first place; and, in the second place, the technology once achieved brings some changes not only in the details of those sustaining attitudes but also in a host of other cultural attitudes and values, usually going well beyond anything envisioned in the first impulse to develop a particular set of technologies. The history of the automobile would sustain that description of the dialectic.

Our society has now become conscious of this dialectic at work in biomedicine, but I believe it has some special features that will sharply distinguish it from that brought about by the development, say, of machinery and industrialization in general. The latter have had the primary effect of changing the external conditions of life, the environment. While it would be foolish to underestimate the impact of that kind of change on human behavior and self-conception, biomedical change can have a very different kind of impact. Biomedical technology intervenes directly into the internal world, first into our bodies and then into our minds and emotions (with of course considerable overlap). The change is direct rather than indirect, unmediated rather than mediated. Whether the change is as simple as reducing infant mortality rates or as complex as psychosurgery, the intervention is straightforward and targeted, and the target is the human body and/or self in one or all of its features. Hence, one can understand both the sense of new power and, here and there at least, the kind of dejection or nervousness that can accompany it. For the dialectic in this case begins in the usual way, attempting to make use of scientific knowledge and technological skill to achieve some desired end; but then, as that end is gradually achieved, it comes to be seen that the changes in attitudes and values it brings with it are of a kind entirely different from what society has become accustomed to when the changes are environmentally introduced. One is working directly with human consciousness from the inside, whether the target happens to be the mind or the body, and that is a very formidable way of dealing with some ultimate values at their source, the mind and its bodily substance itself. One tinkers with a machine or tries to develop a better model in order to effect a different environmental outcome (knowing that this outcome may influence society and thus eventually bring about change and thereby affect the human mind). But in this case, the process is exactly the opposite: we begin with the mind and body and work out from there, changing very drastically the feedback circuitry between intervention and values.

Let me give a simple illustration. Spina bifida is a congenital disorder in which a child is born with an open spinal cord. Ten years ago the fatality rate was approximately 60 percent, and even those who survived were ordinarily permanently and severely crippled and retarded. Here, then, was a perfect target for technological progress, in this instance an advancement in surgical technique; obviously, it was thought, if such a condition could be treated many children would be saved, many parents relieved, and the human condition bettered. Who could argue with that or fail to call it progress? And it happened. It is now possible to save the lives of 90 percent of those children born with spina bifida. Unfortunately, it has not been possible to save those children from a crippled and mentally retarded life, nor may it ever be. Would they be better off dead? Do we really count that technological development as progress?

Those are the obvious questions at one level, and they merely symbolize one by now old and familiar story with technology, that of unintended and undesired consequences. But far more important is the way that intervention into the human body, together with the kind of troubled reflections it has engendered, has set in train (though not by itself, of course) a very different kind of logic of values. Put simply, the process of trying to deal with the dilemma of a procedure that saves lives only to create a new misery has pressed the value discussion back to a still more fundamental question: What is a life worth living and a life worth saving? The apparent answer that is emerging, judging only from scattered clues, moves in the direction of a narrower rather than broader view of a normative "quality of life." Fewer lives are now thought worth saving than was the case before attempts were made to devise surgical cures or ameliorations. Even those who under poorer surgical conditions would have had every effort expended to save them, however terrible their condition and however slight the relief offered, will now be allowed to die. This is increasingly true with spina bifida and even more strikingly with Down's Syndrome (mongoloidism). Where it was once the case that routine simple surgery would have been customarily performed to save the life of a mongoloid, the trend now is not to perform the surgery, even though there are more routine techniques available than before.

Paradoxically, then, the attempt to achieve what can be called "simple" progress—the treatment of a condition universally accepted as bad—led, in the end, to a very fundamental change of values toward defective newborns, with the final result likely to be far fewer defective children being saved now than was the case before the advent of a medical "progress" meant to save more lives.

Now it is unlikely that this kind of change in values has come about in total isolation of other changes taking place in medicine and, no less important, in public attitudes toward health. In the case of spina bifida and mongoloidism it is not just physicians who are changing their thinking about saving the severely defective child; even more, it is the parents of the children. Given a choice, they increasingly elect not to have life-saving surgery performed, a striking and very rapid shift in attitude. It is a very delicate matter to interpret the origin and meaning of the shift, which at its extreme includes a sharp rise in the outright abandonment of defective children by their mothers in hospital nurseries, previously an exceedingly rare event.

I believe the underlying cultural phenomenon here can be traced to some important changes in the concept of "health," in notions of what constitutes a "right to health," and, more generally, to the increased demands upon medicine and biology to solve human problems. The definition of "health" adopted by The World Health Organization in 1946 provides an insight into the historical origin of the changing concept of "health." "Health," the WHO said, "is a state of complete physical, mental, and social well-being and not merely the absence of disease or infirmity." It is a definition worth meditating upon, for not only did it mean to encompass the burgeoning mental health movement, but it also meant—quite literally, it seems from the record of early WHO discussion—to encompass everything that could be included under the heading of human welfare and happiness. It was an ambitious definition, giving medicine an enormous mandate and theoretically excluding no human problem from treatment by medical means or from interpretation in medical or biological categories. That much of the popular moral language of our culture is now cast in terms of deviants—criminals and radical politicians being "sick" rather than just wrong, stupid, or immoral—is a reflection of the power that animated the WHO definition of "health."

Moreover, it is patently the case that the combination of an all-encompassing concept of health together with biomedical advances has created a situation in which nearly anything that anyone wants from medicine can find legitimation as a health need. The abortion reform movement, culminating in the Supreme Court decision to allow abortion on request for the first two trimesters of pregnancy, drew heavily on health and well-being arguments, and the wording of the court's decision made much of putting the final choice jointly in the hands of women and their physicians, as if it were simply a medical matter. The emergence of genetic counseling as a major medical profession has drawn much of its force not only by concentrating on the genetic health of fetuses and neonates but also and simultaneously by concentrating on the mental health of parents faced with the possibility of producing a defective child. The word "suffering" is a common one in the literature of genetic counseling, but it is rarely clear whether the suffering referred to is that of the child, the parents and family, or the society as a whole; they are usually mixed together in ways that make them almost indistinguishable. "Health," now seen as the alleviation of all suffering, provides a very handy basket into which can be thrown both physiological considerations and emotional responses. A similar analysis could be developed from an examination of much of the literature, now mountainous, about the dying patient.

To my mind, the most disturbing aspect of the way in which the concept of "health" is made amenable to any and all human demands is less the ultimate meaninglessness of the term when so employed than the way it so well serves a medicine and society that are highly individualistic in orientation. One major feature of individualism in our society is that it knows no limits: anything may be aspired to, anything may be hoped for, anything may be sought. A very loose concept of health, then, allows people to trade upon the fact that with minor ingenuity any desire can be seen as a health need; and any health need can be legitimated in the name of the right to health. The political system cannot make all of the people happy all of the time, but it is just possible that physician-prescribed psychotropic drugs can. If all of us have a right to happiness, with an equal right to define happiness in our own private terms, why should we not call upon medicine to give us what other institutions cannot?

The central issue, I believe, is what our society will finally make of the "right to health." In that respect, I will present a threefold argument: (1) that the concept of a "right to health" can never be given a full and significant meaning unless, at the same time, we are clear about what the limits to that right are; (2) that the reason we have not managed politically to implement the notion of a right to health in our society in any sensible way is, paradoxically, because we *already* grant the right to health—but in a way which, because that right knows no limits, guarantees a maldistribution of health care; and (3) that for both practical and theoretical reasons, but mainly and crucially the latter, the right to health care is, intrinsically, a limited right.

There are some general premises upon which I will base these arguments:

1. The problem of the right to health care, and especially the limits of that right, currently reflects the more general tension between the tyranny of individualism and the tyranny of survival. Unless that more general problem is solved, it is hardly likely we can solve the right-to-health problem.

The unhealthy tension between the twin tyrannies can be described thus. Survival is a basic drive. In affluent technological societies, acceptable survival (ego- or self-survival) levels are raised very high, particularly under the influence of individualism, which leads people to place high, constantly escalating demands upon life and happiness. One outcome of this process is that such people can be as tyrannized by a perceived threat to survival as those whose survival-demand level is much lower. That the demands of the former are much higher than the latter is less a function of real need than it is of the high demand level to which their individualism (and that of the culture) has led them. The result is a genuinely vicious circle: their individualism pushes them to a higher acceptable survival level, but because that level is higher, they must make more individual demands in order to achieve a sense of safety or security. The only real security lies in having a lower demand level for survival, creating a situation where needs can effectively be met. But the individualism of the culture will not allow that; hence, people never feel secure, no matter how many of their wants are satisfied.

2. The language of "rights" ultimately becomes meaningless when that which is demanded in the name of rights is impossible to achieve in either a real or a plausible world.

In ordinary usage, "the right to health care" has come to mean, in its more modest sense, the right of individuals to equal access to available health care regardless of their ability to pay for that care. The pressure to establish the right to health care developed out of a perception that with laissez faire medicine, the rich could get what the poor could not. The principal value appealed to in that discussion is distributive justice, with an emphasis on the contention that however medical resources are to be distributed, ability to pay provides a wrong, because inequitable, basis for that distribution.

One premise of that line of argument is that health care is, in many respects at least, a scarce resource. One cannot assume that health care exists in such abundance that no problem of distribution exists; thus it is necessary to deal with the problem of equal access, and to deal with that means to invoke the value of distributive justice together with all the political and legal ramifications of that value. Even in its modest sense, then, the right to health care has raised some difficult problems, and they become all the more difficult when one moves into the question of distributing such things as totally implantable artificial hearts, expensive treatment for hemophilia, and kidney dialysis machines.

However, that is not the end of the right-to-health-care issue. As the phrase became more popular, a more extravagant sense began to appear. Not only ought there to be equal accessibility to *available* health resources, but it was asserted that it is also perfectly right and proper for individuals to demand, as a matter of right, that medicine *develop* such new resources as would be required to help them achieve whatever they may desire in the name of health (which in the end becomes indistinguishable from *whatever* they may desire). Thus a claim has been entered that infertile women have a right to in vitro fertilization (and the right to its development) in order to find relief from their infertility. Even more extravagantly, some women demand, also as a matter of right, that in vitro fertilization be developed in order that they may exercise the option not just to have a child but to have a child in the way they choose to have one. In the first instance, the assumption is that there exists a natural right *not* to be infertile—and that society, if that right is to be respected, has the duty to devise ways to implement that right. In the second instance, there is the assumption that the rights of women include the right to have a child in whatever way they may choose to do so—and again, that society has the duty to carry out such research as would be needed to implement that right.

These are, admittedly, rather lurid examples, but they do illustrate what seems to be happening as the concept of "the right to health care" is pressed beyond its original boundaries. It is used to legitimate a claim that there exists a right to have *all* bodily infirmities corrected if scientifically possible or conceivable (and a correlative duty on the part of society to take all necessary steps toward that end) and a right to demand that medical technology be brought to bear (well beyond the narrow boundaries of "illness") to satisfy all desires. Think of the following trends in the logic of the right to amniocentesis (even if it is now a subcurrent): if pregnant women have the right to amniocentesis in order to avoid bearing a Tay Sachs baby or a Down's, why should they not have the right to avoid bearing a child with a cleft palate? And if they should have the latter right, why should they not have the right to avoid bearing a child with a crooked left little finger? But if they should have that choice, why then should they not also have the choice of using amniocentesis in order to have sex selection (if that is what they *want*)? And if they should have the last-mentioned right, does not society have the duty to make amniocentesis available to all women in order that they may gain their rights?

I want to touch on another development of the extravagant sense of the "right to health care": that of the argument—as presented by Bentley Glass et al.—that every child has the right to be born with a healthy mind and body (a variant on the notion that all humans have the right to be free of infirmities); and the correlative argument that, therefore, the way to protect the rights of such a child is to abort it—a really novel notion of a way in which rights can be protected.

With all that by way of preamble, let me return to my three central arguments.

1. The concept of the "right to health care" can never be given a full and significant meaning unless we become clear about what the limits to that right are. This argument can be defended on a number of grounds. First, the word "health" will be meaningless if we do not have a sense of what falls outside the realm of health; if "health" is used to bear on everything to do with human well-being, then the "right to health care" becomes tantamount to a right to happiness—a right, in effect, to everything anyone wants in the name of that which they believe will fulfill them. That is a route which guarantees that the "right to health care" will end up meaning nothing at all—because it will mean anything and everything. Second, even if "health" is given a more circumscribed meaning, the requirements of a manageable circumscription must include (by definition) limitations on the meaning of "health."

Third, the history of discourse and discussion on human rights has always shown (and required) the development of some paradigm of a meaningful limitation of right (e.g. the right to freedom of speech: one can't falsely cry "fire" in a crowded theater). The reason, of course, why such paradigms have proved necessary is that there is more than one human right. Eventually, rights come in conflict and thus, if only to avoid logical absurdity, limitations upon any given right are needed in order that they may not cancel each other out. The "right to health care" has yet to go through that kind of historical process; until it does, there will be no way to keep the right to health from transgressing (at least in principle) all other rights, and no way to establish the relative place of the right to health care in the constellation of other accepted rights. At best, this will mean that it will remain nothing but a slogan; at worst, it could become a monster.

2. One origin of the present maldistribution of health care is the fact that far from actually being denied, the right to health has been granted in practice. But it has been so extravagantly granted and with such an unlimited scope that it has been impossible to deal with the claims of distributive justice. To make this case, one major assumption is needed: I will define as a (de facto) right any claim that any well-placed individual can successfully make without violating an extant law or ingrained social custom. In the case of health, it has been possible for any individual with money and/or clout to demand and frequently to get whatever he has wanted: his face lifted, his infertility treated, his psyche soothed, etc. He cannot get an arm amputated without reason, but beyond that kind of (rare) exception, there is no one who will stand in his way if he calls upon medicine to take care of what ails him (or what he thinks ails him); all he needs is money. That is why I say there exists a *recognized de facto right* to health.

Precisely because that has been the situation, medicine has been prone to develop in a direction where money and/or power have determined how available resources have been distributed. Put another way, because of the recognized de facto right to health, there has been no principle available that would enable the society to say "No" to the person who wants something from medicine, proposes to break no laws, and has the money to pay for it. If every male and female in the country over the age of forty decided that having his or her face lifted was the greatest medical good, and every young doctor decided to become a plastic surgeon to meet the demand for face-lifting, I don't think there is any principle of limitation now available that could deny there was an intrinsic right to face-lifting for all, or that could deny that all physicians would have the right to become plastic surgeons if they chose to do so. We might say that the males and females in question were acting absurdly and that the physicians were acting irresponsibly as a group. But we could put neither group in jail—no law would be broken—and it is hard to see how we could say that any given *individual* physician was acting irresponsibly. If we don't consider it irresponsible for *any* given physician now to become a plastic surgeon, why would it be irresponsible for *all* to become plastic surgeons—particularly if they could show, as a group, that sufficient demand for their services existed?

In short, we are faced with a classic situation. The de facto right to health care has been based on the principle of freedom: anyone can demand anything in the name of health and, if he can pay for it, can have it. When freedom has that much scope, it is hardly surprising that justice can hardly get its foot in the door. Justice is possible only when freedom is limited in some way. But the right to health has (again, de facto) been premised on total freedom; hence, justice has been excluded. If there is to be a just distribution of medical resources, there must be some limitations placed upon the present de facto freedom of individuals (mainly the wealthy and powerful) to get what they want. That, in turn, means that the "right to health care" must eventually be seen as a limited right. Justice is incompatible with absolute individual rights, and a just medical care system is incompatible with unlimited individual health rights.

3. The right to health care will always be to some extent limited by practical considerations, even in the most affluent societies. But more important, there are intrinsic limits to the right. These limits stem from the fact that the human body is a finite material organism, subject to decay and eventual dissolution. Illness is one manifestation of human finiteness. The demand for an absolute "right to health care" is, in the end, a demand to be free of bodily finiteness. One could, I suppose, speculate that medicine may eventually find ways to transcend that finiteness. But I don't think it will ever happen. Finiteness is an intrinsic part of matter and organicity; it may be ameliorated, but it won't be cured. In any event, finiteness is surely a present fact, and our generation and the next (at least) will have to live with that fact. Therefore, in our present situation, the "right to health care" is intrinsically limited.

※ *Chapter 10*

The Right to Health Care and the Anxiety of Liberalism: A Reply to Daniel Callahan

Peter Steinfels

If I were to reduce the propositions argued in the preceding chapter to their general form they would fall into two categories, those I agree with and those I find confusing. That we should be wary of labeling every new development in biomedicine as unqualified "progress"; that there may be unforeseen and extensive consequences of apparently simple and benevolent technological innovation, and that this may be especially the case in the biomedical area; that expectations in regard to health have been increasing and more demands put on biology and medicine to remedy "the ills that flesh is heir to"; that American society in particular as well as our medical practice are characterized by an individualism which makes wise social judgments difficult; that the right to health care, like all other rights, must be limited, first in definition so that it may make sense (when the notion of "religion" in the right to exercise one's own religion, or the notion of "speech" in the right to free speech, becomes wildly extended, the same problems emerge), and then in application so that it does not conflict with other rights; that justice requires restrictions on individual freedom of action; and that human finitude is a fact which must be respected—with none of these propositions do I have any argument.

Addressing myself directly to Callahan's "three central arguments," I am in complete agreement with his first; but, even in their most general terms, the second and third points puzzle me. His thesis that the reason we have not sensibly implemented the notion of a right to health care in this society is that we have already, de facto, granted it, passes beyond paradox to utter confusion of terms. What is this "de facto right to health care"? According to Callahan, it is the ability of "any individual with the money and/or clout to demand and frequently to get whatever he has wanted." This, of course, is precisely what Callahan has earlier defined as the situation *against which* the right to health care has been advocated: "The pressure to establish the right to health care developed out of a perception that, with laissez-faire medicine, the rich could get what the poor could not.... the contention that, however medical resources are to be distributed, ability to pay provides a wrong, because inequitable, basis for that distribution." Having defined as the "right to health care ... in practice" exactly what most people take as more or less the opposite of the right to health care, Callahan can unload on it responsibility for all the ills of laissez-faire medicine. Having defined as the right to health care—"extravagantly granted and with such an unlimited scope," no less!—exactly what the advocates of that right oppose and hope to remedy, namely the dominance of "money and/or clout," Callahan can come up with the conclusion that this newly styled right is responsible for medicine's tendency "to develop in a direction where money and/or power have determined how available resources have been distributed." Not a very remarkable conclusion, given the premise.

This whole exercise strikes me as the equivalent of redefining the right of free speech as censorship (de facto freedom of speech for any individual who hews to the official political or religious orthodoxy), and then attributing to the right of free speech all the disadvantages of censorship (all channels of information would be dominated by those possessing either orthodox opinions or the power to determine orthodox opinions). Pointing out that his regime of money and/or clout could hypothetically result in all medical resources being devoted to face-lifts and that physicians would then be "acting irresponsibly as a group" (presumably because they were not employing their skills for more urgent medical needs), Callahan bemoans the absence of any principle to limit such maldistribution and excess. A less paradoxical thinker might have supposed that the right to health care (in the ordinary sense, not the redefined Callahanian sense) could be the very principle needed here. It would be the grounds for prohibiting the provision of face-lifts to those with money or clout when this deprives everyone else of innoculations and life-saving surgery.

I am similarly confused by the third central argument of the essay, that "intrinsic limits" to the right to health care "stem from the fact that the human body is a finite, material organism, subject to decay and eventual dissolution." I would not challenge the wisdom of recognizing our human finitude, but I am not sure that it has the connection with the right to health care that Callahan asserts but does not demonstrate. It would seem, in fact, that the eventual dissolution of our physical being, a fate which arrives regardless of race, color, creed, socioeconomic class, sexual orientation, etc., would constitute an argument *for* the right to health care. Perhaps Callahan is assuming that the right to health *care* must imply a right to health *cure*—in which case, we can agree, the quest is a futile one, and bodily finiteness poses "intrinsic limits" to the right. But unless one makes this assumption, I do not see why we must speak of "intrinsic limits" that exist beyond, and are "more important" than those "practical considerations"—the availability of resources and the negotiation of conflicts with other rights—which must limit all rights whatsoever.

These are the agreements and the puzzlements that Callahan's propositions provoke in me when they are reduced to general statements. But, of course, his chapter is far more than general statements. His propositions come fleshed out with factual assumptions; and the argument is certainly a whole greater than its summed parts—it represents an emphasis, a mood, a stance. On both these levels, that of fact and that of overall stance, I have serious objections.

The factual issue on which I must part company with Callahan is his assumption, signaled throughout the chapter, that there now exists a widespread and inordinate demand by the public for medical services, and that this rests on a wildly exaggerated concept of health held by the public at large. "It is patently the case," he writes, "that the combination of an all-encompassing concept of health together with biomedical advances has created a situation in which nearly anything that anyone wants from medicine can find legitimation as a health need." "Health," he adds, is "now seen as the alleviation of all suffering." It is true that our standards of health have been increasing, as have our standards of housing and nutrition; and that reliance on medical services is clearly frivolous in some limited areas and perhaps reaching the point of diminishing returns more generally. That the situation deserves to be described in the runaway terms used by Callahan is not at all evident. Consider the rapidly mounting size of the national health budget, the very sort of evidence that would appear to support Callahan's thesis. Between 1965 and 1972 personal health expenditures underwent one of the most dramatic increases ever—jumping from $38.9 billion to $83.4 billion. Nonetheless, it should be pointed out that 52 percent of this increase was due to higher prices. Another 10 percent was due to population growth. The portion due to increased utilization of medical services and the introduction of new techniques is thus limited to the remaining 38 percent. A sizeable portion of that increased use in turn was merely meeting the previously unmet needs of the poor and the elderly who had obtained access to medical care with the introduction of Medicare and Medicaid in 1966—this increase can hardly be attributed to fanciful notions of "health." Another portion, that due to introduction of new techniques, was probably largely determined by the expectations of physicians rather than patients. The role of physicians in this kind of decision-making is well documented. All told, even this dramatic jump in personal health expenditures does not reveal the runaway expectations throughout the general public that Callahan supposes.

But consider Callahan's own evidence. Much has been made in these debates of the World Health Organization's sweeping definition of health. At least in my reading of the WHO record, the purpose of this definition reflected not only post-World War II utopian hopes but also bureaucratic politics—WHO wanted as much of a mandate as possible to cooperate with nonmedical international agencies, especially since many world health problems can be approached best in nonmedical ways. Certainly WHO did *not* want a definition that might restrict its efforts or put it at a disadvantage in jurisdictional disputes. All this is unmistakably expansionist, and whether it has proved dangerous in practice could be determined by examining WHO's history. To assume, however, that the WHO definition provides much of a clue into the public's ideas about "health" is to forget both its political and bureaucratic origins and to neglect the grain of salt we usually apply to political, and especially international, declarations.

Callahan's examples of abortion and genetic counseling also do not strike me as unreasonable cases of demanding increasing services from medicine. One may be morally opposed to the widespread resort to abortion (I am) but nonetheless admit that a procedure mentioned in the Hippocratic Oath (c. 400 B.C.) is a weak instance of a radically new demand placed on medicine. Likewise the emergence of genetic counseling does not appear to mark any sharp break with medical tradition; new knowledge is being applied to alleviate bodily abnormalities that have always been recognized as such, and if the field has its problems of definition, they are similar to those in the rest of medicine. In any case, parents' fear of serious abnormality and mental deficit in their offspring—of sickle cell anemia or Tay-Sachs disease or Down's Syndrome—does not suggest to me an overrefinement of sensibility or an exaggerated, individualistic concern for happiness. Callahan's other examples—demands for amniocentesis to avoid bearing children with cleft palate or "crooked left little finger," for sex selection, for face-lifts, for research to perfect in vitro fertilization and implantation—are worthy topics in themselves for debate; perhaps acquiescing to such demands is even irremediably in the logic of the right to health care. Yet there is no evidence that the public now includes such procedures among those it would want guaranteed by any right; if anything, the opinion is quite to the contrary, and if the right to health care were extended in this fashion, it would be despite, rather than on account of, the public's wishes—just as such extensions presently occur, despite the public's skepticism, in individualistic, laissez-faire medical practice.

The concept of health and the ambitions of medicine have expanded and contracted throughout history. Greek philosophers complained of the power of physicians to define the good life, all the while borrowing medical concepts for their own philosophizing. At the beginning of the twentieth century the concept of health and the role of medicine appeared to contract, as scientific knowledge made it clear what physicians could and could not accomplish. Medical spokesmen argued that doctors should leave to other professions and agencies public health questions that they had previously included among their own tasks. Of course, the birth of psychiatry had already set in motion a countertrend. Our own day sees new claims put forward by branches of medicine like genetics, pharmacological psychiatry, and neurosurgery, while established forms of dynamic psychiatry and even traditional surgery face growing skepticism about their diagnostic and therapeutic reliability, reflected incidentally in the checks and limits written into many national health insurance proposals. In sum, the situation is far more complicated and far less threatening than Callahan supposes. It could be argued, in fact, that the threat is in the other direction. Although it is almost three centuries since John Locke declared that government exists "for the procuring, preserving, and advancing" of men's "civil interests"— that is, of "life, liberty, *health* and *indolency of body* [freedom from pain], and the possession of outward things," no fundamental right to health care is presently recognized by U.S. courts or is about to be; even the obligation of private community hospitals, though operated with public funds, to provide service to patients unable to pay has been barely determined. Recent years have witnessed the constant attrition of the access to medical care belatedly granted the poor and the elderly a decade ago, and the consensus holds that the moving force behind most politically significant discussions of national health insurance is the desire to control costs rather than to expand services.

These differences with Callahan's essay were, I said, on a "factual issue," but clearly "fact," here as elsewhere, has much to do with interpretation. I should pass directly, therefore, to what are perhaps my more important objections, those dealing with his essay's "overall stance." A minor complaint has to do with his tendency, exhibited here as well as in the book to which he refers (*The Tyranny of Survival*), to posit cultural attitudes as the moving forces in history as though they were largely independent of social and economic institutions. He writes of an "underlying cultural phenomenon" that "can be traced to some important changes in the concept of 'health,' in notions of what constitutes a 'right to health care,' and, more generally, to the increased demands upon medicine and biology to solve human problems." He writes that "an all-encompassing concept of health ... has created a situation ... "; that " 'health,' now seen as ... "; that "a more extravagant sense began to appear ... "; that "a claim has been entered ... "; and so on. The language is that of ideas, concepts, notions, demands, and claims apparently acting on their own, or in the passive voice, or more rarely propelled by entities like "society" or "people," and once (but only once) by "some women." Such language, to which only the radical nominalist could object altogether (and then he would lack the terms necessary to framing his objection), is not balanced by any attention to the specific actors and institutions who "socially construct" these attitudes, definitions, and demands. In the case of "health" and the demand for medical services, the result, of course, is to neglect the role that health providers, and the socioeconomic institutional framework in which they operate, play in determining what "society" or "people" or even "some women" want and get. The importance of this role can be gauged if we reconsider Callahan's assertion that for an individual to obtain whatever he wants from medicine, "all he needs is money."

That is not true, at least this side of the Rockefellers. I have an aged relative, for example, who is bedridden, blind, sometimes not lucid—and quite well off economically. If she needed a pacemaker, or even a face-lift, she could probably obtain one with little difficulty. But neither money, nor the strenuous efforts of her sons and daughters, seem capable of obtaining for her the medical care she does need, namely, reliable, thoughtful day-and-night nursing. The fact is that the provision of medical care in this society is organized so that enough pacemakers are available but enough nursing care for the bedridden is not. One can imagine a different system that was short on pacemakers but long on nursing. To leap over the role of institutions is to universalize problems unduly, and mistakenly to take as givens of "society" or "culture" or "people" what could be remedied by redesigning our institutions.

I said this was a minor complaint, but it is not unrelated to my major one. Callahan's chapter is in many ways similar to other essays that have been provoked by the uncertain state of contemporary biomedicine and the recent talk of the "right to health care." All of them reveal what Sheldon S. Wolin has superbly described as the anxiety of liberalism.

For various reasons, including the confusion of liberalism with democratic radicalism, classical liberalism has often been portrayed as the optimistic expression of confidence in the unfettered individual, in the triumph of rationality, in the benevolence of nature and the inevitability of progress. Returning to the sources, Wolin argues that "liberalism was a philosophy of sobriety, born in fear, nourished by disenchantment, and prone to believe that the human condition was and was likely to remain one of pain and anxiety." Hobbes's darker view of man's estate is widely recognized, to be sure, but liberal man as described by Locke, the political economists, and the Mills as well, paid for his expansive energy at tremendous cost.

Liberal epistemology and psychology split the self into reason and desire; we are moved by desires, and reason is their instrument—it cannot establish ends but only calculate means. Rather than believing in an essentially rational man, as later commentators have supposed, the liberal writers emphasized the passions as the mainspring of action. Moral judgments and human purposes were the products of feeling—and thus variable and unconstrained. Unable to truly fathom and satisfy his needs by any act of understanding, liberal man is unendingly driven by his desires, a relentless "uneasiness," according to Locke, due to "some absent good," some "want of happiness." Such uneasiness is "the chief, if not only spur to human industry and action." Happiness is the ever fleeing carrot that dangles out of reach from a pole attached to the donkey's harness; it is the always receding oasis hallucinated by the desert traveler. True, nature's trick "rouses and keeps in continual motion the industry of mankind" (Adam Smith); but this ultimate optimism did not extinguish awareness of the underlying anxiety. The reality of scarcity; the consequent necessity of a human assault on nature, entailing the pain of labor and the alienation of man from his surroundings; the shadow of the law of diminishing returns, making every increment of material progress ever more costly; finally the demand for sexual repression to hold population in check, turning man against his own instincts—Locke, Smith, Bentham, Malthus, the elder and the younger Mill, had all sketched the discontents of civilization in stark outlines long before Freud.

Several conclusions follow from this portrait of liberal man that are pertinent to the discussion of a right to health care and its limits. One is the anxiety, now ours as well as that of the classic liberals and the creature they described, that things are always about to go wildly out of control. Locke, who found, somehow, a greater role for reason in moral judgments than other liberal thinkers, nonetheless wrote of "the lawless exorbitancy of unconfined man." Second, there is the conclusion that constraints are essentially external to the individual—Hobbes's sovereign, the political economists' self-regulating clash of interests, formal rules and regulations, scarcity of resources, the conflict of one right with another—and that such constraints are therefore painful rather than harmonious. To the degree that constraints are "internalized," they have the same effect, namely pain, as do external constraints—they are simply more efficiently enforced. Third, the role of political and ethical philosophy is fundamentally defensive. It does not hold out hopes of renovating society, of plumbing the inner life, of creating ideals and generating new perspectives. It largely accepts the status quo of society as the departure point for cautious reforms. It is prudential, preaching the limits of human capacities rather than attempting to stretch them.

In several critical ways, Callahan might wish not to identify himself with this liberal tradition, but instead to oppose it. He does not share its faith that the human itch for more will redound to the benefit of all. Quite the contrary. Most probably he would want to escape from the division of desire and reason, fact and value, that we inherit from liberalism, and to restore reason to a role in evaluating and choosing human ends as well as calculating means to their achievement. It is eminently clear from his comments on our contemporary plight, our institutionalized escalation of needs, our reckless individualism, that the legacy of liberalism is precisely what haunts him. But just as the liberal image of man, however partial or limiting a reading of human nature, has framed our institutions so as to foster the very type it portrayed, in effect becoming a self-fulfilling description, so too Callahan, by accepting as given the liberal psychology, strengthens the premises on which it is based and resigns himself to struggling within the framework that is the source of the problems he addresses. Certainly he, and writers like him, consider their own suspicion of public expectations, their caution about innovation, and their pessimism about relieving the human condition as a necessary counter to a utopianism they espy as the moving force behind *both* the claims to socially guaranteed health care and the destructive cultural dynamics Callahan describes as the joint "tyrannies" of individualism and survival. They are mistaken. Those dynamics, insofar as political philosophies move or articulate social forces, have been formed or reinforced by an outlook that is not utopian at all but anxious, suspicious, cautious, and pessimistic, precisely as is their own.

What is the alternative? Fortunately a respondent can evade the request for a positive statement, and so I will. It may be anticlimactic, after such a lengthy critique, to confess that I share with Callahan the suspicion that current formulations of the right to health care, language which is also part of the liberal inheritance, may not be the best approach to the entire question. Such talk is hardly beyond correction and qualification, perhaps frontal challenge. But I believe the problem must be boarded in a very different spirit, one with more confidence in human capacities to discern and distinguish levels of need and to create institutions which will minimize excesses and, yes, maximize "physical, mental, and social well-being."

Chapter 11

Freedoms and Utilities in the Distribution of Health Care[a]

Peter Singer

Should the goods and services required to preserve and restore our health be bought and sold in the marketplace, like television sets and haircuts, or should they be provided in some other way? To give a complete answer to this question we would have to take into account a wide variety of considerations. We would need to inquire into the economics of alternative schemes for providing health care. We could not reach a proper decision unless we knew whether one scheme provided health care at a significantly lower cost than another. We would also need information of a sociological nature: who would receive care under the different schemes, and what kind of care? Even after we had all the economic and sociological information that we would reasonably expect to acquire, however, some very fundamental questions would remain. These would be ethical questions. What are our ends or values? What is it that we are trying to achieve in this area? What are the values or principles that should guide our choice between alternative methods of distribution? What is our conception of a good society, and how does this conception affect our choice of method?

It is these ethical questions that I am going to explore in this chapter. They cannot be considered in isolation from economic and sociological issues, and so I shall be referring to these areas in the course of the chapter, but my focus will be ethical.

Ethical questions are notoriously difficult to discuss fruitfully. There are no universally accepted ultimate principles or standards, and many people seem to

---

[a]I am deeply indebted to the late Richard Titmuss, whose writings have provided me with most of the information and ideas that follow.

think that all that can be done is to state your own view as plausibly as you can, and hope that others will accept it. I do not believe that we are always forced to take quite so subjective an approach. In some areas of ethics, at least, argument is possible, and there are the usual standards of good and bad argument, so we do not have to be content with appeals to emotion or intuition. In this chapter I shall concentrate on these areas of ethics, where argument is possible and discussion can be fruitful. So far as health care is concerned, the main issues of this sort are, I believe, those involving freedom and utility. Before I move on to discuss these questions, however, I should first indicate some of the ethical considerations that I am leaving aside; considerations that many people do think are important to the topic. I do not deny their importance, but I do not affirm it either. I am merely concerned to say that they are matters on which people disagree, and about which reasoned argument is scarce and fruitful discussion difficult to achieve.

HEALTH CARE AS A RIGHT

It is very common nowadays for those dissatisfied with the market approach to the distribution of health care to claim that "health care is a right." Thus Senator Abraham Ribicoff, a leading campaigner for health reform in this country and chairman of a Senate subcommittee that has investigated aspects of medical care, argues in his new book that the most basic need is for "a new way of thinking about medical care, a philosophy that states our belief that to receive medical care is the individual's right, but to provide it is the nation's privilege."[1]

It should not be difficult to find other expressions of the idea that health care is a right. The phrase has a forceful ring to it, and it makes a fine slogan. If we interpret the slogan as saying that everyone should have a legal right to obtain health care free of charge, we have no problem in understanding the claim, although of course it needs argument to back it up; but if we try to take the idea that "health care is a right" literally, as if this idea in itself is all the justification needed for making health care a legal right, we will find it difficult to know what to make of this claim.

How are we to establish that health care really is a right? Argument soon comes to a halt. It is impossible to get people to agree on any list of natural or human rights, once we get beyond the right to life, and even that is rarely held to be absolute. Other rights, like the right to vote, depend on a particular political context. So-called "welfare rights," of which the right to health care would be one, are more puzzling still, since they require not merely that others leave me alone or refrain from doing something to me, but also that others take some positive action to provide me with something. So while we can, in almost any circumstances, claim that to kill someone without his consent is to violate his right to life, we can only speak meaningfully of a violation of a right to health care if a society has reached the level of sophistication at which it has the means and knowledge to provide health care for everyone. The fact that the possibility of talking of a "right to health care" depends on available resources suggests, however, that it is a right that must be balanced against other possible uses of those resources—and this suggests that whether we finally do decide to recognize a right to health care will depend on a complex assessment of the benefits of providing free health care, as compared with the benefits of alternative systems of health care distribution. All of which suggests that it is more fruitful to discuss these benefits, and their concomitant drawbacks, than to discuss the abstract philosophical issues of the nature of human rights, and whether health care is one of them.

DISTRIBUTIVE JUSTICE

A second claim that has seemed to some to settle the problem of whether health care should be taken out of the marketplace is the idea that it is obviously unjust to provide health care on any other grounds than those of need. Justice, it is commonly and I think correctly said, demands that we treat like cases alike, except when there is a relevant difference between them. In the case of the distribution of health care, is it not self-evident that the only relevant consideration is how great a person's need for care is? Money, how wealthy a person is, obviously has nothing at all to do with whether he should receive medical care.

This argument appears plausible, but if it is intended to show that health care is a special case, peculiarly unsuited to the market mode of distribution, the argument proves far too much. It can be applied with equal plausibility to other areas. Is it not also obvious that the only relevant considerations governing the distribution of automobiles are considerations like how difficult it would be for a person to get around without one, how well his neighborhood is served by public transport, how much he needs to travel, and so on? How much money a person has is, by these standards, quite irrelevant. In other words, once we embark on this path of distributing goods and services on the basis of what is "obviously" fitting or relevant, there is no stopping place short of Marx's vision of a society governed by the principle "From each according to his ability, to each according to his need."[2] We may, of course, follow the argument where it leads, and say that it is applicable all the way—all goods and services should be distributed on the basis of need, rather than ability to pay. Personally, I think this really is an ideal form of distribution, if it can be made to work, but the fact that it is a quite general principle means that it cannot be invoked by those who claim that health care is *specially* unsuited to the marketplace. If ability to pay is sometimes relevant to how goods or services should be distributed, why is it irrelevant in this particular case? Within the normal assumptions of a market economy ability to pay for a service is a relevant consideration that distinguishes between cases that are otherwise alike. While we may object to these market assumptions, I do not think that a discussion of considerations of abstract justice is likely to help us to understand why people have thought that it is more important to take the distribution of health care out of the market than the distribution of, say, automobiles.

INTRINSIC EVIL

Finally, in this list of unfruitful approaches, there is the idea that it is somehow an intrinsic evil to make a commodity out of something essential for life. The feeling seems to be particularly strong when people discuss such questions as whether human blood should be sold, or whether it is right for medical schools to pay people who will sign over their bodies, when they die, for teaching or research purposes. I am opposed to making a commodity out of human blood; but I am opposed not because I think human blood is intrinsically not a commodity, and it is wrong to make it one, but because I believe the consequences of permitting the sale of human blood are worse than the consequences of not doing so. I do not know how anyone would argue that something is "intrinsically not a commodity." Once again, it seems to me this position is capable of rational defense only if it is made quite general. To say that intrinsically, *nothing* is a commodity seems sound; but how one could argue that food is intrinsically a commodity while blood is not, I have no idea. On the other hand, if we ask why people feel that blood and bodies are not commodities—a psychological question, not a moral one—the answer may have something to do with the consequences of treating them as commodities, in particular the subtle effects that this may have on the nature of the community that so treats them. About this I shall have a good deal more to say shortly.

I now move on to the issues that can be discussed fruitfully.

FREEDOM

The marketplace is most often defended as a method of distributing goods and services, including health care, by those who see themselves as defenders of freedom. F.A. Hayek is one example; Milton Friedman another.[3] The case of health care allows us to examine the assumption that leaving distribution to the market does increase freedom.

In order to make a clear contrast between market and nonmarket systems of distribution in the field of health care, it would be useful to compare the two systems in their pure forms. If we are considering the field of health care as a whole, however, this is not easy to do, since we do not have, in any major industrialized nation, a pure example of a market distribution. Although in debates on whether to introduce some form of national health insurance or national health service in the United States the assumption is often made that the issue is whether to continue to allow the laws of the market to operate in this area, this assumption overlooks the extent to which health care is already protected from the free and open competition that is an essential element of the marketplace.

Kenneth Arrow, in his widely discussed article "Uncertainty and the Welfare Economics of Medical Care," has noted several aspects in which the medical care market in this country differs from the usual commodity markets.[4] First, the demand for medical care is, preventive services apart, irregular and unpredictable, unlike practically every other item of significance in the average household budget. The need for the service may come suddenly, and one may not be in a position to shop around. Nor can the cost of the care that will be needed often be predicted in advance. Next, the ethics of the medical profession make medical care unlike other businesses: physicians do not advertise; there is no open price competition between physicians; when a physician advises further treatment he is supposed to be entirely unaffected by considerations of self-interest; the existence of a medical profession also severely limits the supply of medical care, for practitioners must be licensed—this in itself is not unusual, but in the field of medicine education plays a specially important role in limiting the quantity of physicians available. Limited entry to medical school controls the number of doctors there will be in future years; but these decisions, despite their great influence on the state of the market, are made by nonprofit-making institutions. Thus the supply of medical care is not directly affected by the profitability of providing it, as would be the case in a normal market. A further consequence of this situation is a restriction of the range of quality of care available to the consumer. In a competitive market different qualities of service would be offered at different prices, and the consumer could choose among them. Other differences between medical care and most commodities are that the consumer cannot learn reliably from experience, whether his own or that of friends, whether the care offered by a particular physician or hospital was satisfactory. The factor of care received cannot be isolated from unknowables like the patient's own recuperative powers. Finally, medical care cannot be returned to the seller for a money-back refund; it cannot be taken back for repairs if it goes wrong; nor can one cut one's losses and throw it away.

It is worth noting that many of these differentiating features of medical care are the work of professional bodies such as, in this country, the American Medical Association. Although the A.M.A. strongly opposes any move away from the status quo toward a national health service, the organization is equally firm in its opposition to measures which would be a move towards more open competition and effective consumer choice. A.M.A. officials have sometimes tried to present the doctor as "essentially a small businessman" who sells his services and so "is as much in business as anyone else who sells a commodity."[5] When Ralph Nader's consumer research organization took this idea seriously, however, and tried to compile a consumer's directory of doctors in Prince George County, Maryland, listing fees, doctor's qualifications, office hours, and so on, the County Medical Society sent a letter to its members advising them not to cooperate, and warning of possible sanctions against those who did. (The incomplete survey that resulted revealed some remarkable variations in fees that consumers would have had difficulty discovering for themselves—for example, for sending a throat culture to a laboratory for a standard test, fees ranged from $3 to $16.50)[6]

There can be no freedom without adequate information on which to make a choice. Clearly, there would be an increase in the freedom of the consumer if he were better informed about items like fees. We could also expect that competition of this kind would lead to some reductions in fees. But before we conclude that this move is desirable from the point of view of freedom, we need to take into account the effect that this change could have on medical practice.

In an open market the individual doctor would be less secure, economically, than he is at present. Economic considerations would therefore, become more prominent in the doctor's relationship with his patient. The patient would be aware of this, and might come to suspect self-interested considerations when the doctor advises frequent visits or further treatment. So market considerations could undermine the relationship between the doctor and his patient. The A.M.A. places a great deal of emphasis on this relationship, and I believe it is right to do so. Medical practice would be changed for the worse if a patient could not trust his doctor, confident that the doctor's motivation was exclusively a concern for his patient's well-being.

Let us look at an example of what may happen when the ethical relationship between doctor and patient breaks down. The increasingly impersonal and businesslike nature of medical practice in the United States appears to be reflected in the huge rise in the number of lawsuits. The more people travel around, change their doctors, or see specialists with whom they establish no personal contact, the more likely they are to sue if anything goes wrong.[7] Doctors, of course, insure themselves against malpractice suits. One result of the rising number of cases brought is that premiums for malpractice insurance have now gone sky-high. The premium for a Manhattan general surgeon, for instance, has risen from around $700 ten years ago to over $4000 today. This annual expenditure must be recovered in increased fees from patients. Even at these rates, insurance companies are dropping out of the business because it is unprofitable. In January 1974 the company that had underwritten almost all malpractice insurance for New York State physicians decided to terminate its group policy. Nationally, more than 16,000 suits were filed in 1972, with settlements ranging up to $1 million.[8]

By comparison, in Britain medical practitioners are covered against lawsuits for negligence by a subscription to the Medical Defence Union. In 1973, the most recent year for which I have figures, the subscription was £25 per annum, and the society handled 236 cases of alleged negligence. While there are obviously other important variables between the two countries that could explain this startling variation, it is possible that when the doctor is taken out of the marketplace the patient is less likely to treat him like any other supplier of a commodity who fails to deliver. If this is the case, then to move toward more open competition among doctors would only aggravate the situation in the United States. More open competition would probably lead people to change their doctors more frequently, and this in itself would damage the relationship between doctor and patient.

In the long run, the ordinary consumer suffers most from the high incidence of malpractice suits. It is he who must bear the brunt of the costs. Malpractice suits do not adequately protect him against incompetent doctors, since doctors almost invariably continue to practice after malpractice decisions go against them. Moreover, in order to keep down their premiums, doctors now tend to practice what has been termed "legally defensive medicine," ordering batteries of unnecessary X-rays and other tests, consulting with specialists and other doctors, all in order to cover themselves against possible lawsuits. This causes inconvenience for the patient, and, once again, higher medical fees. The only real beneficiaries of malpractice suits are the lawyers, who may take up to 50 percent of an award if they win. Otherwise individual patients who win cases may gain, but patients as a whole lose.[9]

The upshot of this discussion of malpractice litigation is that an attempt to increase the patient's freedom of choice in one area may, without him knowing it, compel him to accept a type of medical care that he would never have chosen voluntarily. If medical care were to become a commodity like any other the consumer would be able to make a more informed choice between doctors on the basis of fees charged, but he may also be told to have X-rays or other tests that he would not have had, were the doctor not concerned to protect himself against all eventualities. He may be sent to specialists for the same reason. In the end, he will have to pay a greatly inflated medical bill; even if a particular patient has no additional tests he will have to pay higher fees to cover his doctor's insurance premiums; and if he is insured against all these costs, his insurance premium will reflect them. Finally, it is reasonable to suppose that these practices will contribute to the further deterioration of the relationship between the doctor and his patient. The doctor will hardly be able to reveal to his patient the true reason why he is sending him off to see the specialist, or have an X-ray. The patient may fear that more is wrong with him than the doctor has said. Alternatively, he may suspect that the doctor is trying to make money from it all. Any ethical relationship is easier when nothing is hidden.

If consequences anything like those just sketched would flow from a decision to increase competition in medical care—and I freely admit that no link has been proved—we would have to think again before we decided that more competition would mean more freedom for the patient. If no patient would voluntarily choose the more competitive system with its attendant disadvantages, an increase of competition appears to be coercive rather than liberating.

There has been a lot of speculation in what I have been saying up to now. We do not have, in any countries that are even roughly comparable, systems of medical care that represent the extremes of market and nonmarket distribution. There is, however, one aspect of medical care that does allow us to compare systems that come close to being pure forms of market and nonmarket systems. I am referring to systems of obtaining human blood for medical purposes. In Britain, blood is obtained by means far removed from the market. It is neither bought nor sold. It is given, voluntarily and without reward beyond a cup of tea and a biscuit, by ordinary citizens. It is available to anyone who needs it, without charge and without obligation. The donor gains no preference over nondonors in the event of his needing blood—since enough is available for all, he needs no preference. Nor does the donor have any hope of a return favor from the recipient, not even a grateful smile. Although the gift is in one way a very intimate one—the blood that now flows in the donor's veins will soon flow in those of the recipient—the donor will never know whom he has helped. It is a gift from one stranger to another. The system is as close to a perfect example of institutionalized generosity and concern for one's fellows as can be imagined.

In the United States, only about 7 percent of the blood obtained for medical purposes comes from similarly voluntary donations. Around 40 percent is given to avoid having to pay for blood received, or to build up credit so that blood will be available without charge if needed. Approximately half of the blood and plasma obtained is bought and sold on a strictly commercial basis, like any other commodity. So completely commercial, in fact, is the operation of the commercial blood banks that when hospitals in Kansas City chose to obtain blood exclusively from a nonprofit community blood bank rather than from either of two commercial banks operating in the city, the commercial banks complained to the Federal Trade Commission. In due course the commission ruled that the community bank and the hospitals had illegally conspired together to restrain commerce in whole human blood, and ordered them to stop doing so—this despite testimony that the commercially obtained blood carried a greater risk of infecting the recipient with hepatitis.

These contrasting systems of blood collection provide us with the opportunity to ask whether the market leads to greater freedom in this area. I shall also, later, use the comparison to examine other differences between the systems, in terms of the values they further. The important thing about this comparison is that, for once, we cannot only ask the questions, but also try to answer them on the basis of some solid evidence. Thanks to Richard Titmuss's absorbing study of the subject we now have facts and figures, as well as Titmuss's own remarkable insights, to guide us.[10]

Freedom takes a variety of forms. We cannot quantify it, and so there is no immediately obvious answer to the question, "Which system provides the greater freedom?" All I can do is indicate different directions in which freedom is enhanced or diminished.

If we ask, "Under which system does the individual have the freedom to choose whether to give or sell his blood?" the answer must be that this freedom is possible only where there is a commercial blood supply system as well as a voluntary one. This aspect of the situation is the basis of the orthodox economists' claim, defended recently by Kenneth Arrow, that

> since the creation of a market increases the individual's area of choice, it therefore leads to higher benefits. Thus, if to a voluntary blood donor system we add the possibility of selling blood, we have only expanded the individual's range of alternatives. If he derives satisfaction from giving, it is argued that he can still give, and nothing has been done to impair that right.[11]

According to this orthodox economic view of freedom, once we see that the market creates this additional "freedom to sell," we need look no further, so far as the question of freedom is concerned. Why, these economists would argue, should we prevent anyone who chooses to do so from obtaining the market price for his blood, rather than giving it away? Is it not a blatant infringement of the freedom of the individual to prevent him from doing something that harms no one? Moreover, the result of allowing the market to operate freely will be, these economists believe, beneficial in other respects, such as cost and quality of supply.

In reply to this claim that the commercial system provides greater freedom, Titmuss has argued that while a commercial system allows freedom to sell, it denies the citizen his freedom to give. The notion of social rights, Titmuss says, should embrace "the right to give" in both material and nonmaterial ways.[12]

Here it seems to me that Titmuss has not expressed himself with sufficient clarity. Arrow denies the existence of any incompatibility between the right to give and the right to sell, and indeed it is not strictly accurate to say that the existence of a commercial system alongside a voluntary one denies anyone their right to give voluntarily. If we choose to give we may do so, even when others are selling. The simple right to give remains intact.

What is it, then, that Titmuss had in mind when he claimed that the existence of a commercial system denies the right to give? The point is worth exploring, because it reveals the limits of the orthodox economists' notion of freedom.

In the language of orthodox economists, we enlarge a person's freedom if we increase the choices open to him. It does not matter *why* someone chooses as he does. So long as he is able to choose, the choice is regarded as a reflection of his preferences. In fact the economist defines a person's preferences, or "revealed preferences" in terms of what he chooses. This is supposed to make economies a value-free science. Why the individual chooses as he does is something that the economist does not concern himself with. The goal is to give everyone what he prefers; never mind why he prefers what he does, or whether he will be happier once he has what he prefers.

This notion of freedom is superficial in the most literal sense of the term. It refuses to probe beneath the surface. In the particular case we are considering, this notion of freedom is satisfied in the American situation because a person can give his blood voluntarily *if* he chooses to do so. It is, on this notion of freedom, irrelevant to consider that, as Titmuss shows, the existence of a commercial system may discourage voluntary donors. It appears to discourage them, not because those who would otherwise have made voluntary donations choose to sell their blood instead if this alternative is available to them (donors and sellers are, in the main, different sections of the population), but because the fact that blood is available as a commodity, to be bought and sold, affects the nature of the gift that is made when blood is given. If blood is a commodity with a price, to give blood seems merely to save someone money—it has a cash value of a certain number of dollars. As such, the importance of the gift will vary with the wealth of the recipient. If blood cannot be bought, however, the gift of blood is a gift whose value depends on the need of the recipient. Often, it will be worth life itself. Under these circumstances giving blood becomes a very special kind of gift, an act of providing for strangers without hope of reward something that they cannot buy and without which they may die. The gift relates strangers in the community in a manner that is not possible when blood is a commodity.

All this may seem to be removed from the real world of ordinary people and hard facts. It is not. It is something of which ordinary people can be as much aware as the most unworldly philosopher. It is an idea spontaneously expressed by British blood donors themselves, in response to a questionnaire Titmuss gave them which asked why they first decided to become a blood donor. As one woman, a machine operator, wrote in reply:

> You cant get blood from supermarkets and chaine stores. People them selves must come forword, sick people cant get out of bed to ask you for a pint to save thier life so I came forword in hope to help somebody who needs blood.

A company secretary answered, with better spelling but less warmth:

> I feel that with blood it would have to be used for the purposes it was given, no deductions for administrative purposes like so many Charity Organizations. Blood is something which could not come out of the rates.

Other donors expressed a wish to help the National Health Service. In some cases they indicated that they had been helped, either by the Health Service generally, or by blood transfusions specifically, and they now wanted to do something in return. With others, the motivation was that they might themselves once need the assistance of a stranger, and if they were then to have a moral right to receive it, they felt that they should themselves give when they had the opportunity.[13]

The implication of some of these answers is clear: even if these people had had the formal right to give to a voluntary program that existed alongside commercial blood banks, their gift would have lost much of its significance, and they may well not have given at all. The fact that blood is a commodity, that if no one gives it, it can still be bought, makes altruism unnecessary, and so loosens the bonds that can otherwise exist between strangers in the community.

The accuracy of this interpretation of the effect of a commercial blood system on a voluntary one is borne out by statistics on voluntary donations in England and Wales, as compared with countries where commercial systems now exist, like the United States and Japan. In all three countries there has been a sharp rise in the need for blood in recent years. In England and Wales, donations have increased sufficiently to cover this increased demand, and the National Blood Transfusion Board "has never consciously been aware of a shortage, or an impending shortage, of potential donors."[14] In the United States, on the other hand, voluntary donations have not only failed to keep pace with the increased demand, they have actually fallen in absolute terms. In New York, for instance, the only city to have published sufficient figures to indicate a trend, voluntary community donations fell from 20 percent of total supplies in 1956 to 1 percent in 1966. The rise in commercial supplies has not been sufficient to compensate for this fall, and serious shortages have resulted, frequently forcing surgery to be postponed.[15]

In Japan the decline in voluntary donors has been still more abrupt. Apparently donors were not paid until 1951, when the need to supply blood to American forces in Korea led to the introduction of payment. Now 98 percent of all blood is paid for, and the shortage of blood is said to be still more critical than in the United States.[16]

So it appears that where payment for blood does not exist the number of donors has kept pace with the sharp rise in demand; but where the opportunity to give is forced to coexist with the opportunity to sell, the number of volunteers declines and can only with difficulty, if at all, be made good by increases in the amount of blood bought. A reasonable conclusion to draw from these facts is that to make blood a commodity does discourage voluntary donors, while a purely voluntary system fosters altruism in a way that a mixed commercial and voluntary system does not.

The upshot of all this, so far as freedom is concerned, is complex. I have already conceded that the creation of a commercial system alongside a voluntary one allows people to sell their blood, while leaving them formally free to give it voluntarily, if they so desire. But Titmuss's idea that the creation of a commercial system threatens the right to give is not so much mistaken as inadequately developed. The right that Titmuss sees threatened is not the simple right to give, but the right to give "in nonmaterial as well as material ways." This means not merely the right to give money or some commodity that can be bought or sold for a certain amount of money, but the right to give something that cannot be bought, that has no cash value, and must be given freely if it is to be obtained at all. This right, if it is a right—it would be better to say, this freedom—really is incompatible with the freedom to sell, and we cannot avoid denying one of these freedoms when we grant the other.[17]

Even if we discount the value of this "freedom to give in nonmaterial terms" I think the facts I have presented bear out my claim that the orthodox economists' notion of freedom is superficial. What is more important: whether Americans have the formal freedom to give their blood, if they so desire, or whether the conditions under which blood may be given are such as to tap the resources of altruism and community feeling that Americans may be presumed to have to the same degree as Britons? The fact that many people who would otherwise give blood will not do so if it can be bought should not be ignored or brushed aside. To say that this decision is the individual's free choice and that so long as a person can give if he chooses to do so freedom is maximized is to take a naïve view of the nature of choice. We know that social circumstances affect individual choices. Therefore we must either deepen our notion of freedom, so as to recognize that certain kinds of social conditions restrict freedom, or else acknowledge that freedom is an idea with form but no substance. If we take the latter view, it would seem that freedom, considered apart from the circumstances in which it is exercised, is less important than it is usually thought to be. In my opinion it is the former course that is the sounder one. In deepening our notion of freedom, we recognize that the individual does not make his decision in a vacuum, and that the social policies we pursue affect the decisions individuals make. We cannot say that it will determine the decision of any given individual, but we know that statistically it will alter a number of decisions. Knowing this, we cannot pretend we do not know it, and say that by not interfering with the market we are leaving the decision up to the individual. To decide not to interfere is to make a decision that affects individual choices just as the decision to interfere does.

UTILITY

Titmuss's study of blood supply systems helps us to explore other issues apart from that of freedom that are important to the whole area of health care. In particular, it enables us to assess the utility of market and nonmarket systems, and to ask which leads to the greater good in the long run.

Marx suggested that money, by converting human requirements into commodities, degrades and dehumanizes us:

> If money is the bond binding me to human life, binding society to me, binding me and nature and man, is not money the bond of all bonds? Can it not dissolve and bind all ties? Is it not, therefore, the universal agent of separation? . . . Money then appears as this overturning power both against the individual and against the bonds of society, etc., which claim to be

essences in themselves. It transforms fidelity into infidelity, love into hate, hate into love, virtue into vice.... Assume man to be man and his relationship to the world to be a human one: then you can exchange love only for love, trust for trust, etc.[18]

The area of blood supply offers remarkably concrete illustrations of Marx's insight. We have already seen that the market may hamper the expression of a desire to help strangers. It can also be shown, very simply, that the market in this area does indeed turn truth into falsity, virtue into vice, and a life-saving gift into a deadly poison. Not all blood is of the same quality. Some diseases may be passed from donor to recipient in a transfusion. It is possible to test for some diseases in a laboratory, but not for all. Of those that it is not possible to check, by far the most important is serum hepatitis. The only way to eliminate or substantially reduce the risk of serum hepatitis is to ask the donor or seller about his medical history and social habits. When asked these questions, the voluntary donor has no reason to lie. He does not want his gift to harm anyone. His interests and those of the recipient are in harmony. The would-be seller, however, does have an incentive to lie. If he tells the truth he may be unable to sell his commodity. His private interests conflict with those of the recipient of his blood. The resulting lack of truthfulness, combined with the fact that those who sell blood are usually from social groups with a higher incidence of hepatitis than the population as a whole, produces an incidence of hepatitis following transfusions of commercially obtained blood that is many times higher than the incidence following the use of donated blood. One carefully controlled study of patients undergoing cardiac surgery, in which an average of eighteen or nineteen pints of blood are used, showed that a group using commercial blood had an incidence of hepatitis of 55 percent, while a similar group using voluntarily donated blood had no cases at all. Although such exceptionally high rates occur only when a lot of blood is used, only one pint of which needs to be infected, other studies suggest a general rate of infection at least four times as high in the United States as in Britain, while in Japan the situation is still worse.[19] There seems to be no means by which the market mechanism can equal the performance of the voluntary system in this respect.

There are other areas in which the voluntary system works better than its rival. We have already seen that the voluntary system has been able to procure enough blood to meet rising needs, while commercial systems have not. (The United States, incidentally, is now starting to import some of its blood requirements from Latin America, whose inhabitants have a greater need for money than U.S. citizens, but less protein to replace what they give.) The voluntary system also produces blood more cheaply. Titmuss estimates that commercially obtained blood in the U.S. is between five and fifteen times as expensive to the consumer as blood is to the nation in Britain. (To the consumer, of course, it is free.)

In addition to these straightforward advantages, there is also a more subtle one. The nature of a community depends on the nature of the people who make up the community, and this in turn will depend to some extent on the institutions of the community and the attitudes that these institutions foster. Institutions that put a money value on everything, that restrict ways in which strangers can assist each other, and that set the interest of one man against the interests of another, are consonant with a materialistic community in which each looks out only for his own interests. Such institutions are both the product of such a society and a factor in its continuance. Institutions that facilitate the expression of a desire to help others, and distribute goods according to need, are a means of preserving and fostering attitudes of concern for one's fellows. Controlled experiments suggest that people are more likely to behave altruistically when they observe altruism on the part of others;[20] on a personal level I have found that nothing brings out my better impulses as well as being with others who habitually act out of generosity and consideration for others. A society with institutions that foster altruism may therefore expect to reap further benefits. There may be no direct link between the amount of blood donated voluntarily in London and New York, and the crime rates in these cities; but both sets of figures point in the same direction, and they say similar things about human relations in the two cities.

Let us now turn our attention from this particular aspect of health care back to health care in general. Prior to embarking on the discussion of blood supply systems, I drew attention to some of the consequences that might follow from making health care more competitive than it is at present in the United States. I think I have raised sufficient doubts about the desirability of so doing. Should we then take medical care out of the marketplace altogether? Is the British National Health Service a model to follow, as the British National Transfusion Service is? Somewhat different issues are raised by this question.

A NATIONAL HEALTH SERVICE?

A national health service must be financed by taxation. It does, therefore, limit the freedom of the taxpayer to decide for himself how much he shall spend on health, and how much on other items. Of course, other welfare measures like social security do the same, in their own area. There is, however, a prima facie case against such a restriction. What can be said in defense of the restriction in this case?

First, it may be that the community, acting together, can achieve goods that the individual could not achieve, no matter how much he decided to spend on health care. We have already seen examples of this in respect of obtaining cheap, uncontaminated blood and obtaining medical services that have not been distorted by the threat of malpractice suits. There are many other ways in which the special nature of medical care may make it unsuited to market control. For instance, the market's answer to the uncertainty of an individual's need for extensive medical care is private insurance. Private insurance, however, tends to be extremely expensive for ordinary visits to a doctor, because a doctor, in the privacy of his office, is not subject to supervision from his peers or anyone else, and so might prescribe unnecessary treatment in order to increase his remuneration from the insurance company. One consequence of this is that most people are insured for hospital visits, but not for office visits; and a consequence of this is that some medical care now takes place in hospitals that would be done more economically in the patient's home or the doctor's office. The ultimate consequence is that the consumer pays more for his medical insurance.

This difficulty is not one that can be eliminated simply by a system of national health insurance like those envisaged in recent congressional bills. These proposals would retain the principle of paying the doctor for each treatment, and this would leave the system wide open to abuse if it covered office visits, unless there were a huge and expensive system of inspectors. On the other hand, if the scheme does not cover office visits, it will accelerate the trend to increased hospitalization.

This problem can be avoided under a national health service, by paying the doctor on some basis other than the cost of the treatment he prescribes. In Britain, for example, doctors are paid according to the number of patients on their roll, with a lower payment per patient after a certain figure is reached to discourage excessively large rolls, and an absolute ceiling at a higher point, to prohibit unworkably large practices. Admittedly there are drawbacks to this method too, for a doctor gets paid even if he does very little for his patients. A complaints procedure and the possibility of patients transferring to another doctor may curb this tendency. A more important restraint is the bond of an ethical relationship between doctor and patient that has not been eroded by the commercialization of medical practice.

Another frequently cited drawback of proposals for either a national health service or national insurance is that the patient has no disincentive to prevent him visiting a doctor as often as he likes, since he does not pay for it. In fact, British statistics do not bear out this fear; although the figures are not comprehensive enough to give a decisive answer, they do not appear to show any rise in demand per patient since the inauguration of the National Health Service.[21] Perhaps the explanation for this is that the overutilization that one might expect from a few people is compensated for by the practice of preventative medicine. Prevention is, as the saying goes, better than cure, and a patient who goes for a regular checkup, or when he first notices something wrong, may in the end be much less expensive to treat than one who puts off a visit to the doctor until he is seriously ill. One thing that is certain is that Britain spends a smaller percentage of its Gross National Product on health than the United States does, despite the fact that health is free to all in Britain. Quite apart from the question of expense, though, it should be asked how many cases of overutilization are needed to offset one case of a patient who dies because he postponed seeking treatment in order to save money.

Another possible justification for a national health service is that it is an effective means of redistributing income, since it may be paid for by a progressively graduated income tax, and distributed to all irrespective of income. The poorest, especially, are assisted, since they will pay little or no tax, and receive essential services that they could not otherwise afford. It is hardly necessary to describe the distress that a person may feel if he requires medical care but is unable to afford it. The security and peace of mind that arises from knowing that one will never be in this situation is one of the greatest benefits that a society can bestow on its poorer citizens. Indeed, the heights that medical expenses have reached in this country recently mean that it is not only the poor, but also those in the middle income bracket, that require this security. Senator Ribicoff, in *The American Medical Machine*, cites the case of a family that received a bill of $4600 for the four and a half days their father had been in hospital before he died. Medical bills are now a major factor in bankruptcies: in Tulsa, Oklahoma, a survey showed that they account for 60 percent of all bankruptcies.[22]

Conservative economists are not necessarily opposed to some measure of redistribution, especially if it is designed to improve the condition of the very poor. Milton Friedman, in *Capitalism and Freedom*, goes so far as to advocate a negative income tax. This would mean redistribution in cash rather than services. Friedman prefers cash because he thinks it makes for more freedom, leaving it up to the individual to spend his money as he likes. He may choose to spend it on health insurance, or he may choose whatever else he desires.

I have already suggested that the freedom of the individual is limited by the marketplace in subtle ways that Friedman and his likeminded colleagues overlook. Still, we must admit once again that there is *some* truth in what Friedman says here; and if we wish to defend a national health service on redistributive grounds, we should admit that there is an element of paternalism in so doing. If we give benefits to the poor in services rather than cash, it is at least partly because we believe that they will be better off with the services; and that even if they were able to buy adequate medical services with the money we gave them, some at least would spend it less prudently, so as to gain short-term satisfactions at a cost of greater distress and suffering in the long run.

Friedman grants that a paternalist position is internally consistent, but he associates it with dictatorship and insists that "those who believe in freedom must believe also in the freedom of individuals to make their own mistakes." Paternalism, Friedman says, is an arrogant position, while the liberal displays humility in refusing to decide for others what is good for them.[23] The standpoint from which Friedman criticizes paternalism, however, is the same superficial liberalism that we encountered earlier. Friedman does not inquire into the social conditions and circumstances in which the poor decide how to spend their money. He does not consider the effect of being brought up in a family that never had the habit of providing for the future because there was never more than enough to provide for the present. He does not consider that alcoholism, drug addiction, or gambling may be factors in producing poverty. Is the alcoholic free to choose whether to invest his money in health insurance? He is not; and there are many others who for a variety of reasons are scarcely more able to make an informed, carefully considered, long-term choice. How often do we have to watch people do something that they come to regret bitterly when it is too late to do anything about it, before we can say to the next person about to do the same thing that he is making a mistake? Is it really arrogant to claim that we may sometimes know what is in another person's interests better than he does himself? Or is it merely an honest appreciation of a fact that stares us in the face, a fact that could hardly be denied were it not for a prevailing mythology that demands that we do deny it?

The final justification for overriding the freedom of each to spend his income as he prefers is one that relates to a theme that has run through this chapter: the nature of the community that we live in. Here we must consider whether it is not desirable that a community be integrated in certain fundamental areas of life, rather than being divided along lines of class or race. As Brian Barry has noted, the promotion of this value distinguishes a national health service from a system of universal insurance that provides standard sums of money for given treatments, while leaving doctors and hospitals to charge what they will, and the patient to make up the difference if he selects a doctor or hospital that charges above the standard amount. This insurance system would provide a basic level of care for everyone.[24] I do not agree with Barry that this value is the *only* one that distinguishes these two systems of providing health care (I have suggested others in this chapter); but it is true that universal insurance would provide many of the benefits of a national health service, including redistribution and the provision of security for all against the threat of ruinous expenditure on medical care. What the insurance proposal could not do, however, is provide an integrated health service that is used by people of all classes and races. We would still have one standard of care for the wealthy and another for the poor.

How important is integration in the area of medicine? It does not seem to be as important as in education, for it does not determine a person's opportunities for the whole of his life to the extent that education does (although medicine may do this in exceptional cases). Still, there are important reasons for desiring integration in medicine too. As Barry says, "so long as those with money can buy exemption from the common lot the rulers and the generally dominant groups in a society will have little motive for making sure that the public facilities are of good quality." In other words, if we want good public facilities, we have to ensure that those who can complain effectively when standards are allowed to drop use the facilities.

A more fundamental aspect of integration is that it makes a substantial difference to the image that we have of our community. The knowledge that when it comes to vital things like medical care we are all in it together, and your money cannot buy you anything that I am not equally entitled to, may do a good deal to mitigate the effects of inequality in other less vital areas, and create the atmosphere of community concern for all that I have already discussed.

This last consideration is the first one we have encountered that goes beyond even what the British National Health Service has achieved. Private medicine does exist in Britain, and very wealthy people do sometimes get treatment that the National Health Service does not provide. Money may allow one to go down to London and be operated on by an outstanding surgeon, while a person who could not afford this would have to accept the general level of surgery in the area in which he lived. Yet this is not a major problem. Because of the generally high standard of treatment that the National Health Service provides at no cost, and the high costs of private medicine, only a very few people avail themselves of private treatment. Of those who do, by no means all actually do receive treatment that is superior to that offered by the National Health Service. So long as private medicine remains such a minor part of health care as a whole, it does not seem necessary to take the step of prohibiting it altogether. Allowing private medicine to exist, can, as Barry suggests, be seen as a reasonable compromise between the values of freedom and integration.

Notes to Chapter Eleven

1. Abraham Ribicoff, *The American Medical Machine* (New York: Harrow Books, 1972), p. 10.

2. Karl Marx, *Critique of the Gotha Programme*, various editions.

3. F.A. Hayek, *Constitution of Liberty* (Chicago: University of Chicago Press, 1960); M. Freidman, *Capitalism and Freedom* (Chicago: University of Chicago Press, 1962).

4. Kenneth Arrow, "Uncertainty and the Welfare Economics of Medical Care," *American Economic Review*, vol. 53, 1963, 941-73. See also R.M. Titmuss, *Commitment to Welfare* (New York: Pantheon Books, 1968), pp. 145-47.

5. Dr. F.G. Dickenson, Head of the A.M.A. Bureau of Medical Economic Research, quoted in Titmuss, p. 249.

6. *Village Voice* (New York), February 21, 1974.

7. Ribicoff, p. 116. For a fuller account, see the report of the Senate Subcommittee on Executive Reorganization and Government Research, *Medical Malpractice: The Patient versus the Physician*.

8. *New York Times*, January 8, 1974.

9. Ribicoff, ch. 5. See also R.M. Titmuss, *The Gift Relationship* (London: Allen and Unwin, 1970), pp. 167-70.

10. R.M. Titmuss, *The Gift Relationship*. I have previously discussed some of the issues that follow in "Altruism and Commerce: A Defense of Titmuss against Arrow," *Philosophy and Public Affairs*, Vol. 2, 1973, pp. 312-20.

11. Kenneth Arrow, "Gifts and Exchanges," *Philosophy and Public Affairs*, Vol. 1, 343-62.

12. Titmuss, *The Gift Relationship*, p. 242.

13. Ibid., pp. 226-36.
14. Ibid., p. 120.
15. Ibid., pp. 39-40, 59, 96.
16. Ibid., p. 156.
17. I did not fully recognize this incompatibility in the work referred to in n. 10, above.
18. Karl Marx, *The Economic and Philosophic Manuscripts of 1844*, trans. by M. Milligan, ed. D.J. Struik, New York, International Publishers, 1967, pp. 167-69.
19. Titmuss, *The Gift Relationship*, ch. 8.
20. A summary of some experiments that lead to this conclusion may be found in D. Wright, *The Psychology of Moral Behavior* (London and Baltimore: Penguin Books, 1971), pp. 133-39. Arrow, in "Gifts and Exchanges," writes of the risk that we will "use up recklessly the scarce resources of altruistic motivation," but he offers no support whatsoever for the view that altruism is, like oil, a commodity of which the more we use the less we have.
21. R.M. Titmuss, *Essays on 'The Welfare State'* (London: Unwin University Books, new ed., 1963), p. 174. Titmuss notes also that the introduction of "Major Medical Expense Insurance" in the United States did apparently lead to an increase in demand for treatment.
22. Ribicoff, pp. 11, 12.
23. Friedman, pp. 187-88.
24. Brian Barry, *Political Argument* (New York: The Humanities Press, 1965), ch. VII.

**Part II:
Ethics and Allocating
Scarce Medical
Resources**

PREAMBLE

The fundamental ethical issues of the conflict between the individual and society, the competing interpretations of justice, and the right to health care must have an impact on a national health care policy. In addition to the global questions, they give rise to more specific questions of allocation of scarce resources. The chapters in this part of the volume explore the problems of resource allocation, first looking at the process of allocation itself and then at one specific and dramatic example.

James Childress asks the question "Who Shall Live When Not All Can Live?" After exploring alternatives for distributing scarce, life-saving medical resources on the basis of criteria such as medical acceptability, social worth, and various methods of random allocation, he argues for the principle "first come, first served" after a group has been established who would be "medically acceptable patients." Frederic B. Westervelt responds to Childress's proposal, offering what he calls a "view from within." He rejects the Childress position in favor of the view that triage decisions should remain the responsibility of those running the medical program—that is, the physicians and medical administrators. "The key to responsible actions," he claims, "lies with the responsible physician."

The next chapter in this part of the book is an excerpt from a study by a government advisory panel established to examine the dramatic policy question raised by the possibility of producing a totally implantable artificial human heart. With demand running perhaps as high as 50,000 per year in the United States alone, the totally implantable artificial human heart could well become the medical device that either breaks the health care system or forces the society to redefine its health care priorities. The excerpt selected first presents the factual background and then poses the policy problems: Can we afford the billions of dollars required? Can we set criteria for selection of a privileged group of recipients? Can we permit anyone to have this life-saving device if all cannot have it? Can we choose a cheaper nuclear power source for the heart if it exposed nonrecipients to additional radiation exposure risk? The artificial heart is only one of a large number of expensive, scarce, life-saving medical technologies. It is presented here as a case study of allocation problems to come.

The final chapter of this part of the volume is a criticism by Clark C. Havighurst of the artificial heart report. As a member of the assessment panel, he accuses the panel members as a body of not giving sufficient attention to a conceptual framework for making ethical choices. In particular he believes an artificial heart policy could be justified while still appealing to "a pure utilitarian approach," where potential net gains are made to exceed potential net losses. He extends this criticism to the panel's rejection of the nuclear-powered artificial heart, concluding that the panel's basis for rejecting the nuclear-powered heart violates the principles of justice.

※ *Chapter 12*

Who Shall Live When Not All Can Live?

James F. Childress

Who shall live when not all can live? Although this question has been urgently forced upon us by the dramatic use of artificial internal organs and organ transplantations, it is hardly new. George Bernard Shaw dealt with it in *The Doctor's Dilemma:*

> Sir Patrick. Well, Mr. Savior of Lives: which is it to be? that honest decent man Blenkinsop, or that rotten blackguard of an artist, eh?
> Ridgeon. It's not an easy case to judge, is it? Blenkinsop's an honest decent man; but is he any use? Dubedat's a rotten blackguard; but he's a genuine source of pretty and pleasant and good things.
> Sir Patrick. What will he be a source of for that poor innocent wife of his, when she finds him out?
> Ridgeon. That's true. Her life will be a hell.
> Sir Patrick. And tell me this. Suppose you had this choice put before you: either to go through life and find all the pictures bad but all the men and women good, or go through life and find all the pictures good and all the men and women rotten. Which would you choose?[1]

A significant example of the distribution of scarce medical resources is seen in the use of penicillin shortly after its discovery. Military officers had to determine which soldiers would be treated—those with venereal disease or those wounded in combat.[2] In many respects such decisions have become routine in medical circles. Day after day physicians and others make judgments and decisions "about allocations of medical care to various segments of our population, to various types of hospitalized patients, and to specific individuals,"[3] for example, whether mental illness or cancer will receive the higher proportion of available funds. Nevertheless, the dramatic forms of "Scarce Life-Saving Medical Resources" (hereafter abbreviated as SLMR) such as hemodialysis and kidney and heart transplants have compelled us to examine the moral questions that have been concealed in many routine decisions. I shall not attempt in this chapter to show how a resolution of SLMR cases can help us in the more routine ones that do not involve a conflict of life with life. Rather I shall develop an argument for a particular method of determining who shall live when not all can live. No conclusions are implied about criteria and procedures for determining who shall receive medical resources that are not directly related to the preservation of life (e.g. corneal transplants) or about standards for allocating money and time for studying and treating certain diseases.

Just as current SLMR decisions are not totally discontinuous with other medical decisions, so we must ask whether some other cases might, at least by analogy, help us develop the needed criteria and procedures. Some have looked at the principles at work in our responses to abortion, euthanasia, and artificial insemination.[4] Usually they have concluded that these cases do not cast light on the selection of patients for artificial and transplanted organs. The reason is evident: in abortion, euthanasia, and artificial insemination, there is no conflict of life with life for limited but indispensable resources (with the possible exception of therapeutic abortion). In current SLMR decisions, such a conflict is inescapable, and it makes them morally perplexing and fascinating. If analogous cases are to be found, I think that we shall locate them in moral conflict situations.

ANALOGOUS CONFLICT SITUATIONS

An especially interesting and pertinent one is *U.S. v. Holmes.*[5] In 1841 an American ship, the *William Brown*, which was near Newfoundland on a trip from Liverpool to Philadelphia, struck an iceberg. The crew and half the passengers were able to escape in the two available vessels. One of these, a longboat, carrying too many passengers and leaking seriously, began to founder in the turbulent sea after about twenty-four hours. In a desperate attempt to keep it from sinking, the crew threw overboard fourteen men. Two sisters of one of the men either jumped overboard to join their brother in death or instructed the crew to throw them over. The criteria for determining who should live were "not to part man and wife, and not to throw over any women." Several hours later the others were rescued. Returning to Philadelphia, most of the crew disappeared, but one, Holmes, who had acted upon orders from the mate, was indicted, tried, and convicted on the charge of "unlawful homicide."

We are interested in this case from a moral rather than a legal standpoint, and there are several possible responses to and judgments about it. The judge contended that lots should have been cast, for in such conflict situations, there is no other procedure "so consonant both to humanity and to justice." Counsel for Holmes, on the other hand, maintained that the "sailors adopted the only principle of selection which was possible in an emergency like theirs,—a principle more humane than lots."

Another version of selection might extend and systematize the maxims of the sailors in the direction of "utility"; those are saved who will contribute to the greatest good for the greatest number. Yet another possible option is defended by Edmond Cahn in *The Moral Decision.* He argues that in this case we encounter the "morals of the last days." By this phrase he indicates that an apocalyptic crisis renders totally irrelevant the normal differences between individuals. He continues,

> In a strait of this extremity, all men are reduced—or raised, as one may choose to denominate it—to members of the genus, mere congeners and nothing else. Truly and literally, all were "in the same boat," and thus none could be saved separately from the others. I am driven to conclude that otherwise—that is, if none sacrifice themselves of free will to spare the others—they must all wait and die together. For where all have become congeners, pure and simple, no one can save himself by killing another.[6]

Cahn's answer to the question "who shall live when not all can live" is "none" unless the voluntary sacrifice by some persons permits it.

Few would deny the importance of Cahn's approach, although many, including this writer, would suggest that it is relevant mainly as an affirmation of an elevated and, indeed, heroic or saintly morality that one hopes would find expression in the voluntary actions of many persons trapped in "borderline" situations involving a conflict of life with life. It is a maximal demand that some moral principles impose on the individual in the recognition that self-preservation is not a good that is to be defended at all costs. The absence of this saintly or heroic morality should not mean, however, that everyone perishes. Without making survival an absolute value and without justifying all means to achieve it, we can maintain that simply letting everyone die is irresponsible. This charge can be supported from several different standpoints, including society at large as well as the individuals involved. Among a group of self-interested individuals, none of whom volunteers to relinquish his life, there may be better and worse ways of determining who shall survive. One task of social ethics, whether religious or philosophical, is to propose relatively just institutional arrangements within which self-interested and biased men can live. The question then becomes: which set of arrangements—which criteria and procedures of selection—is most satisfactory in view of the human condition (man's limited altruism and inclination to seek his own good) and the conflicting values that are to be realized?

There are several significant differences between the *Holmes* and SLMR cases, a major one being that the former involves *direct* killing of another person, while the latter involve only *permitting* a person to die when it is not possible to save all. Furthermore, in extreme situations such as *Holmes*, the restraints of civilization have been stripped away, and something approximating a state of nature prevails, in which life is "solitary, poor, nasty, brutish and short." The state of nature does not mean that moral standards are irrelevant and that might should prevail, but it does suggest that much of the matrix that normally supports morality has been removed. Also, the necessary but unfortunate decisions about who shall live and die are made by men who are existentially and personally involved in the outcome. Their survival too is at stake. Even though the institutional role of sailors seems to require greater sacrificial actions, there is obviously no assurance that they will adequately assess the number of sailors required to man the vessel or that they will impartially and objectively weigh the common good at stake. As the judge insisted in his defense of casting lots in the *Holmes* case: "In no other than this [casting lots] or some like way are those having equal rights put upon an equal footing, and in no other way is it possible to guard against partiality and oppression, violence, and conflict." This difference should not be exaggerated, since self-interest, professional pride, and the like obviously affect the outcome of many medical decisions. Nor do the remaining differences cancel *Holmes*'s instructiveness.

CRITERIA OF SELECTION FOR SLMR

Which set of arrangements should be adopted for SLMR? Two questions are involved: Which standards and criteria should be used? and, Who should make the decision? The first question is basic, since the debate about implementation, e.g. whether by a lay committee or physician, makes little progress until the criteria are determined.

We need two sets of criteria, which will be applied at two different stages in the selection of recipients of SLMR. First, medical criteria should be used to exclude those who are not "medically acceptable." Second, from this group of "medically acceptable" applicants, the final selection can be made. Occasionally in current American medical practice, the first stage is omitted, but such an omission is unwarranted. Ethical and social responsibility would seem to require distributing these SLMR only to those who have some reasonable prospect of responding to the treatment. Furthermore, in transplants such medical tests as tissue and blood typing are necessary, although they are hardly fully developed.

"Medical acceptability" is not as easily determined as many nonphysicians assume, since there is considerable debate in medical circles about the relevant factors (e.g., age and complicating diseases). Although ethicists can contribute little or nothing to this debate, two proposals may be in order. First, "medical acceptability" should be used only to determine the group from which the final selection will be made, and the attempt to establish fine degrees of prospective response to treatment should be avoided. Medical criteria, then, would exclude some applicants but would not serve as a basis of comparison between those who pass the first stage. For example, if two applicants for dialysis were medically acceptable, the physicians would *not* choose the one with the *better* medical prospects. Final selection would be made on other grounds. Second, psychological and environmental factors should be kept to an absolute minimum and should be considered only when they are without doubt critically related to medical acceptability (e.g., the inability to cope with the requirements of dialysis, which might lead to suicide).[7]

The most significant moral questions emerge when we turn to the final selection. Once the pool of medically acceptable applicants has been defined and still the number is larger than the resources, what other criteria should be used? How should the final selection be made? First, I shall examine some of the difficulties that stem from efforts to make the final selection in terms of social value; these difficulties raise serious doubts about the feasibility and justifiability of the utilitarian approach. Then I shall consider the possible justification for random selection or chance.

Occasionally criteria of social worth focus on past contributions, but most often they are primarily future-oriented. The patient's potential and probable contribution to the society is stressed, although this obviously cannot be abstracted from his present web of relationships (e.g., dependents) and occupational activities (e.g., nuclear physicist). Indeed, the magnitude of his contribution to society (as an abstraction) is measured in terms of these social roles, relations, and functions. Enough has already been said to suggest the tremendous range of factors that affect social value or worth. (I am excluding from consideration the question of the ability to pay, because most of the people involved have to secure funds from other sources, public or private, anyway. Legislation in 1972 provided payment for most persons who need kidney dialysis or transplantation.) Here we encounter the first major difficulty of this approach: How do we determine the relevant criteria of social value?

The difficulties of quantifying various social needs are only too obvious. How does one quantify and compare the needs of the spirit (e.g., education, art, religion), political life, economic activity, technological development? Joseph Fletcher suggests that "some day we may learn how to 'quantify' or 'mathematicate' or 'computerize' the value problem in selection, in the same careful and thorough way that diagnosis has been."[8] I am not convinced that we can ever quantify values, or that we should attempt to do so. But even if the various social and human needs, in principle, could be quantified, how do we determine how much weight we will give to each one? Which will have priority in case of conflict? Or even more basically, in the light of which values and principles do we recognize social "needs"?

One possible way of determining the values that should be emphasized in selection has been proposed by Leo Shatin.[9] He insists that our medical decisions about allocating resources are already based on an unconscious scale of values (usually dominated by material worth). Since there is really no way of escaping this, we should be self-conscious and critical about it. How should we proceed? He recommends that we discover the values that most people in our society hold and then use them as criteria for distributing SLMR. These values can be discovered by attitude or opinion surveys. Presumably if 51 percent in this testing period put a greater premium on military needs than technological development, military men would have a greater claim on our SLMR than experimental researchers. But valuations of what is significant change, and the student revolutionary who was denied SLMR in 1970 might be celebrated in 1990 as the greatest American hero since George Washington.

Shatin presumably is seeking criteria that could be applied nationally, but at the present, regional and local as well as individual prejudices tincture the criteria of social value that are used in selection. Nowhere is this more evident than in the deliberations and decisions of the anonymous selection committee of the Seattle Artificial Kidney Center, where such factors as church membership and Scout leadership have been deemed significant for determining who shall live.[10] As two critics conclude after examining these criteria and procedures, they rule out "creative nonconformists, who rub the bourgeoisie the wrong way but who historically have contributed so much to the making of America. The Pacific Northwest is no place for a Henry David Thoreau with bad kidneys."[11]

Closely connected to this first problem of determining social value is a second one. Not only is it difficult if not impossible to reach agreement on social value, but it is also rarely easy to predict what our needs will be in a few years and what the consequences of present actions will be. Furthermore it is difficult to predict which persons will fulfill their potential function in society. Admissions committees in colleges and universities experience the frustrations of predicting realization of potential. For these reasons, as someone has indicated, God might be a utilitarian, but we cannot be. We simply lack the capacity to predict very accurately the consequences which we then must evaluate. Our incapacity is never more evident than when we think in societal terms.

Other difficulties make us even less confident that such an approach to SLMR is advisable. Many critics raise the specter of abuse, but this should not be overemphasized. The fundamental difficulty appears on another level: the utilitarian approach would in effect reduce the person to his social role, relations, and functions. Ultimately it dulls and perhaps even eliminates the sense of the person's transcendence, his dignity as a person that cannot be reduced to his past or future contribution to society. It is not at all clear that we are willing to live with these implications of utilitarian selection. Wilhelm Kolff, who invented the artificial kidney, has asked: "Do we really subscribe to the principle that social standing should determine selection? Do we allow patients to be treated with dialysis only when they are married, go to church, have children, have a job, a good income and give to the Community Chest?"[12]

The German theologian Helmut Thielicke contends that any search for "objective criteria" for selection is already a capitulation to the utilitarian point of view which violates man's dignity.[13] The solution is not to let all die, but to recognize that SLMR cases are "borderline situations" which inevitably involve guilt. The agent, however, can have courage and freedom (which, for Thielicke, come from justification by faith) and can

> go ahead anyway and seek for criteria for deciding the question of life or death in the matter of the artificial kidney. Since these criteria are ... questionable, necessarily alien to the meaning of human existence, the decision to which they lead can be little more than that arrived at by casting lots.[14]

The resulting criteria, he suggests, will probably be very similar to those already employed in American medical practice.

He is most concerned to preserve a certain *attitude* or *disposition* in SLMR—the sense of guilt that arises when man's dignity is violated. With this sense of guilt, the agent remains "sound and healthy where it really counts."[15] Thielicke uses man's dignity only as a judgmental, critical, and negative standard. It only tells us how all selection criteria and procedures (and even the refusal to act) implicate us in the ambiguity of the human condition and its metaphysical guilt. This approach is consistent with his view of the task of theological ethics: "to teach us how to understand and endure—not 'solve'—the borderline situation."[16] But ethics, I would contend, can help us discern the factors and norms in whose light relative, discriminate judgments can be made. Even if all actions in SLMR should involve guilt, some may preserve human dignity to a greater extent than others. Thielicke recognizes that a decision based on any criteria is "little more than that arrived at by casting lots." But perhaps selection by chance would come the closest to embodying the moral and nonmoral values that we are trying to maintain (including a sense of man's dignity).

THE VALUES OF RANDOM SELECTION

My proposal is that we use some form of randomness or chance (either natural, such as "first come, first served," or artificial, such as a lottery) to determine who shall be saved. Many reject randomness as a surrender to nonrationality when responsible and rational judgments can and must be made. Edmond Cahn criticizes "Holmes' judge" who recommended the casting of lots because, as Cahn puts it, "the crisis involves stakes too high for gambling and responsibilities too deep for destiny."[17] Similarly, other critics see randomness as a surrender to "non-human" forces which necessarily vitiates human values. Sometimes these values are identified with the process of decision-making (e.g., it is important to have persons rather than impersonal forces determining who shall live). Sometimes they are identified with the outcome of the process (e.g., the features such as creativity and fullness of being that make human life what it is are to be considered and respected in the decision). Regarding the former, it must be admitted that the use of chance seems cold and impersonal. But presumably the defenders of utilitarian criteria in SLMR want to make their application as objective and impersonal as possible so that subjective bias does not determine who shall live.

Such criticisms, however, ignore the moral and nonmoral values that might be supported by selection by randomness or chance. A more important criticism is that the procedure that I develop draws the relevant moral context too narrowly. That context, so the argument might run, includes the society and its future and not merely the individual with his illness and claim upon SLMR. But my contention is that the values and principles at work in the narrower context may well take precedence over those operative in the broader context, both because of their weight and significance and because of the weaknesses of selection in terms of social worth. As Paul Freund rightly insists, "The more nearly total is the estimate to be made of an individual, and the more nearly the consequence determines life and death, the more unfit the judgment becomes for human reckoning.... Randomness as a moral principle deserves serious study."[18] Serious study would, I think, point toward its implementation in certain conflict situations, primarily because it preserves a significant degree of *personal dignity* by providing *equality* of opportunity. Thus it cannot be dismissed as a "nonrational" and "nonhuman" procedure without an inquiry into the reasons, including human values, which might justify it. Paul Ramsey stresses this point about the *Holmes* case:

> Instead of fixing our attention upon "gambling" as the solution—with all the frivolous and often corrupt associations the word raises in our minds—we should think rather of *equality* of opportunity as the ethical substance of the relations of those individuals to one another that might have been guarded and expressed by casting lots.[19]

The individual's personal and transcendent dignity, which on the utilitarian approach would be submerged in his social role and function, can be protected and witnessed to by a recognition of his equal right to be saved. Such a right is best preserved by procedures which establish equality of opportunity. Thus selection by chance more closely approximates the requirements established by human dignity than does utilitarian calculation. It is not infallibly just, but it is preferable to the alternatives of letting all die or saving only those who have the greatest social responsibilities and potential contribution.

This argument can be extended by examining values other than individual dignity and equality of opportunity. Another basic value in the medical sphere is the relationship of trust between physician and patient. Which selection criteria are most in accord with this relationship of trust? Which will maintain, extend, and deepen it? My contention is that selection by randomness or chance is preferable from this standpoint too.

Trust, which is inextricably bound to respect for human dignity, is an attitude of expectation about another. It is not simply the expectation that another will perform a particular act, but more specifically that another will act toward him in certain ways—which will respect him as a person. As Charles Fried writes:

> Although trust has to do with reliance on a disposition of another person, it is reliance on a disposition of a special sort: the disposition to act morally, to deal fairly with others, to live up to one's undertakings, and so on. Thus to trust another is first of all to expect him to accept the principle of morality in his dealings with you, to respect your status as a person, your personality.[20]

This trust cannot be preserved in life-and-death situations when a person expects decisions about him to be made in terms of his social worth, for such decisions violate his status as a person. An applicant rejected on grounds of inadequacy in social value or virtue would have reason for feeling that his "trust" had been betrayed. Indeed, the sense that one is being viewed not as an end in himself but as a means in medical progress or the achievement of a greater social good is incompatible with attitudes and relationships of trust. We recognize this in the billboard which was erected after the first heart transplants: "Drive Carefully. Christiaan Barnard Is Watching You." The relationship of trust between the physician and patient is not only an instrumental value in the sense of being an important factor in the patient's treatment. It is also to be endorsed because of its intrinsic worth as a relationship.

Thus the related values of individual dignity and trust are best maintained in selection by chance. But other factors also buttress the argument for this approach. Which criteria and procedures would men agree upon? We have to suppose a hypothetical situation in which several men are going to determine for themselves and their families the criteria and procedures by which they would want to be admitted to and excluded from SLMR if the need arose.[21] We need to assume two restrictions and then ask which set of criteria and procedures would be chosen as the most rational and, indeed, the fairest. The restrictions are these: (1) The men are *self-interested*. They are interested in their own welfare (and that of members of their families), and this, of course, includes survival. Basically, they are not motivated by altruism. (2) Furthermore, they are *ignorant* of their own talents, abilities, potential, and probable contribution to the social good. They do not know how they would fare in a competitive situation, e.g., the competition for SLMR in terms of social contribution. Under these conditions which institution would be chosen—letting all die, utilitarian selection, or the use of chance? Which would seem the most rational? the fairest? By which set of criteria would they want to be included in or excluded from the list of those who will be saved? The rational choice in this setting (assuming self-interest and ignorance of one's competitive success) would be random selection or chance since this alone provides equality of opportunity. A possible response is that one would prefer to take a "risk" and therefore choose the utilitarian approach. But I think not, especially since I added that the participants in this hypothetical situation are choosing for their children as well as for themselves; random selection or chance could be more easily justified to the children. It would make more sense for men who are self-interested but uncertain about their relative contribution to society to elect a set of criteria that would build in equality of opportunity. They would consider selection by chance as relatively just and fair.[22]

An important psychological point supplements earlier arguments for using chance or random selection. The psychological stress and strain among those who are rejected would be greater if the rejection is based on insufficient social worth than if it is based on chance. Obviously stress and strain cannot be eliminated in these borderline situations, but they would almost certainly be increased by the opprobrium of being judged relatively "unfit" by society's agents using society's values. Nicholas Rescher makes this point very effectively:

> a recourse to chance would doubtless make matters easier for the rejected patients and those who have a specific interest in him. It would surely be quite hard for them to accept his exclusion by relatively mechanical application of objective criteria in whose implementation subjective judgment is involved. But the circumstances of life have conditioned us to accept the workings of chance and to tolerate the element of luck (good or bad): human life is an inherently contingent process. Nobody, after all, has an absolute right to ELT [Exotic Lifesaving Therapy] —but most of us would feel that we have "every bit as much right" to it as anyone else in significantly similar circumstances.[23]

Although it is seldom recognized as such, selection by chance is already in operation in practically every dialysis unit. I am not aware of any unit that removes some of its patients from kidney machines in order to make room for later applicants who are better qualified in terms of social worth. Furthermore, very few people would recommend it. Indeed, few would even consider removing a person from a kidney machine on the grounds that a person better qualified *medically* had just applied. In a discussion of the treatment of chronic renal failure by dialysis at the University of Virginia Hospital Renal Unit from November 15, 1965 to November 15, 1966, Dr. Harry Abram writes: "Thirteen patients sought treatment but were not considered because the program had reached its limit of nine patients."[24] Thus, in practice and theory, natural chance is accepted, at least within certain limits.

My proposal is that we extend this principle (first come, first served) to determine who among the medically acceptable patients shall live or that we utilize artificial chance such as a lottery or randomness. "First come, first served" would be more feasible than a lottery since the applicants make their claims over a period of time rather than as a group at one time. This procedure would be in accord with at least one principle in our present practices and with our sense of individual dignity, trust, and fairness. Its significance in relation to these values can be underlined by asking how the decision can be justified to the rejected applicant. Of course, one easy way of avoiding this task is to maintain the traditional cloak of secrecy, which works to a great extent because patients are often not aware that they are being considered for SLMR in addition to the usual treatment. But whether public justification is instituted or not is not the significant question; it is rather what reasons for rejection would be most acceptable to the unsuccessful applicant. My contention is that rejection can be accepted more readily if equality of opportunity, fairness, and trust are preserved, and that they are best preserved by selection by randomness or chance.

This proposal has yet another advantage since it would eliminate the need for a committee to examine applicants in terms of their social value. This onerous responsibility can be avoided.

Finally, there is a possible indirect consequence of widespread use of random selection which is interesting to ponder, although I do *not* adduce it as a good reason for adopting random selection. It can be argued, as Professor Mason Willrich of the University of Virginia Law School has suggested, that SLMR cases would practically disappear if these scarce resources were distributed randomly rather than on social worth grounds. Scarcity would no longer be a problem because the holders of economic and political power would make certain that they would not be excluded by a random selection procedure; hence they would help to redirect public priorities or establish private funding so that life-saving medical treatment would be widely and perhaps universally available.

In the framework that I have delineated, are the decrees of chance to be taken without exception? If we recognize exceptions, would we not open Pandora's box again just after we had succeeded in getting it closed? The direction of my argument has been against any exceptions, and I would defend this as the proper way to go. But let me indicate one possible way of admitting exceptions, while at the same time circumscribing them so narrowly that they would be very rare indeed.

An obvious advantage of the utilitarian approach is that occasionally circumstances arise that make it necessary to say that one man is practically indispensable for a society in view of a particular set of problems it faces (e.g., the president when the nation is waging a war for survival). Certainly the argument to this point has stressed that the burden of proof would fall on those who think that the social danger in this instance is so great that they simply cannot abide by the outcome of a lottery or a first come, first served policy.

Also, the reason must be negative rather than positive; that is, we depart from chance in this instance not because we want to take advantage of this person's potential contribution to the improvement of our society, but because his immediate loss would possibly (even probably) be disastrous (again, the president in a grave national emergency). Finally, social value (in the negative sense) should be used as a standard of exception in dialysis, for example, only if it would provide a reason strong enough to warrant removing another person from a kidney machine if all machines were taken. Assuming this strong reluctance to remove anyone once the commitment has been made to him, we would be willing to put this patient ahead of another applicant for a vacant machine only if we would be willing (in circumstances in which all machines are being used) to vacate a machine by removing someone from it. These restrictions would make an exception almost impossible.

While I do not recommend this procedure of recognizing exceptions, I think that one can defend it while accepting my general thesis about selection by randomness or chance. If it is used, a lay committee (perhaps advisory, perhaps even stronger) would be called upon to deal with the alleged exceptions, since the doctors or others would in effect be appealing the outcome of chance (either natural or artificial). This lay committee would determine whether this patient was so indispensable at this time and place that he had to be saved even by sacrificing the values preserved by random selection. It would make it quite clear that exception is warranted, if at all, only as the "lesser of two evils." Such a defense would be recognized only rarely, if ever, primarily because chance and randomness preserve so many important moral and nonmoral values in SLMR cases.[25]

Notes to Chapter Twelve

1. George Bernard Shaw, *The Doctor's Dilemma* (New York, 1941), pp. 132-33.

2. Henry K. Beecher, "Scarce Resources and Medical Advancement," *Daedalus* (Spring 1969), 279-80.

3. Leo Shatin, "Medical Care and the Social Worth of a Man," *American Journal of Orthopsychiatry*, 36 (1967), 97.

4. Harry S. Abram and Walter Wadlington, "Selection of Patients for Artificial and Transplanted Organs," *Annals of Internal Medicine*, 69 (September 1968), 615-20.

5. *United States v. Holmes*, 26 Fed. Cas. 360 (C.C.E.D. Pa. 1842). All references are to the text of the trial as reprinted in Philip E. Davis, ed., *Moral Duty and Legal Responsibility: A Philosophical-Legal Casebook* (New York, 1966), pp. 102-18.

6. *The Moral Decision* (Bloomington, Ind., 1955), p. 71.

7. For a discussion of the higher suicide rate among dialysis patients than among the general population and an interpretation of some of the factors at work, see H.S. Abram, G.L. Moore, and F.B. Westervelt, "Suicidal Behavior in Chronic Dialysis Patients," *American Journal of Psychiatry*, 127 (1971):

1119-1204. This study shows that even "if one does not include death through not following the regimen the incidence of suicide is still more than 100 times the normal population."

8. Joseph Fletcher, "Donor Nephrectomies and Moral Responsibility," *Journal of the American Medical Women's Association*, 23 (December 1968), 1090.

9. Leo Shatin, pp. 96-101.

10. For a discussion of the Seattle selection committee, see Shana Alexander, "They Decide Who Lives, Who Dies," *Life*, 53 (November 9, 1962), 102. For an examination of general selection practices in dialysis see "Scarce Medical Resources," *Columbia Law Review* 69:620 (1969) and Abram and Wadlington.

11. David Sanders and Jesse Dukeminier, Jr., "Medical Advance and Legal Lag: Hemodialysis and Kidney Transplantation," *UCLA Law Review* 15:367 (1968), 378.

12. "Letters and Comments," *Annals of Internal Medicine*, 61 (August 1964), 360. Dr. G.E. Schreiner contends that "if you really believe in the right of society to make decisions on medical availability on these criteria you should be logical and say that when a man stops going to church or is divorced or loses his job, he ought to be removed from the programme and somebody else who fulfills these criteria substituted. Obviously no one faces up to this logical consequence" (G.E.W. Wolstenholme and Maeve O'Connor, eds. *Ethics in Medical Progress: With Special Reference to Transplantation*, A Ciba Foundation Symposium [Boston, 1966], p. 127).

13. Helmut Thielicke, "The Doctor as Judge of Who Shall Live and Who Shall Die," *Who Shall Live?* ed. by Kenneth Vaux (Philadelphia, 1970), p. 172.

14. Ibid., pp. 173-74.

15. Ibid., p. 173.

16. Thielicke, *Theological Ethics*, Vol. I, *Foundations* (Philadelphia, 1966), p. 602.

17. Cahn, op. cit., p. 71.

18. Paul Freund, "Introduction," *Daedalus* (Spring 1969), xiii.

19. Paul Ramsey, *Nine Modern Moralists* (Englewood Cliffs, N.J., 1962), p. 245.

20. Charles Fried, "Privacy," in *Law, Reason, and Justice*, ed. by Graham Hughes (New York, 1969), p. 52.

21. My argument is greatly dependent on John Rawls's version of justice as fairness, which is a reinterpretation of social contract theory. Rawls, however, would probably not apply his ideas to "borderline situations." See "Distributive Justice: Some Addenda," *Natural Law Forum*, 13 (1968), 53. For Rawls's general theory, see "Justice as Fairness," *Philosophy, Politics and Society* (Second Series), ed. by Peter Laslett and W.G. Runciman (Oxford, 1962), pp. 132-57 and *A Theory of Justice* (Cambridge, Mass., 1971).

22. Occasionally someone contends that random selection may reward vice. Leo Shatin (op. cit., p. 100) insists that random selection "would reward socially disvalued qualities by giving their bearers the same special medical care opportunities as those received by the bearers of socially valued qualities. Personally I do not favor such a method." Obviously society must engender

certain qualities in its members, but not all of its institutions must be devoted to that purpose. Furthermore, there are strong reasons, I have contended, for exempting SLMR from that sort of function.

23. Nicholas Rescher, "The Allocation of Exotic Medical Lifesaving Therapy," *Ethics*, 79 (April 1969), 184. He defends random selection's use only after utilitarian and other judgments have been made. If there are no "major disparities" in terms of utility, etc., in the second stage of selection, then final selection could be made randomly. He fails to give attention to the moral values that random selection might preserve.

24. Harry S. Abram, M.D., "The Psychiatrist, the Treatment of Chronic Renal Failure, and the Prolongation of Life: II" *American Journal of Psychiatry* 126:157-67 (1969), 158.

25. I read a draft of this paper in a seminar on "Social Implications of Advances in Biomedical Science and Technology: Artificial and Transplanted Internal Organs," sponsored by the Center for the Study of Science, Technology, and Public Policy of the University of Virginia, Spring 1970. I am indebted to the participants in that seminar, and especially to its leaders, Mason Willrich, Professor of Law, and Dr. Harry Abram, Associate Professor of Psychiatry, for criticisms which helped me to sharpen these ideas. Good discussions of the legal questions raised by selection (e.g., equal protection of the law and due process) which I have not considered can be found in "Scarce Medical Resources," *Columbia Law Review*, 69:620 (1969); "Patient Selection for Artificial and Transplanted Organs," *Harvard Law Review*, 82:1322 (1969); and Sanders and Dukeminier, op. cit.

Chapter 13

The Selection Process as Viewed from Within: A Reply to Childress

Frederic B. Westervelt

The concept of triage—the selective utilization of medical resources inadequate to cope with all those in need—has always evoked expressions of regret from those responsible for its execution and of dismay from those witnessing its impact. Implicit in this concept is the provision of treatment to restore to effectiveness (i.e., a useful life worth living) the greatest possible number of patients according to the experience and judgment of those responsible for providing care, and within the constraints of the system. It is axiomatic that the effort expended upon each individual will have bearing upon each individual within the treatment sphere, be he (in current parlance) "provider" or "consumer."

The advent of hemodialysis and kidney transplantation, which in their beginning were of uncertain therapeutic applicability and extreme scarcity, led to triage of an almost purely investigative sort in the effort to assure suitable candidates from the medical standpoint, explore the impact of such procedures on patients and their families, and develop appropriate technology. Later the goal became a record of efficacy (an "image") sufficient to foster the desire within and without professional ranks to develop and extend programs such that these techniques would be of therapeutic importance to a significant segment of the population, not merely isolated phenomena.

It was understandably, and I believe correctly, held that the "image" would best be served by combining an acceptable degree of technical success—dependent in large measure upon the patient's medical status—with the demonstration that the considerable effort (in the broadest sense) did more than merely prolong individual lives. The return to the community of its more visible, articulate, and contributory members in exchange for its current or projected large expenditures became a secondary goal.

It must be clear that in these earlier days, as today, "selection procedures," however effected, emphasized the candidate's freedom from significant or threatening illness other than his kidney disease, and sought to ascertain that he could comprehend, cope with, and benefit from his treatment program. The latter signified not merely "staying alive" but also returning to a reasonably happy life, useful to himself and to others. The "social" considerations, so deplored by some, seemed inextricably interwoven with these circumstances, if only indirectly.

Motivation, intelligence, "the need to prevail," ability to adhere to broad therapeutic premises with interpretive flexibility or to adhere to rigid restrictions faithfully, the capacity early to recognize and report deviations from the usual, all these attributes tend to be found in these persons who because of these same attributes are vocationally and socially "successful." There is, of course, no single scale of success. One may be a successful carpenter, clergyman, executive, mother, engineer, or taxi driver, and these are not to be judged of different merit. In essence, we refer to effectiveness within the individual's appropriate sphere.

Similarly, access to adequate general medical care, with its corollaries of early prevention and treatment of intercurrent illness as well as earlier detection and attempted control of the ultimately lethal kidney failure and its consequences, is more likely to lead to referral for dialysis or transplantation before irreversible "complications" can supervene. Those higher in the socioeconomic order are more likely to fall in this category than are their less fortunate brethren. While this latter state of affairs is to be deplored, it is nonetheless largely true, and the responsibility for it should not fall upon the selection process as a form of protest.

Thus, in general, selection for dialysis and transplantation has not so much been prejudicial *against* the socially disadvantaged as prejudiced *in favor of* those persons who have, in the eyes of those responsible for triage, certain attributes of "survival value" and who coincidentally exhibit the "social values" that lead to controversy.

Perhaps clarification of the social value concept is in order. While at its basest this could imply racial or ethnic considerations, neither Mr. Childress nor I is discoursing at this level. Indeed, if somewhere selection is thus influenced, it is unlikely that the controlling interests will submit to any alteration of their strategem. It is equally incorrect to speak only of abstract "society," to imply social standing, influence, or prominence, or to think only in terms of grand-scale contribution to the community, nation, or world.

Value judgments exist at all levels, for limitless reasons, and by common consent. So long as man is relating to man this relationship is influenced by values, and I am not persuaded that this is unethical. One might argue that all lives are of equal value, and that by virtue of being alive all persons have an equal right to continue to live. This premise accepted, perhaps it becomes self-canceling on either side of the biologic equation, and that which remains can be meaningful.

It is noteworthy that as experience accumulates so does confidence and flexibility. Just as the concept of dialysis and transplantation has evolved toward a position of increasing permissiveness as regards "acceptable" candidates, so does each institution's or community's program briefly recapitulate this trend from conservative to liberal selection, in terms of both medical and ancillary criteria. This evolution is facilitated by a diminishing of the limelight, as well as by technical and intellectual maturation such that factors previously accorded importance, objectively or by implication, have been found to be less relevant. In a sense, the "pressure to make good" is relieved, realism replaces idealism, and an investigational concept has become operational.

This is not to say that the need for triage has ceased to exist; demand still vastly exceeds supply. More widely available dialysis facilities, both institutional and in the home, shorter periods of dialysis while awaiting transplantation because of regional kidney-sharing programs, and the decreasing number of transplant recipients returning to dialysis because of graft rejection have only marginally lessened the disproportion. The problem is perhaps less severe with each passing year (not in a cumulative sense, however, for last year's unsuccessful applicants have not lived to become part of this year's pool); but still less than 10 percent of the needy can be provided care. Each patient entering a dialysis-transplant program exerts some influence upon those undergoing therapy, those under consideration at or near the same time, and those to follow. He influences also those directly and indirectly responsible for his care and, albeit almost intangibly, the attitudes and sense of conscience of his society. How can we conduct triage in the most satisfactory manner from the medical, ethical, and social viewpoints within existing limitations?

With apologies for this lengthy preamble, let us address ourselves to Mr. Childress's thoughtful and eloquent proposal, and several of its assertions. Attractive in its apparent simplicity and in its appeal for equal consideration of all candidates by means of random selection, the proposal nonetheless entails certain operational difficulties that deserve mention. Foremost among these is the inordinate emphasis upon "social value" judgments, which he implies are a prime function of selected committees. I submit that this is not the proper definition of the dilemma, although to an extent it is deserving of criticism.

I shall not dwell upon the considerable difficulties inherent in specifying "medical suitability," which Mr. Childress would like to believe to be a single-stage, yes-no judgment prefatory to second-order lottery selection. Often this is true, of course, although the nosologic criteria for suitability change with experience. Further, medical criteria may legitimately differ, depending upon whether in-center or home dialysis, or transplantation, is the available resource.

Lastly, if we examine medical suitability in its most universal sense as a determinant of ultimate effectiveness of therapy, we are including the psychological, motivational, familial, intellectual, and vocational factors that move us perilously close to "social value judgments." After all, these are inherent in the "quality of life" with which medicine as a profession tries, not always successfully, to contend. A selection process would be derelict if it did not seek the "most suitable" of those suitable, for such is a continuum. Medical criteria must not, of course, serve as a façade behind which other manipulations take place.

The acceptance of patients on a "first come, first served" basis is, Mr. Childress contends, a random chance procedure. This is true and ethically reasonable only if one is very arbitrary. For instance, when is "first?" The earliest patient referred for consideration of dialysis may be the latest to require such therapy. Other means of therapy may significantly defer, for months or even years, the need for dialysis and transplantation so long as therapeutic advice is followed. Would a patient follow such advice if he thought this would jeopardize his "place in line"? If not, would this behavior constitute grounds for psychiatric unsuitability? The need for dialysis in a given instance is defined largely by the inability of the uremic patient to function with reasonable effectiveness and safety while undergoing more "conservative" means of therapy (diet, medication, etc.). How does one interpret the symptoms of a patient who may be "not doing well" in an attempt to maintain his priority?

The lottery or coin-tossing approach is presumed to be advocated when two equally suitable individuals (without regard to "social value") are competing simultaneously for a single program vacancy, a photo-finish circumstance of exceeding rarity. Or should it also apply to all candidates, even if the "adversary" is not yet visible? Perhaps the problem of serial randomization could be solved by the acceptance of patients with even hospital record numbers, a code which when broken would permit the odd man ample time to seek a haven elsewhere. (Record numbers are permanently assigned when a patient first presents for medical care for whatever reason, including birth.) These approaches would avert the difficulties of "first come, first served" and maintain an unparalleled "equality of opportunity," yet do not fulfill our needs.

Mr. Childress's assumption that men would agree upon a chance method of selection if their own, or their children's, lives were at stake is a compelling one. While some prefer playing bridge to rolling dice, lives are not generally in the balance and one can always "fold" if the stakes become unacceptably high. Quite possibly he has perceived a fundamental truth, that those customarily involved in this sort of triage, lay or professional, probably feel relatively secure, even if subconsciously, of their successful competitiveness and are hence convinced of the rectitude of the system in which they are participants. His conclusion that chance selection is a prelude to a trusting relationship (note the bidirectional term) is hard to follow, however. Not long after the fact only those who remain are of overt concern to each other, and whatever trust was engendered in the rejected candidate and his family has likely been replaced by resentment or dismay, not to be countered by the knowledge that he was treated fairly. He who was found suitable would, I should think, be more secure and possibly positively motivated by the knowledge that he survives because of his own attributes. Might he otherwise not be concerned that subsequent important decisions are to be made by coin-tossing rather than with objectivity? Agreed, we cannot now cope with these concepts in utilitarian fashion, but we can recognize man's need to try.

Another consideration comes to mind, one which may seem parochial but which has some relevance. The physician long has been accorded the privilege, even the legal right, of determining to whom he shall and shall not render care, just as the patient may select his own physician. This stems from a recognition of the phenomenon, hardly unique to medicine, that there may exist personal, behavioral, or even professional incompatibilities that would thwart an effective therapeutic relationship. During a brief period of contact, as in an acute, limited illness, both parties may rise above such incompatibility. The dialysis-transplantation context, however, is prolonged, at times complicated, occasionally desperate, and frequently more stressful for the "team" than is generally realized. At such times, as well as during smooth sailing, a firm, positive, and (again) trusting relationship is often of immense importance to the outcome. The factors responsible may not be so intangible as they are undefinable. I do not refer to petty prejudices or differences, but to such that lead to a sense of responsibility, respect, and a conviction that the task is worthwhile, all leading to the needed capacity for extra effort. It is this all-too-human trait, perhaps, that may render a chance selection process unfortunate.

On occasion a medically suitable candidate finds unacceptable the conditions to be imposed on him in the conduct of his treatment. I refer not only to medical or technical considerations, but also to travel or dislocation requisites, economic impact, the inability to adapt to an existence of some uncertainty, or the prospect of a degree of disability. This aspect of self-selection might not seem to be the committee's responsibility, yet the perceptive group will recognize and contend with these factors as early as possible, and thus may avert the unnecessary rejection of another candidate.

To some extent the physician must consider the impact of a patient upon the program—his potential relations with other staff, his need for unusual or time-consuming care, and possibly his relationship with other patients. Seldom of predictable importance, this aspect of group interaction may hit hard at morale, stability, and equitable distribution of time and effort when applied to a group as close as are dialysis patients and their staff.

Medicine has been accused of being too impersonal. This is certainly not the arena in which to justify that accusation. The point can be overdrawn, of course; the circumstances are unusual, the judgments often final, and the need for deep contemplation extreme. But that subjectivity may properly exist cannot be ignored.

The allocation of limited life-prolonging resources remains a complex issue, possibly such that there is no universally satisfactory solution. Mr. Childress presents a cogent, compelling theoretical argument with certain merits deserving of wide discussion; possibly his is the way of the future. It is my position, however, that triage should remain the purview of those answerable for the program, who must avail themselves of all relevant sources of information, opinion and guidance. The key to responsible action lies with the responsible physician. So long as his decisions, however effected, are forthright, conscionable, subject to discussion, and consonant with his obligation to individual and group, these difficulties can be met. If otherwise, far more is in jeopardy than the patient with failing kidneys.

Chapter 14

The Totally Implantable Artificial Heart: Economic, Ethical, Legal, Medical, Psychiatric, and Social Implications

**The Artificial Heart Assessment Panel,
National Heart and Lung Institute**

THE PANEL AND THE PROBLEM

The Magnitude of the Assignment

The Artificial Heart Assessment Panel was established in July 1972 by the National Heart and Lung Institute. It was charged with "detailing the economic, ethical, legal, medical, psychiatric and social implications of clinical application of a totally implantable artificial heart." NHLI's interest in these issues reflects in part its own active involvement over a number of years in the research and development effort that may, in the not-too-distant future, make the artificial heart ready for use in human patients. In addition, the recent experience with heart transplantation, which took the world—including NHLI—by surprise and drew attention to numerous unresolved moral, legal, and other problems, revealed the importance of anticipating developments. Moreover, increasing recognition of the frequency of unanticipated consequences of technology in general, and government-supported technology in particular, has also stimulated early evaluation of technological programs, and the appointment of the panel may be seen as an exercise in "technology assessment."

Implantable Artificial Heart. If heart disease reaches the stage of intolerable levels of cardiac output and pressure, survival may depend on complete cardiac replacement, i.e., a mechanical or transplanted heart. Since cardiac transplantation is not within the purview of the present report, only the mechanical replacements will be considered. Moreover, "replacement" will be considered in the broad sense of replacing function rather than of replacing anatomy. Three categories of pump systems are currently being developed in the attempt to achieve satisfactory mechanical replacement for the function of the natural heart: 1) an implanted left and a right assist heart, leaving the patient's own heart in situ; the implanted pumps, using external power, then assume the function of the heart in perfusing the lungs and the systemic circulation; 2) an implanted four-chambered pump with external power and controls as a substitute for the patient's heart; modifications of this approach have included an implanted pump and actuator but with external energy and controls; and 3) an implanted four-chambered pump that is a complete package, including pump, energy source, and controls.

Although as considerable volume of data has been generated in short-term animal experiments using these types of devices, only one human trial has been performed to date, and that involved an implanted four-chambered heart with external power and control.

State of the Art

At the present time, only a prototype of the totally implantable artificial heart exists. The prototype is complete with power and controls, and its components have been extensively tested with respect to engineering performance. It has been only tentatively evaluated with respect to physiological performance in animals. The prototype has a mechanical efficiency comparable to that of the natural heart, and is capable of changing its output on demand. As yet, the models under test are larger and heavier than the natural heart, but newer models approximate the natural heart in size and weight.

Although most experts agree that development of a clinically acceptable totally implantable artificial heart is feasible, the panel believes that trial of such a device in man is not an immediate prospect. Predictions of the earliest date for clinical trials range from a little less than ten years to considerably longer than ten years. However, it is expected that partially implantable devices, such as an internal pump, driven and controlled from without the body, may be available for clinical trials at an earlier date.

Since development of the artificial heart is still in the pre-clinical phase, it may be instructive to review briefly some of the obstacles that remain to be overcome.

Biomaterials. Synthetic materials invariably injure blood components after a few hours of perfusion. Many new materials are currently under investigation. Most promising of these is a pump lining composed of living, self-regenerating intima. However, at present there is still no synthetic lining that can reliably be used as a basis for a totally implantable artificial heart.

Control System. Control systems are now widely used in circulatory assist devices and are being tested for the totally implantable artificial heart. Preliminary bench trials and observations in a few animals suggest that considerable flexibility can be achieved with respect to variations in cardiac output. However, control systems have yet to be evaluated in chronic experiments.

Energy Systems. A number of alternative approaches have been considered for providing an implantable energy source to power the artificial heart. These can be categorized as follows:

The Biological Fuel Cell. An implanted device would utilize energy derived from various muscles of the body or from bioelectric potentials of body materials. Although such a system may someday become technically feasible, many difficult problems remain to be solved, and it seems certain that such an energy source will not be available for many years.

The Electrical System. In this system, the artificial heart would be powered from external electrical sources transmitting energy across intact skin. This energy might be delivered directly to the implanted motor from a source that is easily worn (e.g., a belt or a vest) or carried (e.g., in an attaché case) by the recipient. In addition, there might be a small implanted rechargeable battery for the storage of energy so that the recipient could be free from the external source for limited periods of time. Alternatively, energy might be provided from larger implanted batteries that could be recharged periodically across the intact skin. Such systems involve the obvious disadvantage of dependence on external energy sources and the necessity for a periodic recharging of the battery or the external mobile source. Moreover, present technology limits the life of rechargeable batteries. The panel has been informed by experts in battery technology that it is presently within technological possibility to implant a battery of acceptable weight and size that could power an artificial heart reliably for a two-year period, with no more than four brief recharging periods per day. Obviously, for an artificial heart to sustain life for a longer period of years, it would be necessary, once each two years, to remove and replace the implanted battery. This in itself involves added expense, risk, and inconvenience to the patient. It should be noted that such procedures are commonplace in the case of the battery-powered cardiac pacemaker. However, information provided by the battery experts suggests that within the next five years battery technology can be improved to the point that implanted batteries would have a five-year reliable life period.

The Plutonium-238 System. The third system involves the use of an implanted fuel capsule containing Plutonium-238 that would provide a reliable source of energy without need for external resupply, for a ten-year period. Such a system appears presently within technological capabilities. Although this system would obviously be optimal from the standpoint of reliability and convenience to the patient, there are also disadvantages relating to cost and to the risk to the patient and to those around him created by the radioactive characteristics of Plutonium-238. In addition, the use of Plutonium-238 in artificial heart systems would be subject to substantial government regulation to ensure the health and safety of the public. This topic is considered at greater length in Chapter IV of this Report [pp. 232-236 in this volume].

Surgical Techniques. The techniques that would be required to implant an artificial heart and to make appropriate hemodynamic measurements are within the scope of skilled cardiovascular surgeons who have been performing open-heart surgery.

Potential Candidates for Implantation

The panel has attempted to arrive at a reasonable estimate of the potential number of candidates for an artificial heart, recognizing from the outset that any such estimate must be largely speculative since the totally implantable artificial heart will become available for use in man only at some time ten years or so hence, at the earliest. During the intervening period, many medical advances can be expected, including possible alternatives such as cardiac transplantation, more effective prophylactic therapies, and new forms of surgical treatment. Moreover, at such time as the artificial heart may become a reality, indications for this drastic intervention will have to be weighed against the inevitable problems that will attend the surgical introduction of a prosthesis as a substitute for the natural heart.

Estimated Number of Potential Candidates. As a result of the introduction of cardiac transplantation, the National Heart Institute in 1968 appointed the Ad Hoc Task Force on Cardiac Replacement to consider problems relating to the replacement of the human heart. In contrast to this panel, heart transplants were the primary concern of the Ad Hoc Task Force, even though it also gave consideration to replacement of the natural heart with an artificial heart. In its report (p. 7), the Ad Hoc Task Force estimated that the number of potential candidates for heart replacement would range between 11,736 and 32,168 per year. Most of these potential candidates were patients who would otherwise die of ischemic (coronary) heart disease during the year. However, not all patients dying of such disease were regarded as candidates for heart replacement.

Since the focus of this panel is specifically on the artificial heart, and not on heart transplants, considerations relating to immunosuppression and donor availability do not limit the number of potential candidates. Moreover, dramatic surgical advances since 1969 in coronary artery and congenital heart disease and improvement in artificial valves have increased the pool of prospective candidates for heart replacement by prolonging the length and improving the quality of life of cardiac patients. Finally, in contrast to the Ad Hoc Task Force, this panel has enlarged the category of prospective candidates by including patients over sixty-five years of age.

Table 14-1 shows the estimated number of potential candidates per year for artificial heart implantation. Table 14-1 corresponds to Table 7 in the 1969 Cardiac Replacement Report, but has been modified to include older candidates (65 to 74 years) with ischemic heart disease and to reflect more recent data (i.e., the use of 1969, rather than 1967, data on deaths from heart disease).[a] The potential number of candidates for implantation of a clinically acceptable artificial heart is predicted to range from about 16,750 to 50,300 per year. This increase over the figures used in the 1969 Cardiac Replacement Report is primarily attributable to the inclusion of patients aged 65 to 74 in the pool of

Table 14-1. Potential Candidates for an Artificial Heart Among Persons Dying of Heart Disease, United States, 1967[a]

Heart Disease Diagnosis	Deaths in 1969	Potential Candidates			
		High Estimate		Low Estimate	
		Percent	Number	Percent	Number
Total	363,999	13.8	50,336	4.6	16,749
Ischemic heart disease without hypertension, under age 65	151,948	16.4	24,919	3.8	5,774
Ischemic heart disease without hypertension, age 65-74	157,494	11.2	17,639	2.6	4,075
Ischemic heart disease with hypertension, under age 65	20,376	10.0	2,038	10.0	2,038
Other hypertensive heart disease, under age 65	3,622	10.0	362	10.0	362
Rheumatic heart disease, under age 65	8,978	25.0	2,245	15.0	1,347
Congenital heart disease, under age 65	7,884	5.0	394	5.0	394
Other heart disease, under age 65	13,697	20.0	2,739	20.0	2,739

[a]This table corresponds to Table 7 of the October 1969 Report on Cardiac Replacement, with certain modifications. Because this table includes patients 65-74 years old, and because the criteria for artificial heart implantation are somewhat different than those for transplantation, the fraction of patients who are candidates for artificial hearts has been (1) increased from 5 to 10 percent for patients dying of hypertensive diseases, (2) increased from 10 to 25 percent for patients dying of rheumatic heart disease, and (3) decreased from 25 to 5 percent for patients dying of congenital heart disease.

[a]Table 14-1 also predicts that fewer congenital heart disease patients will be candidates for artificial hearts than were estimated for heart replacement in the 1969 Report. This discrepancy stems from the realization that most deaths from congenital heart disease occur in infancy and early childhood, thereby imposing the formidable complication of miniaturizing the artificial heart followed by successive implantations of larger artificial hearts as the child grows. Finally, since 1969 it has become apparent that many rheumatic heart patients cannot be helped by heart valve surgery, and therefore, such patients become prime candidates for artificial hearts.

candidates. The panel believes that, if the artificial heart can be developed to meet the objectives and expectations of its sponsors, the number of candidates for implantation is more likely to approximate the higher, rather than the lower, end of this estimated range.

Quality of Life. Another factor considered by the panel has been the quality of life that would be enjoyed by recipients of the artificial heart. One of the objectives of implanting an artificial heart is to extend the meaningful and productive life of the recipient. Assuming, therefore, that implantation of an artificial heart eliminates any major disability resulting from cardiac disease, it is necessary to consider the extent to which the recipient may suffer disability from other chronic medical conditions. Table 14-2 shows that chronic disabling illness is present in 5 percent of the population under 45; in 19 percent of the population age 45 to 64; and in 46 percent of the population over 65. If artificial heart implantations completely excluded disabling heart disease, an appreciable number of artificial heart recipients would suffer disability from diseases other than heart conditions. This is particularly true in the case of patients who are 65 years of age or older, about 35 percent of whom will have disabilities caused by conditions other than heart disease. In contrast, only 16 percent of those in the 45-to-64-year-old group would be expected to suffer from chronic, non-heart disability.

Quality of Death. In considering the quality of life, it is also relevant to consider the quality of death. How will implantation of an artificial heart affect a person's life expectancy and his chances of dying from causes other than heart disease? In considering this question, we assume that implantation of an artificial heart will eliminate the possibility that the recipient will die of heart disease for ten years, and that without the implantation death would occur within a very short time.

Figure 14-1 shows the expected mortality within a ten-year period for persons age 40, 50, 60, and 70 in the general population, as well as for those of

Table 14-2. Prevalence of Chronic Disabling Conditions By Age (in percents)

	Under 45	45-64	65 & over
No chronic conditions	62	29	14
No limitation in activity	34	52	40
Limited in activity (all causes)	5	19	46
Limited in activity (all causes other than heart disease)	(4)	(16)	(36)

Source: National Center for Health Statistics; National Health Interview Survey, July 1965 to June 1967.

The Totally Implantable Artificial Heart 225

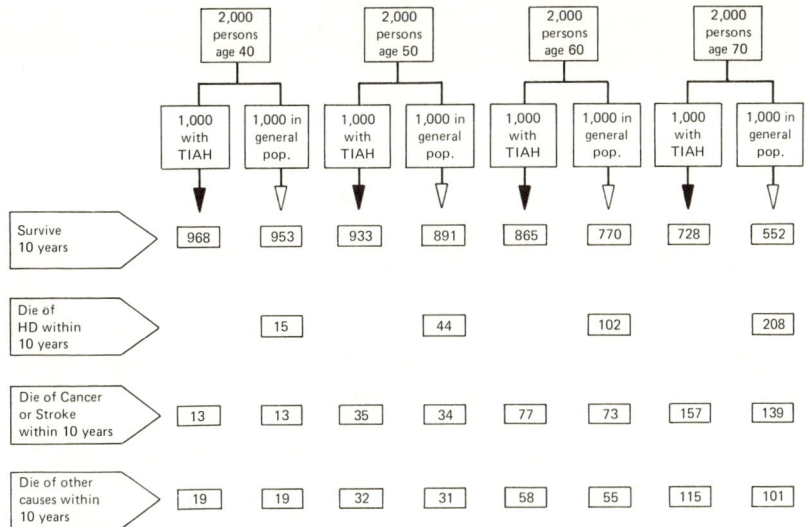

Source: National Heart and Lung Institute: Computed from data in "United States Life Tables by Cause of Death: 1959-1961," Public Health Service Publication Number 1252, Vol. 1, No. 6, May, 1968.

Figure 14-1. Expected Mortality Within Ten Years for 1,000 Persons With An Artificial Heart Compared to 1,000 Persons in the General Population.

each of these ages who have an artificial heart implanted. For example, a person 60 years of age who has an artificial heart implanted increases his chances of survival for ten years from zero (since it is assumed he would otherwise face imminent death) to 865 out of 1000. For the general population, the chance of ten-year survival of persons age 60 is only 770 out of 1000 (heart disease will claim 102 of each 1000 lives).

If, however, the 60-year-old artificial-heart recipient does die within the ten-year period, there is a 77 out of 1000 chance that he or she will die of cancer or stroke. Although this probability of death from cancer or stroke is only slightly greater than for the general population, recipients of the artificial heart will accept a significant probability, as a price of extending their lives, that they will suffer a death (from cancer or stroke) that may be painful and lingering, as contrasted with death from heart disease, which frequently is fast and without prolonged suffering.

In considering the mortality risks shown in Figure 14-1, it should be noted that, because artificial heart recipients will be patients who do not have other diseases which might make them unsuitable candidates, the probability of their survival for the ten-year period may be greater than is shown. On the other hand, since cardiac disease warranting replacement of the natural heart is generally a complication of atherosclerosis, and since atherosclerosis is a generalized process, it is likely that the risk of death from some other complication of atherosclerosis (i.e., stroke) is greater than indicated in Figure 14-1.

Costs and Benefits to Society and Individuals. There are numerous ways in which the artificial heart can affect society as a whole and each of us in his capacity as a member. We may benefit because the group whose lives are saved includes many highly productive individuals whose services have value above and beyond what they consume. On the other hand, we may be disadvantaged taxpayers by the costs of supplying the artificial heart under possible government medical insurance schemes or by increased Social Security taxes needed to support recipients who survive into retirement. As life insurance policy holders, we might enjoy reduced premiums, but health insurance rates would rise. As users of scarce environmental resources, we might find that the larger population resulting from the use of the artificial heart implies more air pollution or higher heating oil prices. The energy source adopted might generate greater demand and higher prices for electricity, or it might produce radiation hazards. These are but a few of the advantages and disadvantages that arise because our complex economic and social system is, to a considerable and probably increasing degree, an integrated whole. The existence and functioning of individuals who are complete strangers to us impinge upon our lives and the lives of millions of other persons, and when the probability that they will continue to exist and function is altered, as it would be by the use of the artificial heart, the probability and extent of these effects are also altered.

The impact of the artificial heart on society as a whole will of course depend to a large extent on the quality of life which its recipients are able to enjoy. First of all, this factor would dictate the extent of use of the device. Second, it is likely to make a considerable difference to society as a whole whether a recipient of the artificial heart is able to live a more or less normal life or is instead condemned to the status of an invalid.

If the artificial heart is successful in restoring the greater number of its recipients to productive lives, society as a whole will benefit because of the preservation of large investments in the education, experience, and skills of persons who would otherwise die or be disabled from heart disease. Since heart disease affects large numbers of individuals during their most productive years, the potential gains are substantial. It is, of course, impossible to predict the number of persons who could be given the capacity for continuing productive careers and the number who, even though they had such capacity, would nevertheless elect to withdraw from their employment or reduce their output. Clearly, the quality of the device will have a major impact on productivity.

If the artificial heart should disappoint expectations in a large number of cases, the cost to society could be quite high. If recipients of the artificial heart were to become a burden not only to themselves but also to their families and the community, the benefits of prolonging their lives might be exceeded by the burdens created for others, with a substantial toll in terms of general welfare. Perhaps the worst possible outcome would be for the device to work just well enough to induce patients to want it—so they could see their grandchildren grow up, for example—but not well enough to prevent the typical recipient from substantially burdening others. In this event, although the welfare losses would exceed the gains, society might balk at any explicit decisions which would deny life to those for whom it could be technologically preserved. If there were not good reason to hope that the quality of life made possible by the artificial heart would be better than this, society might well elect to restrict development.

Decisions on Government's Role in Making the Artificial Heart Available to Patients. Against this background, the dollar costs of the artificial heart can be seen as raising some particularly difficult societal problems. ... There may be as many as 50,000 candidates for artificial heart implantation annually. Adopting a more conservative estimate of 20,000 implantations per year, and conservatively estimating the total costs of each implantation at $25,000, aggregate costs would be on the order of $500 million per year for this single medical procedure. Because of the probability that most of these costs will be borne socially, through Medicare or other public or private means of insuring or financing health care, patients will be encouraged to employ the artificial heart even though life of the quality to be anticipated might not be worth to them the publicly incurred cost of the medical treatment, or would not warrant the non-financial burdens imposed on others. A dilemma is thus potentially created as society faces the possible need to limit very large but unproductive expenditures without seeming to deny the sanctity of human life. As health care becomes more and more a public responsibility, it may become politically difficult to allow people to die when there is an available alternative, however costly or imperfect it may be. While the humanitarian concern thus manifested cannot be faulted, the cost of preserving the myth of the infinite value of human life could in these circumstances be very high.

Indeed, the confrontation with the cost of honoring the sanctity of life may already have begun, as our society examines the recent decision to cover sufferers from kidney disease under Medicare. Despite the relatively poor quality of life enjoyed by many dialysis patients and recipients of renal transplants, and despite the burdens frequently imposed on their families and the community, some patients are kept alive "at all costs." In some cases these costs, both monetary and psychological, were borne strictly within the family itself. Now, however, nearly all of the financial costs are to be borne by society at large. If the artificial heart device turns out to be effective, we may see a repetition of the experience with the kidney transplant and kidney dialysis patients, whose political power proved to be as great as their appeal was strong. Victims of catastrophic diseases have the capacity to become potent pressure groups, challenging indeed to society's pretensions of humanitarianism. Public officials concerned about their own humanitarian images may find it difficult to oppose their claims.

If the artificial heart works well, the demand for it may be so great that society will find itself hard pressed to supply the device to all who want it. Even assuming that an adequate supply would be forthcoming at some price so that rationing would not be necessitated by absolute scarcity, society might be unwilling to supply the device at public expense to all needful patients. Convicted criminals, drug addicts, and perhaps other persons viewed as noncontributing members of society might be seen as candidates for exclusion. But any such governmental process of rationing life on the basis of the value of individual members to society would take a heavy toll in public values. On the other hand, the choice of universal availability, while entailing substantial expense, would produce no added societal benefits aside from preserving the appearance of humanitarianism—which may of course be worth the price. The challenge is to design economically realistic and acceptable financing and allocation arrangements that will not require sacrifice of humanitarian values....

Population Impacts. A particularly important societal impact of the artificial heart will appear in the form of an expanding elderly population. Persons who would have died young will live longer and may be substantially more productive in their older years than they would have been without the artificial heart. Moreover, elderly patients who are otherwise in good health should surely not be denied the right to an artificial heart—at public expense, if that is the way things go. The result of enlarging the older population will be to exacerbate the problems which our society is already experiencing in trying to provide a meaningful existence for its senior citizens. Many older people who are in all respects, both physical and mental, the equal of many younger people are treated as if their ability to make any useful contribution to society had long since ended. For those who are less well off, the need to supply decent and dignified living conditions is also not being met. The costs and human challenges are very great already, but the artificial heart will add to both. One is entitled to wish that technology could be applied with as much promise to this heart-rending problem as it is being applied to the organ on which longevity so much depends.

Still another population impact is worth note. Some cardiac disease is of genetic origin. To the extent that the artificial heart will enable carriers of such cardiac disease, who would otherwise not be able to reproduce, to have children, this would tend to increase the prevalence of genetic cardiac disease in the population. In this sense it might be said that use of the artificial heart in itself may generate additional candidates for its use in future generations.

Evaluating the Advantages and Disadvantages

Having identified the advantages and disadvantages which the panel believes are of potential importance, we shall now consider how the advantages and disadvantages can be evaluated and compared.

Methodologies for Evaluation and Comparison. At the outset it must be observed that all of the many advantages and disadvantages that we have discussed are qualitatively different, and many are not, at least in the first instance, expressible in quantitative terms. They are non-commensurable apples and oranges, which cannot simply be added to or subtracted from one another. We therefore require a set of value-weights which will quantify them and make them commensurable. If such weights can be assigned to each advantage and disadvantage, it would be possible to add up the various positive and negative value weights (for advantages and disadvantages respectively) to determine net value (or net benefits). But how can these weights be obtained?

In practice, social decision-making almost never involves the use of explicit value weights for all relevant effects. Introspection and intuition have been and will continue to be important elements of the evaluation process. But few would disagree[b] that the quality of intuitive judgments can be improved by reliance on additional information gained from nonintrospective processes. In particular, there is good reason for seeking information on the value weights that would be assigned to various advantages and disadvantages by the individuals to whom they accrue. The significance of these weights for our decision is that they serve as quantitative measures of the extent to which each advantage (disadvantage) contributes to (detracts from) individual well-being. If the sum of any individual's value weights for the advantages arising from a particular action were greater than the sum of his (negative) value weights for the disadvantages, we could conclude that the action will improve his well-being.

Given that effects on individual well-being are our fundamental concern, the desirability of an explicit valuation process for obtaining information on individuals' value weights seems obvious. This information is, however, sometimes very difficult if not impossible to obtain. The best we can hope for, in considering an issue as complex as the use of artificial hearts, is to obtain some

---

[b]Professor Green, Dr. Jonsen, and Dr. Katz dissociate themselves from this entire section. In their view, it is neither possible nor useful to attempt to quantify advantages and disadvantages in a manner that will contribute meaningfully and properly to public policy decision-making in a democratic society. They regard this kind of exercise as a numbers game through which the subjective values of the public can easily be subordinated to the conclusions reached by elite groups on what is "best" for society. Professor Kaplan is in essential agreement with the view expressed by Professor Green, Dr. Jonsen, and Dr. Katz. Dr. Smythe believes that an attempt to either quantify the unquantifiable or to emphasize the quantitative over the qualitative is unlikely to help in the determination of what is truly best for society.

very crude "ballpark" figures. The reason for this difficulty is easy to understand. For example, each of us would have great difficulty attaching a value weight to the principal advantage of the artificial heart, increased life expectancy. These difficulties are especially severe in view of the unfamiliarity of the condition in which we might find ourselves as recipients. The problem is further complicated by the fact that the artificial heart is still only hypothetical, so that assigned value weights would not now reflect either experience or knowledge.

What information on individual value weights can, in fact, be obtained? One principal source of such information is the price system. At least as a crude approximation, the value to individuals of the goods and services which must be foregone in order to make artificial hearts available (the opportunity costs of the artificial heart) can be measured in monetary units by the dollar costs of the resources used to provide artificial hearts.

While the price system provides some (admittedly imperfect) information about individual value weights for the opportunity costs of the artificial heart, similar information on most of the advantages and disadvantages is not readily available. An alternative approach to get around this difficulty would be to ask a "representative" sample of individuals to state explicitly their value weights for specific advantages or disadvantages which the artificial heart is expected to yield. The most common technique used in other areas has been the "willingness-to-pay" survey, in which individuals are asked to state their value weights in monetary terms. (The use of monetary value weights in this context is dictated by convenience rather than principle.) It is encouraging to note that willingness-to-pay surveys have recently been applied, with at least limited success, to the evaluation of reductions in the probability of death, a type of advantage quite relevant in the present context.

Another approach to determining individual value weights for advantages such as increased life expectancy or reduced morbidity relies upon price-system information rather than survey information. This information, commonly termed the "economic benefits" of medical programs or the "economic costs" of illness, is typically presented in two parts—the medical expenses eliminated by reduction in illness and the earnings losses due to illness or death that are averted. The difficulty with the economic-benefits approach to determining individual value weights is that they may not correspond very closely with the true weights expressed by informed individuals. There is reason to believe that this approach substantially underestimates these true weights in most circumstances.

The currently available information on value weights for the various advantages and disadvantages of the artificial heart is extremely limited. Although we discuss resource costs in the next section, the uncertainty attached to these figures is substantial. Information on other types of advantages and disadvantages is even less adequate. The panel therefore recommends that efforts be made to generate additional information relevant to evaluation by both the survey and "economic benefits" approaches.[c] In the case of the former, development and testing of basic techniques should be carried out on a limited scale to determine potential usefulness. In the case of the latter, at least crude data should be developed on the socioeconomic and demographic characteristics of potential recipients, on the direct medical costs saved by the use of artificial hearts, and on the ability of recipients to return to productive lives after treatment. Some of these calculations will, of course, involve the difficult problem of predicting the availability, costs, and effectiveness of other modes of prevention and treatment now being developed.

We recognize that even such additional information will not aid in dealing with many of the difficult problems of evaluation, especially those relating to impacts on social institutions and values. As noted above, there will always be a need for informed introspection and intuition in the evaluation process.

The Dollar Costs of the Artificial Heart. As noted above, it is not feasible, at least on the basis of present knowledge, to attempt to reduce the overall advantages and disadvantages of the artificial heart to quantitative terms. What can be said, however, on the benefit side, is that a totally implantable artificial heart that will prolong, for an estimated ten-year period, the productive lives of cardiac patients who would otherwise face imminent death, and that would enable seriously incapacitated cardiac patients to enjoy ten years of life of a substantially better quality, involves immense benefits to society. Indeed, even without the ability actually to compare quantified benefits and costs, it is apparent on an intuitive basis that the benefits appear to outweigh the costs by a substantial margin. Since, however, it is possible to discuss in dollar terms the potential costs of implanting the artificial heart, even if only crudely, and since these costs are substantial and appear to raise important issues of social policy relating to resource use, the panel believes it would be appropriate to consider existing information on these costs.

At the outset, the speculative nature of our information about costs of clinical application must be clearly recognized. Future technological breakthroughs may profoundly affect the magnitude of these costs, but we are obviously incapable of making cost projections which take these into account. Specific numerical projections made by various experts in the engineering, design, and testing of devices reflect a degree of disagreement and uncertainty which must be frankly acknowledged. However, agreement on order-of-magnitude figures appears sufficient to warrant a very brief recounting of these figures.[d]

The costs per patient include costs of initial operative and postoperative treat-

---

[c]Dr. Smythe dissociates herself from this recommendation. In her view, the potential value of further evaluation is dubious, particularly since much of the basis for judgment is nonquantifiable and unrelated to economic benefits.

[d]Dr. Salkever has prepared estimates based on more specific projections. These estimates and a description of the methodology employed are presented in Appendix B of the original report.

ment, costs of the device, and costs of the energy system. Medical and hospitalization expenses for surgery and subsequent treatment are expected to be of the order of $15,000 to $25,000 (in current purchasing power). Device costs are expected to fall in the $1500 to $6000 range, depending to some extent on the number of recipients, since economies of large-scale production are anticipated. Energy costs, because they depend upon a host of technical performance parameters, are very difficult to predict. The present value of energy costs for the nuclear system, assuming a ten-year patient lifetime, might be as low as $3000 or $4000 under very favorable circumstances, or four times as great under unfavorable circumstances; but the uncertainty of these estimates is substantial, and we cannot confidently predict that actual cost will fall within even this broad range. The energy costs of battery systems will probably be less than those for the nuclear system, but it is difficult to concoct even very crude projections of the extent of this difference. Furthermore, internal battery systems may also entail additional treatment costs for replacement of batteries. Recognizing that this estimate may well be on the low side, the panel has decided, for purposes of exposition, to use the range of $15,000 to $25,000 as its order of magnitude estimate of the total cost of each artificial heart implantation.

ISSUES IN THE USE OF THE CLINICALLY ACCEPTABLE DEVICE: ALTERNATIVE POWER SOURCES

There are now essentially three alternative modes for providing the energy necessary for operation of the totally implantable artificial heart. The most attractive of these appears to be the biological fuel cell, which would utilize energy derived from the skeletal muscles, the respiratory system, and/or biolectric potentials to power the artificial heart system. Unfortunately, however, the present state of technology is such that a biological fuel cell is not available to provide an adequate level of power, adequately controlled, for an adequately long period of time to make this a realistic alternative. Although research and development with respect to the biological fuel cell concept are proceeding, the panel has been informed that it is highly unlikely that a satisfactory biological fuel cell can be developed within the time period in which a totally implantable artificial heart will otherwise be available for clinical application. Accordingly, the realistic alternatives at the present time appear to be the battery system and the nuclear system. As will be described below, significant implications—i.e., advantages and disadvantages—flow from the choice between these two alternative systems. In the following discussion, the panel relies heavily on scientific and technical information that it has received from various experts on the subjects discussed.

Relative Advantages of the Nuclear System

It appears at the present time that, from the standpoint of purely technical considerations, the nuclear system is optimum. It is presently within technological capability to implant a fuel capsule containing Plutonium-238, as part of an artificial heart system, which would provide a reliable source of energy for a period of ten years. Such an energy system has the obvious advantage of enabling the artificial heart to function reliably for the ten-year period without any necessity for action to be taken by the recipient to maintain the availability of the energy.

In contrast, the battery system is far less satisfactory from the technical standpoint. In order to maintain an adequate level of energy, it would be necessary for the recipient periodically to recharge the battery through transmission of electro-magnetic energy across the intact skin from an external recharging unit into an internal receptacle placed near the skin. The battery could be recharged directly from an ordinary electrical outlet or from a portable source of stored energy contained in an attaché case or a vest worn by the recipient. When convenient, the recipient could plug into an electrical outlet in his home or place of work; under other circumstances, he could use the portable device for recharging, thereby enabling a high degree of mobility. Unfortunately, however, the rechargeable battery has a limited life, the length of which is dependent in large part on the number of recharging cycles. The panel has been informed by experts knowledgeable in battery technology that it is presently within technological capability to provide a battery system requiring no more than two hours of recharging per day, with no more than four recharging operations per day, that will reliably power an artificial heart system for a two-year period. The panel has also been informed by these experts that there is a good possibility, given an adequate level of research and development, that within a five-year period a battery with a life of five years will be available. This means, if the objective of the artificial heart is to extend life for a period of ten years, that the recipient will be required to undergo surgery, at intervals dependent on the battery life, to replace the battery. Thus, given present battery technology, a recipient, in order to live ten years with an artificial heart, would probably require four subsequent operations for replacement of the battery. If the technology is improved as predicted by the experts so that a five-year battery is available, only one subsequent operation would be necessary during the ten-year period. Although the battery would be located in the abdominal cavity, easily accessible for removal with minimum risk, each surgical procedure would, of course, involve some risk to the recipient's life. It should be noted, however, that similar procedures, although involving less risk, have been required for some time in the case of patients in whom battery-powered cardiac pacemakers have been implanted.

It is obvious that, from the technical and practical standpoints, the nuclear system is far superior to the battery system. Not only does the nuclear system provide a longer-term, more reliable source of energy from the artificial heart, but it also is self-functioning and imposes no requirement on the recipient to think or worry about, and remember, the inexorable necessity for recharging. It also frees the recipient from dependence for his very life on external sources of energy and from the burdens and risks of periodic replacement surgery. Finally, unlike the battery system in which the necessity and apparatus for recharging serve as constant reminders to the recipient's associates that he has an artificial heart, i.e., is "different," the nuclear system is without any tangible external manifestations. In these respects, in short, the nuclear system is far more advantageous to the recipient in terms of his sense of well-being and personal convenience.

Disadvantages of the Nuclear System

There are, however, conspicuous disadvantages to the nuclear system. In considering these disadvantages, it should be recognized that they are characterized as disadvantages in terms of the existing state of technology and the existing state of scientific knowledge. It is, of course, possible that technological advances, as well as future experience, may minimize or eliminate these factors which presently appear to be disadvantageous. At the same time, it is possible, even with improved technology, that future scientific research and experience may indicate that the disadvantages are greater than presently are estimated. Accordingly, it should be understood that the following discussion is based on present circumstances, and that the validity of the panel's statements should be subject to reconsideration in the light of future developments.

Disadvantages Relating to Radiation Exposure. Given present technology, the nuclear-powered artificial heart may, in normal day-to-day operation, involve a health hazard to the recipient himself, to his family and close associates, and to the public generally because of its emission of radiation. There is no way to eliminate completely this emission of radiation, the amount of which is a function of the quantity of plutonium in the fuel capsule, of the purity of the plutonium, and of the manner in which the plutonium is shielded. It is anticipated that exposures can be reduced as systems become available that will operate with less Plutonium-238 than required in present systems, and as further improvements are made in plutonium purity. Significant reductions in exposure by more shielding are impracticable because of added weight and volume.

A fundamental moral question is raised by the possibility that implantation of nuclear-powered artificial hearts in specific individuals in order to prolong their lives will result in injury to other members of the population, including future generations. It should be noted that even though the number of individuals who might sustain manifest injury may be statistically very small, the injury sustained by such few persons may be substantial (e.g., leukemia, cancer, genetic death or defects).

A traditional mode of analysis in deciding whether society should acquiesce in the use of a technology capable of inflicting harm has been the balancing of aggregate benefits to society against the aggregate risks. In this analysis, there would be reckoned as benefits the direct benefit to recipients and their families, and also the substantial benefits to society as a whole of the preservation of the productive capacity of the recipients. In addition, moreover, the availability of the nuclear-powered artificial heart must be regarded as a benefit to all members of society, since even if they now do not need the artificial heart, there is a statistical probability that they may require one to prolong their lives at some future date. These benefits would appear to outweigh what appear to be the low risks. Some members of the panel have serious doubt that a decision based on such a benefit-risk analysis can be ethically justified when measures to improve the health and extend the lives of specific individuals pose a risk to the health and lives of the population generally, including unborn future generations.

The issues discussed in the preceding paragraph are simplified when consideration is given to the fact that there exists an alternative to the nuclear-powered artificial heart.... Although the battery-powered system is less convenient than the nuclear system, and the requirement for surgery to replace the battery subjects the recipient to additional risk—thereby making the battery system less beneficial than the nuclear system—the battery system does not involve any known risk to the health and lives of other persons. Accordingly, the panel concludes that it is ethically unjustifiable, regardless of the benefit-risk balance, when (we are informed by experts) the battery-powered alternative is available, to subject the population at large to any significant degree of risk as a consequence of extending or improving the lives of particular recipients. Whatever may be the burdens and risks, it is appropriate that they fall upon those who are directly benefited rather than involuntarily on random members of society who benefit at best only potentially and indirectly.

In view of the foregoing, the panel recommends that the nuclear-powered artificial heart not be implanted in human beings until such time as it is established scientifically that there will be no significant risk of injury involuntarily imposed on other persons. Consistent with this, the panel recommends that greatly increased effort be devoted to development of more adequate battery and biological fuel cell systems. Recognizing the obviously superior performance characteristics of the proposed nuclear-powered system, we emphasize our hope that technological advances and increased understanding of the effects of radiation on life will in time enable a determination that the nuclear-powered artificial heart can be used without significant risk to society. Meanwhile, we urge continuing effort, including experiments in animals, looking towards perfection of both the nuclear and battery systems and development of the biological fuel cell. We recognize that important information could be gained from implanting a nuclear-powered artificial heart in a limited number of human beings on an experimental basis. We oppose such experimentation solely on the basis of our doubt that, if the experiments prove successful, it will be possible to hold the line against more widespread use of the nuclear system.

ISSUES IN THE USE OF THE CLINICALLY ACCEPTABLE ARTIFICIAL HEART: ALLOCATION AND REGULATION

Financing Mechanisms

By any standard, the total costs for implantation and maintenance of an artificial heart will be quite substantial, raising a question as to how broadly available the artificial heart will be to persons who need one. The extent to which the cost of an artificial heart would be a deterrent to implantation in a patient whose family will have to absorb the costs out of their own resources will be dependent upon the particular circumstances in each case. Where the patient faces imminent death unless the artificial heart is implanted, his family will in all likelihood be willing to make whatever financial sacrifice is necessary to save his life. There will, of course, be poor families that will simply be unable to bear costs of this magnitude, and in such cases, even if the patient faces imminent death, implantation would be dependent upon the willingness of the medical center and physicians to do the operation without expectation of payment. On the other hand, where the patient is not desperately ill, or does not face imminent death, but where the risk of a cardiac event in the near-term is sufficiently great to justify implantation, the substantial costs may operate as a significant deterrent. Moreover, in some cases the physician's knowledge that the patient is unable to afford the procedure, or that the procedure would impose great financial burden, may lead the physician not to consider or recommend implantation of an artificial heart.

Fortunately, the harsh realities of the costs of clinical implantation of artificial hearts are expected to be somewhat mitigated by the broad availability of medical insurance. Most American families are presently covered by hospitalization insurance, either individually or through employment-related plans. Unfortunately, however, this coverage involves gaps related to income level. While all but 8 percent of families with income over $10,000 have hospitalization coverage, 22 percent of those with incomes of $5000 to $7000, and 43 percent with incomes between $3000 and $5000, are without such coverage. Persons in unskilled occupations or those employed in very small businesses or service occupations are less likely to be covered than are workers in steadier, better-paying jobs. At the same time, individual insurance, theoretically available to cover the gaps, is too expensive for families of lower or lower-middle incomes.

Even where medical insurance is available, there may be gaps with respect to the artificial heart. Medical insurance covers only procedures that are regarded as genuinely therapeutic, as adjudged by the American Medical Association. Thus, in the early stages of the use of artificial hearts, while the procedure is still experimental, it is likely that insurance coverage will not be available. On the other hand, it is likely that most of the costs incident to the experimental phase will be borne under NIH grants. Another gap might exist if the artificial heart is regarded as a "prosthetic device," since some plans exclude expenses of such devices. Also, in this connection, there may be some question as to whether the power source will be regarded as a medical item. There appears, however, to be a trend toward liberalization of medical insurance policies in these respects. Finally, some policies have limitations on total dollar coverage or on the total period of covered hospitalization. The latter limitation does not appear to be a significant obstacle, since the hospitalization required for implantation and recovery is not expected to be notably longer than for other major surgical procedures. The dollar limitation may result in less than full coverage under many policies if the total costs are in the range of $35,000 to $100,000.

The 1970s have seen considerably increased concern for the modern health needs of the population at large, and old assumptions and restraints are beginning to be challenged by more creative approaches to health care delivery. Insurance companies are in a position to offer virtually any kind of plan demanded by a subscriber, provided that experience ratings can be calculated. A 1972 survey of twelve of the largest writers of group health insurance by the Health Insurance Association of America gave ample evidence that dollar maximums need not be a problem in the near future: four of the companies already have unlimited maximums (and a fifth expects to join them shortly); five have $250,000; one $100,000; and two (one of which will shortly join the unlimited group) $50,000. Although the very high maxima are not yet characteristic of health insurance plans, they indicate the direction of current developments in providing for catastrophic illness.

Although the gaps described above are likely to be overcome, in terms of policy definitions and design, it will still be possible for persons who need to have the device implanted to be uncovered because of interstitial inadequacies; e.g., a person temporarily between jobs is no longer covered by his former employer's plan, nor yet that of his future employer; and a dependent student of twenty-four can no longer be covered by his parents' insurance, yet he may not be automatically covered by another plan. Not all persons have access to employment-related plans, and the confusing variety of possibilities may make the choice of appropriate private arrangements exceedingly difficult for one not experienced in the field of health insurance, even if money is available to pay the premiums. Average consumers have little understanding of the complex terms of their health-care insurance and are in a poor position to evaluate in advance its suitability to their needs.

In short, even though it appears that medical and hospitalization plans may be adequate for financing the artificial heart in the case of a large proportion of those Americans who might need one, it is likely that various gaps will leave uncovered a significant portion of the population. It is possible in the light of the precedent established in Public Law 92-603, which brought renal dialysis and transplants within Medicare coverage, that there will be new legislation bringing artificial heart implantations within the coverage of the social security laws.

In general, therefore, we believe it likely that, through either private or government insurance mechanisms, the implantation of artificial hearts will be brought within a system of cost-sharing whereby a portion of the financial burden of implantation of artificial hearts will be shifted from individual recipients to nonrecipients. Although the dramatic aspects of artificial heart technology, as well as public funding of its development, make the artificial heart a special case, it should be recognized that cost-sharing in this area is merely a logical extension of the general trend in our society in the direction of ensuring that all persons have appropriate medical care and of protecting individuals against the consequences of catastrophic medical expenses.[e]

Patient Selection Criteria

It is possible, at one or more points in the evolution of the artificial heart, that there will be a short supply of artificial heart resources so that the demand for implantation is in excess of supply. Such scarcity may be attributable to a limited supply of the device itself, to a shortage of qualified medical personnel and facilities, or, in the case of the nuclear-powered system, to a shortage of Plutonium-238. Such scarcity is most likely to exist in the early stages of initial experimentation and second-generation use, before the point of clinical application is reached, by which time, of course, mass-production of the system could be anticipated.

If the artificial heart works well in the sense of extending life and giving recipients a reasonable quality of postimplantation life, it is to be expected that patients may be clamoring for the opportunity to have the life-extending and -enhancing artificial heart. If there is a situation of scarce resources, how will decisions be made as to who will and will not be chosen for implantation? There are three basic alternative means for determining who shall have priority: (1) decisions based on appropriate medical criteria, i.e., providing the artificial heart to those with the most urgent need; (2) decisions based on estimates of "social worth"; and (3) decisions based on some form of random selection.

The Panel believes that the optimum criterion for establishing priorities is the decision based on medical need. Under this system, a medical center would

---

[e]Separate statement by Professor Kaplan: If cost-sharing is to be considered, it should meet three desiderata not sufficiently detailed in the present discussion. (1) All costs, including such items as transportation, family expenses away from home while the patient is hospitalized, etc., should be included; (2) the amount of sharing, if any, must take into account the total family situation, including short- and long-range effects on all concerned; (3) given the current trend of rising costs, some effort must be made by the society as a whole to examine and control some of the costs instead of leaving them to a monopolistic situation which is sometimes mislabeled as a "free" market. I believe that the whole question of costs and cost sharing merits far more study and attention for a much more extended period of time than was possible for our panel.

determine, strictly on medical criteria, which of the candidate patients being treated by the medical center have the greatest need for implantation of the artificial heart and are suitable candidates (e.g., can withstand the trauma of surgery, etc.). Unfortunately, however, this system is not without complexities. Considerations as to ability to pay, which is in itself a form of "social worth" criterion, may consciously or subconsciously affect decisions as to medical need. Moreover, use of this system may produce a number of candidates with roughly equal medical need under circumstances when available resources are not sufficient to take care of all.

A persuasive case can be made for the second alternative, the position that "society is entitled to minimize its losses by saving those who can contribute most by rewarding past performance and, thus, encouraging future good performance by others."[1] The belief in differential social worth is familiar to us; and the easy game of nominating groups of obviously questionable characters is a tempting one: convicted criminals, Bowery "bums," drug addicts, confirmed alcoholics, psychotics, syphilitics, hunchbacks, paralytics, epileptics, the severely handicapped of other varieties, the mentally retarded, the senile. Even if one avoids more controversial additional categories (the chronically unemployed, hippies and other nonconformists, political extremists of the right or the left, draft dodgers, members of unpopular ethnic or religious minorities, functional illiterates, people on welfare, eccentrics of a range of descriptions, people in debt, residents of Appalachia), it is obvious that there are conflicting value systems at work.

There are alternatives to setting up machinery to determine social worth: first, permitting matters to operate without conscious direction, thus letting power, individual preference, and social pressures make the determination as they now do in the absence of a deliberate decision in favor of individual equality of well-defined social criteria; second, a form of random selection, such as taking earlier applicants in preference to later ones or conducting some type of lottery.

In the current tendency to absolve persons of responsibility for the unintended effects of their unconscious decisions and actions, it is simpler and easiest to avoid decision-making and let fate determine who lives and who dies. Could we be comfortable with a system of allocation which provided little access for minorities or poor persons, and which allowed for frivolous use of a scarce health resource by persons of wealth? Would it be moral, for example, for a wealthy eccentric to be able to buy an artificial heart for a beloved pet when a thirty-five-year-old parent of three children must be denied?

Moreover, when such a resource is developed largely at public expense, what is the stake of the average taxpayer in its use?

Some will argue that any laissez-faire arrangement for allocating the artificial heart is bound to result in a form of social worth assessment, since ability to pay and power in general are themselves viewed by some as rough measures of social value. Some would argue that to deny social worth judgments is dishonest; it fails to face our constant differentiation among people. Shatin[2] notes our unembarrassed drawing of distinctions in providing medical care for veterans, allocating public funds for special disease categories (e.g., mental illness, cancer, tuberculosis), selecting patients for kidney dialysis in the years when there was a shortage of facilities, and fund drives for specific illnesses (e.g., muscular dystrophy, birth defects, mental retardation). He argues for a high standard of basic medical care for all, regardless of ability to pay; only beyond this level would social value (not power or wealth) enter into judgments as to whether it is in society's interest to make a substantial investment in an expensive new or scarce procedure in a particular case.

So far the argument for social evaluation has a persuasive logic: it is what we do, anyway; is it not more honest to say so and examine fully and critically the ways of setting standards and agree upon a method which can be publicly supported for establishing and applying criteria?

Unhappily, our record in this area is not encouraging. The openness and fortitude required for dealing with complex and painful social concerns is in short supply; people may logically agree that it is cruel to prolong the dying agony of a cancer victim, but they do not want to be involved in the act of terminating his life—they want someone else to do it. When the artificial kidney was new and there were not enough machines to treat all those whose lives equally depended on immediate treatment selection was necessary—but no one wanted the job. In the only well-documented case in the literature, the Admissions and Policies Committee of the Seattle Artificial Kidney Center at Swedish Hospital[3] agreed to serve from a sense of duty, rather than enthusiasm for the job, and insisted upon keeping their identities secret (they also avoided learning the names of the patients they screened). That committee disbanded with alacrity—and relief—when treatment facilities increased and the number of patients who could be accommodated came close to the number who could be considered medically suitable. While we have today federally-financed treatment for kidney patients unable to finance it for themselves, there is still more than a suggestion of social value assessment in the allocation of treatment. Persons involved in patient-selection processes have noted instances in which decisions to treat borderline cases were simply postponed until the patient died or was too ill to be treated, so reluctant was anyone to make a clearcut negative decision.

Let us look more closely at the matter. If we accept Shatin's assumption that society's first duty is to provide a high standard of basic medical care for all, then the investment in more exceptional and expensive kinds of resources need not be made at the expense of the higher priority case, and could logically be presented as a purchase of exceptional resources at society's expense for the purpose of obtaining the further services of persons of high social value (or of rewarding such persons for past services, thus motivating others to give such services).

What is high social value? What are the criteria for judgment? By whom and how can they be applied? How absolute can they be in a changing society? What mechanisms would be necessary to assure periodic revisions? These questions are difficult, perhaps even impossible, to resolve in a satisfactory manner. It is difficult enough to define the criteria for judgment and even more difficult to provide a mechanism for implementing them in an even-handed and objective manner. Moreover, the very essence of making decisions based on "social worth" runs counter to basic principles of equality in our society. Accordingly, the Panel recommends against any system of priorities for implantation of artificial hearts based on consideration of relative "social worth."

The third alternative, random selection, also has much to commend it. We do not, however, believe that a principle of random selection should override medical criteria. It may be appropriate, once priorities have been established using medical criteria, to choose among candidates with roughly equivalent need on the basis of random selection. Random selection could be implemented either by lottery or by a system of first-come first-served.

The Panel does not have the competence to lay down a set of criteria or rules for ascertaining priorities. We prefer to state our position in terms of general principles. We reject completely the concept of a "social worth" criterion. We believe that disparities in ability to pay—which disparities hopefully will be eliminated through insurance or governmental measures—should not influence the decision, when implantation would appear to be beneficial, as to who will receive the artificial heart and who will be denied it. And, finally, we believe that random selection, as among equally necessitous patients, is a desirable principle.

The primary mission of the Panel, as stated in our charge, has been to detail the economic, ethical, legal, medical, psychiatric, and social implications of clinical application of a totally implantable artificial heart. A summary of these implications follows below. We do not believe it is meaningful, or perhaps even feasible, to isolate potential implications and characterize them as "economic," "legal," "social," etc., since some do not fit neatly in any such single category and some involve more than a single category. We are reluctant, moreover, to hazard firm predictions as to what specific situations will arise, and, therefore, prefer to state some of our conclusions in terms of issues that we believe will be raised by clinical application of the artificial heart.

We believe that clinical application, and the process of achieving clinical application, of the totally implantable artificial heart will have the following impacts on society.

1. Successful development and use of the totally implantable artificial heart will provide a useful and important therapy for treating various serious cardiac diseases, and for prolonging and improving the quality of life of many patients. If all of the expectations of its sponsors are realized, its benefits to society will be immense.

2. Successful accomplishment of the artificial heart program may establish

an important precedent for development of goal-directed, technologically sophisticated solutions to public health problems.

3. Unless implantation of an artificial heart is covered under insurance programs, its use would involve very substantial monetary burdens to the families of recipients.

4. The high costs of clinical application of the artificial heart may force consideration of means (e.g., private or governmental insurance coverage or direct government funding) for making implantation available to all who need it, without regard for ability to pay, and may lead to broader reconsideration of the financial mechanisms for delivery of health services generally.

5. Clinical application of the artificial heart may, particularly if implantation is generally available without financial constraints, lead to a potentially enormous commitment of health resources specifically related to the artificial heart.

6. Given the obvious benefits of the totally implantable artificial heart and the risks to the recipient (inherent in the surgical procedure, the fallibility of the device, and the radiation effects in the case of a nuclear-powered system) and to others (in the case of a nuclear-powered system), questions are raised about the manner in which societal interests should be reflected in decisions on the use of the device at the initial human experimentation stage and thereafter.

7. Application of the artificial heart may raise questions as to the respective values to be assigned to mere extension of life as opposed to the quality of the extended life; this will be especially true when its application involves older members of society.

8. Use of the artificial heart may necessitate consideration of the ethical, religious, and legal issues pertaining to decisions by recipients, their families, and/or physicians with respect to turning the artificial heart off under various circumstances.

9. The totally implantable artificial heart will undoubtedly stimulate discussion as to the extent to which artificial devices should be substituted for vital organs or functions of the human body, leading ultimately to the question of mechanical brains.

10. Application of the nuclear-powered artificial heart may raise fundamental ethical and policy issues pertaining to the balance between its use for extending the life of specific recipients and the risks thereby imposed on other individuals and on society in general.

11. Recipients of the artificial heart and their families may develop psychological stresses because of the recipient's dependence for life on a machine and his possible dependence on external sources of energy. In the case of a nuclear-powered artificial heart, there may be other stresses because of concerns relating to the possibility that the recipient may cause radiation injury to his family and to others. These possibilities are relevant to questions of the acceptability of the artificial heart, the quality of informed consent, and the quality of life.

12. Reactions of family members, associates, and other persons to the presence of an artificial heart in a recipient may also have a bearing on the quality of the recipient's life. This possibility is particularly great in the case of the nuclear-powered artificial heart, because of concern about the risks of exposure to the recipient's radiation emanations.

13. Clinical application of the nuclear-powered artificial heart will result in an increase in radiation in the environment. Public concern about the consequences of exposure to radiation from nuclear-powered artificial hearts may operate as a constraint on other radiation-producing technologies such as nuclear power.

14. Application of the artificial heart may require redefinition of legal and medical criteria for determining the time of death.

15. It may be necessary to enact legislation relating to the requirement for post-mortem removal of nuclear fuel sources and for ready identification of bearers of nuclear-powered artificial hearts in order that such removal may be ensured.

16. Although the risks to society as a whole involved in the use of a properly designed and constructed nuclear-powered artificial heart each of whom bears substantial quantities of plutonium that could cause substantial damage if released, has obvious environmental implications. It is likely that any decision by the AEC to license the widespread use of Plutonium-238 in artificial hearts would have to be preceded by compliance with the National Environmental Policy Act. In addition, it may be necessary to regulate the activities of recipients in order to minimize ambient radiation exposures and the possibility of accidental rupture of the fuel capsule, and consequent danger to life and the environment in general.

17. In addition to extending the productive life of younger and middle-aged members of society, clinical application of the artificial heart may increase the number of older, and perhaps the number of medically dependent, individuals in our society, and should intensify concern about means for improving the quality of life enjoyed by such persons generally.

18. The process of moving forward from the present developmental stage of the technology to the point of clinical application involves important issues pertaining to the relationship between experimentation and therapy, selection of patient-subjects, conditions for human experimentation, and informed consent. These problems are not unique to the artificial heart, but their early consideration provides an opportunity for thoughtful planning to ensure that appropriate decisions are made.

19. If the feasibility of the totally implantable artificial heart is demonstrated in human experimentation, there may be a substantial demand for implantation of the device in seriously ill patients who otherwise would face imminent death. Pressures may result to use the artificial heart too broadly before adequate data are available as to its technical performance and potential consequences. Demand for implantation of the artificial heart may exceed available artificial

heart resources, necessitating judgments as to who shall have and who shall be denied implantation.

20. The continued development of very costly forms of medical intervention, such as the artificial heart, may lead us to examine critically basic values about the preciousness of human life, and to consider the potentially broad ethical, legal, and social implications of changes in these values.

The Panel recommends:

1. In light of the information that the Panel has received, we believe that development of the totally implantable artificial heart should proceed. The scope and direction of the program should, of course, be periodically reconsidered relative to other programs directed towards prevention and treatment of cardiac disease.

2. Every effort should be made to develop more satisfactory non-nuclear energy systems.

3. Further steps in the development, testing, and use of the artificial heart should involve adequate consideration of the kinds of societal implications of the artificial heart that are discussed in this report. The National Heart and Lung Institute should consider establishment of a permanent, broadly interdisciplinary, and representative group of public members to monitor further steps and to participate in the formulation of guidelines and policies.

4. There is a need for careful advance planning to minimize the possibility that artificial heart resources will be in short supply.

5. In the event artificial heart resources are in scarce supply, decisions as to the selection of candidates for implantation of the artificial heart should be made by physicians and medical institutions on the basis of medical criteria. If the pool of patients with equal medical needs exceeds supply, procedures should be devised for some form of random selection. Social worth criteria should not be used, and every effort should be exerted to minimize the possibility that social worth may implicitly be taken into account.[f]

6. Particularly in view of the substantial commitment of public funds for development of the artificial heart, implantation should be broadly available, and availability should not be limited only to those able to pay. This objective can be accomplished through either private or government insurance mechanisms. It is important, however, that financing mechanisms be constructed in such a manner as not to result in inefficient or inappropriate use of the artificial heart.[g]

---

[f]Professor Havighurst accepts these recommendations as advice to providers, but would object to the use of governmental compulsion to realize these ethical objectives. He also doubts that some implicit use of social worth criteria is necessarily destructive.

[g]Professor Sapolsky wishes to point out that investment of public funds in the development of particular technologies does not in itself require government intervention in the application of those technologies, nor would the absence of such investments prohibit government intervention. In addition, he is concerned that the panel's recommendation will

7. In view of the risks (based on the present state of the technology and the present state of scientific knowledge concerning the effects of low-level radiation exposures) to the families and associates of recipients, and to the public and the environment generally, the nuclear-powered artificial heart should not be implanted in human beings until it has been scientifically determined that such a device can be used without significant risk to other persons. Meanwhile, however, development of the nuclear-powered artificial heart, including tests in animals, should proceed. But for its doubt that it would be possible to hold the line against broader use if the experiments were successful, the Panel would not be opposed to experimental use of the nuclear-powered artificial heart in a limited number of human patients.

8. If the nuclear-powered artificial heart is used, licensing and regulation with respect to the health and safety of the public should be by the federal government rather than the states.

9. Every effort should be made to inform the public of developments with respect to the artificial heart and to engage the public in consideration and discussion of the artificial heart's potential impact on society. Such effort is particularly necessary with respect to the nuclear-powered artificial heart in view of the fact that this system may have a broad impact and may involve risks, beyond the circle of the individuals directly involved in its clinical use. If a decision should be reached contrary to the Panel's recommendations against use of the nuclear-powered artificial heart in human beings under present circumstances, implementation of such decision may be highly controversial. This controversy may impede introduction of the device, or may create a social environment making its use unattractive to many potential recipients and their families. If such a controversy should develop, it is important that it involve debate based on realistic and factual allegations, and not on distortions or "old wives' tales." The government should take the lead in presenting the issue to the public at an early date with full and candid disclosure of both the benefits and the costs and risks.

Notes to Chapter Fourteen

1. Jesse Dukeminier, Jr., and David Sanders, "Legal Problems in Allocation of Scarce Medical Resources: The Artificial Kidney," in *Arch. Intern. Med.*, V. 127 (June 1971), 1133-37 at 1134.

---

be taken as implying that potential recipients of artificial hearts deserve to be singled out for special financial assistance in obtaining what will be only one of many expensive life-saving therapies. Equity considerations, he believes, demand that the financing of health care be approached in a more comprehensive manner. Since the panel did not examine the financial implications of a comprehensive health care system, he feels that the panel should remain silent on the matter of financing the artificial heart. Professor Havighurst associates himself with Professor Sapolsky's statement. Professor Kaplan believes that the wording of the panel's recommendation implies broad availability to those able to pay, with the admonition that the device should not be limited only to this group. His own value preference would have been to state that it should be broadly available according to medical need irrespective of the ability to pay.

2. Leo Shatin, "Medical Care and the Social Worth of a Man," *American Journal of Orthopsychiatry*, V. 36 (1966), pp. 96-101.

3. Shana Alexander, "They Decide Who Lives, Who Dies," *Life*, V. 53, No. 19 (November 9, 1962), pp. 102-25.

❇ *Chapter 15*

Separate Views on the Artificial Heart

Clark C. Havighurst

The panel has written an interesting and occasionally provocative document, but on some issues, in my view, the report [of the Artificial Heart Assessment Panel] fails to reflect the application of a coherent conceptual framework for evaluating the "economic, ethical, legal ... and social implications" of the artificial heart. The job of disciplined analysis, it appears, must be left to others, using the extensive information provided by the panel as a starting point from which to probe the profound issues presented by the artificial heart and by other similar developments in medical technology.

In my view, the panel's difficulties resulted primarily from an excessive fascination with the technical aspects of the artificial heart, on which it could make no useful judgments, and an underestimate of the time required to write a report which came to grips with all of the broader implications of the subject. It is interesting, for example, that, of all the experts whose testimony and opinions were obtained, none directly addressed the issue of the appropriate criteria for public decision-making or the economic, ethical, legal, and social issues. By the time writing of its report began, there was little opportunity to develop principled arguments for many of the positions taken, and, in the final assessment, the panel members were left pretty much to their own disciplines and biases in reaching their judgments. Some important problems connected with financing were never addressed at all.

The purpose of this separate statement is simply to suggest some of the analytical tools that might have been employed and to identify some of the issues that I believe have been poorly handled or obscured by the report. Each subhead is keyed to a particular portion of the report, but the first two should be read together.

UTILITARIANISM AND JUSTICE

This section of the report explores "advantages and disadvantages" of the artificial heart and the problems of comparing costs and benefits. In a single paragraph on page 61, the panel notes that it does not explore the ethical limitations of the utilitarian approach that it seems to employ. By failing to develop at this point any neutral principles for use in making public choices, the panel has opened itself to criticism concerning the basis of its judgment on the nuclear-powered artificial heart and on financing questions.

Making social choices solely on the basis of whether advantages or disadvantages predominate is ethically unsatisfying, for it involves an assumption that it is just for some to gain at the expense of others. Thus, the classical utilitarian principle of "the greatest good for the greatest number," often employed in making public choices, has been criticized for seeming to override scruples about inequality of impact and to sanction majoritarian impositions on minorities. Philosopher John Rawls, in *A Theory of Justice*, criticizes utilitarianism from this perspective, and the panel alludes to the problem.

Whether the panel could have been expected to resolve this philosophical dilemma is of course doubtful, but a theoretical construct is available that can be usefully employed in correcting the apparent shortcomings of utilitarianism and arriving at a satisfying ethical judgment about particular issues. This construct is the economist's perfect world, in which all interactions are costless and all conflicts among individuals can therefore be resolved in voluntary transactions rather than through governmental intervention. Beginning from this construct, government can be seen as compensating for the existence of prohibitive transaction costs in the real world and as facilitating the achievement of arrangements roughly similar to those efficient ones which would be produced by cost-free bargaining among citizens having the best available information and bargaining power appropriately distributed. Viewing the matter in this way, one can perhaps see the ethical importance of compensating the losers in any social action—exercise of the power of eminent domain, for example—and of preventing the gainers from enjoying windfalls at others' expense. Utilitarianism, however, appears to ignore the importance of compensation, even though, if the advantages in fact exceed the disadvantages as viewed by the individuals affected, the gainers would be willing to pay the losers (if they could be identified); by hypothesis, the gainers would still enjoy a net benefit.

It is useful to observe that, whatever public choices are made with respect to the artificial heart, there will be both individual gainers and individual losers. Thus, if the device is developed and used in spite of some existing disadvantages, there would be a windfall to heart patients unless they could be made to compensate the disadvantaged portion of the community. Or, less obviously, if a decision were made to prohibit the artificial heart on the basis of overriding disadvantages, the would-be recipients could claim they had been injured—indeed, condemned to death—by the majority, who, again, should be willing to compensate the losers. But of course, even though justice issues (other than those relating to wealth inequalities generally) would disappear if the gainers could always be required to compensate the losers, compensation for such "spillover" effects is very often impossible to arrange. The question then presented is what we should do in that event.

But, since there are losers whichever way the decision goes, private activities or public projects yielding net benefits should not be prohibited or given up just because there would be uncompensated losers; by hypothesis, there would be greater harm done by such a negative choice. Nevertheless, fairness requires that we do the best we can, within the limits of practicality, to do justice to the losers in any particular case. Thus, the law provides numerous means of redressing or controlling the major spillover effects of both public and private activity—by compelling compensation, prohibiting nuisances, regulating behavior, and so forth. Moreover, justice may require special compensation arrangements—welfare programs, perhaps—if one group of citizens seems to come out losers more often than gainers in the sum total of public and private decisions having uncompensated spillovers. Thus, although many private actions as well as many of society's collective choices will necessarily impose unreimbursed costs on some and result in windfalls for others, the law governing private arrangements and the structuring of public programs should take account of these effects and provide compensation, directly or indirectly, wherever possible.

Sometimes, because the social arrangements being made today for the future do not benefit specific individuals at the expense of identifiable others, it may be possible to justify a pure utilitarian approach by viewing the stakes of individuals probabilistically, making each a possible gainer as well as a possible loser. Thus viewed, if potential gains exceed potential losses, the action might be deemed appropriate without concern for compensation of the actual losers. Difficulties remain, of course, if the advantages (disadvantages) are likely to accrue only to the more (less) affluent or to some other group to which all do not have a roughly equal expectation of belonging. But even if compensation is impossible in such circumstances and injustice therefore inevitable, it may still be unjust not to take the action, since that would be to impose uncompensated costs (in the form of benefits denied) on the would-be beneficiaries. Justice demands not that perfect justice be done (for that is impossible), but that every effort be made to design public programs and the legal environment of private activities—if they are justified because the benefits outweigh the costs—so that uncompensated harms are minimized. It is hard to conceive of circumstances when it would not be wrong to require that a large benefit be foregone in order to avoid imposing a small harm.

Perhaps because it was presented to them inexpertly and without time for full exploration and development, this analytical framework seemed to offend some members of the Panel, especially as it might be applied to matters involving life and death, as in the case of the artificial heart. The stumbling block appeared to be their sense that it is inhumane to contemplate bargaining over these questions, even hypothetically. Nevertheless, in the absence of any other disciplined way of looking at the problems presented, I believe the model suggested could have been harmonized with the compunctions expressed had time permitted fuller consideration. Indeed, the challenge of developing such a framework for analysis is exciting; I regret that the panel was unable to accept it.

The omission of a conceptual framework does not loom large in Chapter IV of the report because the benefits of the hypothetical artificial heart there discussed seem to outweigh the costs by a considerable margin; and, indeed, the losses from artificial heart development—aside from dollar costs—seem likely to be small, largely transitional in character, and so widely spread as to be inconsequential from a justice standpoint. The main costs appear in direct and indirect impacts on societal values, and these issues seem more readily discussed in abstract or intuitive terms than as costs capable of being lumped with surgeons' fees or rental charges for Plutonium-238. Nevertheless, the absence of a conceptual framework leads the panel into more serious difficulties in later discussion.

THE NUCLEAR-POWERED ARTIFICIAL HEART

Although I share the panel's belief that too much emphasis may have been placed on the nuclear-power source in developmental work, my grounds for so believing differ fundamentally from those expressed by the panel. As I understand it from the discussion in the report, the panel rejects the utilitarian calculus altogether on this point and would not permit the nuclear device, whatever its value to recipients, to be used so long as it might do harm, however slight, to others. (Interpretation on this point is difficult, but I believe the panel clearly excludes comparison of costs and benefits.) In my view, the panel has fallen into error because it has substituted impulse for analysis. For want of a better one, I follow here the analytical framework suggested above, and conclude that the panel's position violates principles of justice.

The radiation hazard that is presented to the general population by the nuclear-powered artificial heart does raise serious ethical issues, which must be addressed by practical solutions. Theoretically, there would be no issue at all if the recipient of the artificial heart could purchase the right to emit radiation in voluntary transactions with all persons who would come into contact with him. This is of course impossible, but, as discussed above, hypothesizing such transacting (by parties who are well informed and not excessively necessitous) enables us to visualize the nature of ethically appropriate outcomes and to structure regulation or other legal controls to achieve them. Indeed, as a substitute for the unworkable "market," regulation makes appropriate room for paternalistic judgments about how people should construe their own welfare and can eliminate some of the complications introduced by discrepancies in wealth. The question raised by the panel's report is whether, in view of the impossibility of buying and selling the right to emit, the right should be denied altogether or its exercise regulated in particular ways.

Legally, the bearer of a nuclear-power source probably has no affirmative "right" to expose others to a radiation hazard without their consent (although the absence of an effective remedy is sometimes seen as creating a right). Regulation may preempt the legal remedies of individuals, however, freeing the licensed radiation source from the need to compensate others for maintaining a "nuisance" in their midst on the ground either that the radiation is certified to be harmless or that the risk is tolerable in view of the public benefits derived (as in the case of nuclear generation of electrical energy, for example). Individuals actually injured by the radiation would probably have a legal right to recover damages if they could prove the cause and the extent of their injury, but, since such proof would usually be impossible, the public would in fact be unprotected by a damage remedy that could be relied upon to discourage excessive or unwise use of the nuclear device.

Lacking the means of controlling use of the nuclear-powered artificial heart either by voluntary transactions or by legal liability for unconsented-to harms, the society may choose other remedies for dealing with the problem. One possibility is an absolute prohibition of the nuclear device on the basis that no warrant can be found for exposing unknown persons to ill-defined hazards for which compensation cannot be paid. The availability of an electrical device as a less hazardous alternative and the general public apprehension about radiation provide some support for such a prohibition. Moreover, some members of the panel appear to believe that, ethically, individuals have no right to impose life-threatening risks on others without their consent.

Prohibition of the nuclear device has ethical implications of its own, however, for it denies a possibly valuable benefit to potential users. Even assuming the availability of an adequate nonnuclear power source, the quality of the recipient's life may be greatly improved if he is freed of the need to recharge the battery regularly and of visible dependence on external supports. It would be ethically wrong to argue that once the patient's life has been saved, the improved quality of life provided by the nuclear device is a luxury or an amenity to be lightly regarded. To view the nuclear device merely as a frill would be to make the common mistake of viewing life-saving as an imperative irrespective of the quality of life achieved. Although I think the panel may have fallen into this trap, it goes even further, acknowledging that there would be in fact some added risk to the life of the artificial-heart recipient in requiring him to use the electrical device.

In its public choices, the society appears to reserve the right to devalue some individual preferences, not according them their face value in utilitarian calculations because of overriding ethical considerations. Minimum-wage and child-labor laws can be viewed as examples of ethically inspired incursions on freedom of contract, as can prohibitions against voluntary euthanasia, marijuana use, and abortion. (Perhaps even these matters can be seen in utilitarian terms by counting the majority's moral outrage or psychic discomfort among the external costs of otherwise private transactions, but I believe the majority is in fact less dispassionate than this, and inclined to devalue the preferences of others as a kind of moral judgment.) Whether a prohibition of the nuclear-powered artificial heart can perhaps be justified by such ethical judgments about individual preferences needs to be considered. Indeed, I see no ground for supporting the panel's conclusion other than some kind of moral judgment that the preference of a person with heart disease for a higher quality of life, even if costs are imposed on others, is somehow immoral. But it seems to me that the panel's willingness to impose large costs on such patients for the protection of society as a whole against very small risks is itself anything but moral, for I can see no colorable principle—either in the nature of nuclear radiation or in the nature of heart disease—which warrants devaluing the possible preference of a heart patient for a nuclear-powered artificial heart.

Thus, it seems to me that the panel uses different standards to weigh the patient's decision to expose society to risk, on the one hand, and the society's decision to expose the patient to risk and a poorer quality of life on the other. Of course the panel may simply have attached great weight to the public's fears of radiation or to the uncertainties about possibly catastrophic effects, but, if that was its intention, there was no need to reject the utilitarian calculus. Moreover, the fact that "cost-benefit analysis" has come to have a bad name because of a tendency of its practitioners to count only quantifiable items is likewise no reason to adopt an unjust principle for public decision-making. Finally, I would ask why the panel seems to have reversed the normal societal tendency, noted elsewhere in the report, of valuing highly an identifiable life in jeopardy and devaluing "statistical lives." The panel has clearly done more than rectify the imbalance previously noted, explicitly counting statistical risks more heavily than those to aspirants for a nuclear-powered artificial heart.

Absolute prohibition of the nuclear device might, of course, be ultimately warranted by an ethically informed estimate of gains and losses—that is, a calculus that attaches substantial though not infinite value to the preservation of life and gives some recognition to the quality thereof. Such a prohibition would have the result of denying the rich man (who, after all, "can't take it with him") the right to improve the quality of his life slightly at the expense of the death of others. But, if a prohibition cannot be justified on utilitarian grounds, there is no reason why the disadvantages flowing from the impracticability of both voluntary transactions and legal enforcement of a right to be free of radiation should fall on would-be users of the nuclear device rather than potential recipients of radiation. Less sweeping measures seem likely to be more attractive and more in keeping with the objective of maximizing human welfare.

In recognition of the hazards accompanying the nuclear device, its greater cost should not be prevented from operating as a rationing mechanism to deter its use somewhat. The higher price will restrict use, however, only if insurance plans do not pay the full amount of the difference. Thus, it might be necessary to regulate insurance plans to prevent or limit their subsidization of the nuclear device. Although complete prohibition of insurance coverage might be unfair to those who wished to choose a "Cadillac" plan, it might still be justified on the basis of the hazards that are involved. In any event, the hazards connected with the nuclear device may suggest that major public subsidies toward its purchase would be inappropriate, at least if a nonnuclear alternative is available. Indeed, a case could be made for imposing an added cost, in the form of a tax, on the use of plutonium, both as a gesture toward exacting compensation for the possible harm to others in the society and as a means of further discouraging use of the nuclear device; some might think it essential to earmark the proceeds of such a tax either for reducing radiation from other sources or for treating leukemia and other forms of cancer as a way of indirectly compensating the specific victims of radiation, if any.

Another important device for dealing with the radiation hazard would be regulatory curbs on the activities of bearers of the nuclear device. If one thought that bargaining of the kind hypothesized earlier would lead the bearer of the device to live in a rural environment and to avoid crowds, regulation might seek similarly to control the place of residence and activities of the bearer. Regulation might also require disclosure of the presence of the device to the bearer's close associates. A variety of other precautions could also be imposed by regulation, including limitations on the types of employment that could be undertaken. Thus, the bearer of a nuclear device might be prohibited from teaching school. Again, the object of regulation should be to approximate the outcome that would occur in an ideal "market" in which emitters of radiation and persons exposed to its hazards could work out their conflicts to the best advantage of all.

For these reasons, I must reject the panel's ground for recommending against implantation of the nuclear device in human beings. Since this recommendation is apt to be the most widely noted and controversial one in the report, I have felt it necessary to demonstrate the weakness of its ethical premises at some length.

FINANCING AND PATIENT SELECTION

I find this portion to be disappointing in its superficiality, particularly in its avoidance of difficult issues, some of which are mentioned elsewhere in the report but deserve full attention here. The following paragraphs express just some of my reservations and concerns:

1. Some principled judgment must be reached on why we should, or should not, as a society, provide expensive life-saving technology to all who want it. The panel, it would seem, accepts uncritically the life-saving imperative after earlier observing the potentially high cost of maintaining the myth of life's infinite value. Yet financing issues are profoundly influenced by the difficulties that both government and providers face in attaching less than absolute importance to the preservation of life "at all costs." Furthermore, the panel does not set forth the high cost of covering all possible recipients, though this cost is alluded to, and no effort is made to calculate the cost of covering other catastrophic diseases that are equally good candidates for governmental subsidy. Moreover, the panel does not recognize that unlimited government financing will call forth many more expensive technologies, and its discussion of possible inappropriate use induced by insurance coverage may understate the seriousness of the problem. For example, the assumption appears at several points that the nuclear-powered device, if available at all, will be subsidized, even though the added advantage for a particular patient may not warrant the added cost and the radiation hazard may not be negligible. The dilemma presented by the high potential cost should have been discussed, and possible ways of dealing with it or of limiting government's commitment should have been investigated.

2. Government frequently assuages the pangs of society's conscience and maintains its own and the society's humanitarian image by doing such things as spending large amounts to save lives placed in jeopardy, or to supply a highly visible benefit to the poor. Provision of artificial hearts to the poor is a possible case in point. But, given the probable high cost of artificial hearts, does it make sense to provide them to poor people if we have not been willing to give them other things—adequate food and shelter, color TVs, etc.—that they would value more? I have no trouble with, and indeed favor, providing basic health care in kind (preferably through a voucher system) to the poor and near-poor, but unlimited benefits do not seem appropriate unless more basic needs are also satisfied. In value terms, is salving the conscience of society, or relieving providers of charitable burdens, more important than allowing the poor to express their own preferences about the kinds of benefits they enjoy at public expense?

3. Do we want to see government put in a position of either explicitly denying life to some or picking up a very large bill? If not, how can government's assumption of increased responsibility in health care be structured so as to strain the society's humanitarian self-image as little as possible? For example, in which of the following cases is the government most (least) deeply implicated in a human death: When it occurs because a legislatively set benefit limit is exceeded? When charitable resources, available for some, are not made available in a particular case? When a publicly established selection system, random or otherwise, turns the patient down? When, even though the patient was able to pay from his private resources or from insurance which he had

purchased, a public selection process gave the only available treatment to a patient whose treatment was supported by the taxpayers? When a large side payment, or the physician's perception of social worth, leads to preferring one patient over another who is poorer or less socially prominent? The issue is whether some forms of governmental involvement might be ethically more satisfying (less troubling) than others, and perhaps also whether government has an obligation to right all wrongs.

4. At some point, is it undesirable for professionals, as dispensers of charity, to shift their ethical and charitable responsibilities to the government? Is there an ethical difference between decisions by providers to reward social worth by affirmative charitable actions and the use of social-worth criteria to deny governmentally provided treatment to those found less worthy? These questions look toward a stronger role for charity than is sometimes contemplated—perhaps national health insurance with a fixed upper limit—and thus a limited government role in life-death decisions. The panel has commented on the provider's role in such a system, but neglects to face the issue when financing and choice come up for discussion.

5. Professor Guido Calabresi of the Yale Law School has observed that society, in making "tragic choices," tends to move continually from one imperfect solution to another as a means of preserving and regularly reasserting its humanitarian self-image. Thus, the use of social-worth criteria (e.g., draft deferments), lotteries (e.g., the Vietnam War draft), and market systems (e.g., the volunteer army) are alternately chosen as particular ethical objections and discontent with each solution are asserted. Calabresi observes that this instability and the opportunity for frequent change, allowing regular reassertion of whatever value was sacrificed by the previous system, permit all values to be recognized in turn so that none of them is totally denied. This is an intriguing model for appreciating the dynamics of social response to moral dilemmas, and it is unfortunate that the panel failed to elaborate on it and on possible alternative ways of doing business in the midst of conflicts over deeply held ethical beliefs. Another alternative, already noted, would be to structure institutions to minimize direct governmental involvement in the making of hard choices, so that death from catastrophic disease would continue to seem more an act of God than of the legislature.

**Part III:
Ethics and Health Policy
Planning**

PREAMBLE

Delivering health care poses another kind of ethical dilemma in addition to allocating scarce resources. The health policy-planning process itself is a controversial one. Some of the problems are technical: who has the skills to provide the data to project birth and death rates, costs of alternative systems of health care, and social impacts? Other questions, however, are ethical. To introduce some of these social ethical questions a chapter by Rashi Fein looks at how we have measured the economic benefits of health programs historically, and some of the ethical problems raised. He reveals not only that it is difficult to measure the benefits of health programs, but that serious policy problems emerge if we make the attempt. Some outputs are difficult or impossible to measure. Those which can be assigned numbers—economic outputs, for instance—are likely to be given undue weight. Even more basic, he finds that it is dangerous, inconsistent with our social values, to measure a person's worth in terms of his productive contribution. At the least it fails to take into account considerations of equity. Health planning based on judgments of benefits, especially economic benefits, will discriminate against the young, those with relatively little earning power, possibly ethnic and racial groups, and especially the elderly. Fein challenges the notion that economics is a "value free" technique for health planning. Cost-benefit analysis, a technique growing in importance in health policy planning over the past decade, must be explored for its value presuppositions. Fein argues that it is a technique that is too important to be left to analysts or economists.

In addition to health care planning at the national level, local health policies are now more and more open to public scrutiny. One controversial method of local health policy planning is the establishment of community boards in local hospitals to advise, participate in, or dominate health care policy planning. (Whether the local boards advise on or control local policy is itself a crucial part of the debate.) Laurelyn Veatch has studied community boards now required in New York City's municipal hospitals. The first report of her findings is included here.

The final chapter moves from the general question of health policy planning to a more specific example: technology assessment in the area of genetics. LeRoy Walters examines in depth the use of an emerging policy analysis technique (technology assessment) to one of the most controversial health policy questions of our day. While all the ethical conflicts of this one particular kind of technology assessment may not transfer directly to other health assessments, the social and ethical dilemmas raised by the technique itself are directly relevant. Walters gives us one concrete example of how the social and ethical aspects of biomedical technologies must become an integral part of the health policy planning process.

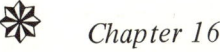 *Chapter 16*

On Measuring Economic Benefits of Health Programs

Rashi Fein

EARLY HISTORY

> When the sentimentalist and the moralist fails, he will have as a last resource to call in the aid of the economist, who has in some instances proved the power of his art to draw iron tears from the cheeks of a city Plutus.[1]

Economic data and analysis have long been used in efforts to influence program and expenditure decisions in the public sector. Those who have favored particular policies have sought allies and supporting arguments for their positions. Particularly appealing have been the arguments that were cast in economic terms, and this has, perhaps, been especially the case in areas involving programs with clear, visible, and direct impact on people. This appeal would appear to have been based on two factors. The general attractiveness of economic arguments has, at least in part, derived from the belief that economics is value free, neutral, and objective. Thus, economic arguments relying on the hard criteria of the market, on "profit" and on "loss" carried a special weight (a weight that was, perhaps, increased by the fact that economists use data, jargon, and methodology that are somewhat mysterious to the uninitiated). The specific attractiveness of economic arguments in social areas (for example in the case of programs that deal directly with people) is increased by the fact that these fields generally lack rigorous monetary guidelines for decision-making. In Chadwick's terms, these are the areas favored by "the sentimentalist and moralist." Therefore, to find that economic criteria were not at variance with humanitarian considerations seemed to be especially useful. Chadwick was correct when he suggested that the economist could prove a useful ally.

The power of the economic argument that the proponents of social programs found useful was not derived from the literary quality with which the arguments were offered, or from the elegance of the economist's prose. Nor, as will become clear, did it result from the fact that the analytical methodology was so refined and the data so exact that disagreement with the conclusions was impossible. Rather it was because the economic argument embodied an appealing pattern of thought and a way of looking at a problem: the economic rationale for various social programs was presented in investment terms. Ill health, ignorance, disability, and death caused by war were costly to an economy. Investment in medical care, public health, education, and the pursuit of peace brought significant economic rewards in increasing the value of human capital. Such investment concepts were looked upon with favor at a time when economic progress was seen as deriving from capital growth brought about by investment.

Thus, the early literature of economics, as well as articles in applied areas of public policy, contains references to the economic value of an education, of acquired skills, of better health, and the economic costs and gains of war, emigration, and immigration. These subjects were examined at irregular intervals by persons concerned with practical policy matters. Unfortunately none of these contributions developed a general theory and methodology concerning the economic value of a human being. They were not integrated into the main body of the economic literature, remaining on, if not beyond, the fringe. Furthermore, because they were derived from a specific interest in a particular applied problem, there was little attempt to generalize or to show the usefulness of the approach to other problems. Those writing on the economic value of an immigrant seemed unaware that a similar type of problem was examined by persons concerned with the economic value of an education; those writing on the economic loss suffered through emigration seemed unaware that other scholars were concerned with the economic loss caused by disease or by casualties in war.

This situation, I might note, makes the examination of early references to human capital a fascinating but time-consuming task. Some years ago, in undertaking just such an examination, I found that in order to locate useful examples of the quantitative application of the concept of human capital, one had to consider the various fields in which such a concept might be used and then search for articles, bibliographies, and references in these applied fields. General indexes were hardly useful, since they contained no classification heading called "human resources" or "human capital." Even titles of articles could be, and were, misleading.

Perhaps the first estimate of the money value of a person were offered by Sir William Petty, writing in the latter decades of the seventeenth century. At various times Petty offered estimates of the value of a person residing in England, ranging between £60 and £90. In his *Political Arithmetick*, for example, Petty calculates the value by deriving the productive contributions of labor (£26 million), multiplying by 20 ("The Mass of Mankind being worth Twenty Years purchase"), and by dividing by 6 million (the population of England). Thus "... makes about £80. Sterling, to be valued of each Head of Man Woman and Child ...: from whence we may learn to compute the loss we have sustained by the Plague, by the Slaughter of Men in War, and by the sending them abroad into the Service of Foreign Princes."[2] Petty then used estimates of the value of human capital to derive a number of policy implications. He asked: "From whence it follows, that 100,000 persons dying of the Plague, above the ordinary number is near 7 Millions loss to the Kingdom [this was based upon an estimate that each person was worth £69]; and consequently how well might £70,000 have been bestowed in preventing this Centuple loss?"[3] In another work he asked: "The value of 140^m people at £90. per head is 12 millions 600^m pounds; soe as the Question seems to be what sum of money, and Meanes ought to be prudently ventured for the probable cutting off 3 fifths of this Calamity."[4] In Petty's plan, dated 7 October 1667, "Of Lesening ye Plagues of London," he attempted to provide an answer to the question. He estimated that, given the value of an individual and the cost of transporting people outside of London and caring for them for three months, thus increasing the probability of survival, every pound expended would yield a return of £84.[5] Here, then, was an economic argument, cast in monetary terms, in favor of a course of action to prevent deaths and thus to increase the value of the nation's human resources.

Petty also used the concept of human capital in advocating lying-in hospitals for illegitimate children. He calculated that the cost of thirty days in childbed would only be 30s. Since the value of mankind was some £70, "a new born Child, bread up to fair and hard work for 25 yeares, will be very well worth 3 times 30 Shillings, as may be seen in the price of Negros Children in the American plantations."[6] It is not without interest to note that Petty advocated lying-in hospitals in order to increase the population. Perhaps, however, to insure that the government receive a direct return on its investment, he also advocated that the child should be the servant of government for twenty-five years. Today, with the growth of income taxation, the argument is not often made in terms of the direct returns to government resulting from the increase in tax revenue.

Some twenty-one years earlier, in 1676, in a lecture on anatomy, Petty noted that the state should intervene to assure better medicine. The value of better medicine, he felt, was that it could save 200,000 subjects a year. Even valued at only £20, the lowest price of slaves, this was a large sum and better medicine, therefore represented a sensible state expenditure. "Wherefore it is not in the Interest of the State to leave Phisitians and Patients (as now) to their own shifts."[7] Almost three hundred years later, the same arguments are presented (though the data are more refined) to advocate similar policies.

It is also of interest that not only was Petty the precurser of present discussions of investment in health activities, but he also presented arguments analogous to those used today in discussions concerning migration and economic development policies. Petty argued that an individual in England was worth £90; in Ireland only £70. This differential value led to the conclusion that transplantation would be economically wise."[8]

Over a century passes before the economic-value-of-man concept reappears again in a major way in the literature. Edwin Chadwick, in his *Sanitary Report* for 1842, estimated that the loss due to excessive sickness and premature disability and death, including the loss of productive power, equaled £14 million.[9] In 1844 he argued that bad sanitation increased the proportion of dependent hands to workers and that sanitation could be viewed "as an economical question of production."[10] He also suggested that it could be shown "how much, by expenditure in well-executed measures, directed by engineering science, they may gain in the reduction of existing pecuniary burdens alone, that are entailed by an excessive mortality."[11] Chadwick, of course, was particularly interested in sanitation, and a number of his many articles contain references to the economic value of sanitation and to the costs that society bears in "excessive sickness, excessive death-rates and funerals, and premature disablement and lost labour" due to poor sanitation.[12]

In 1862, Chadwick argued, "as the artist for his purpose views the human being as a subject for the cultivation of the beautiful—as the physiologist for the cultivation of his art views him solely as a material organism, so the economist for the advancement of his science may well treat the human being simply as an investment of capital, in productive force."[13] He then presented detailed estimates of the value of a person based on the cost of rearing a child, taking account of the factor of death before becoming productive (at age eleven!) and the number of productive years. He used these estimates to derive the costs associated with poor housing and sanitation, and offered additional comments related to the value of human capital. Suggesting that economists should strive to unite personal and pecuniary motives, he defended education on economic grounds and, in words that remain applicable today, argued:

> It is well to subscribe to reformatories as to hospitals for the treatment of the sick, but giving exclusive attention to them is like giving exclusive attention to the foundation and maintenance of hospitals for the alleviation of marsh and foul air diseases, without regard to the drainage of the marshes, or to the removal of the sources of the foul air whence the diseases arise.[14]

Lemuel Shattuck, in the *Report of a General Plan for the Promotion of Public and Personal Health*, presented in 1850, also viewed the public health measures from an economic perspective. In arguing for preventive sanitary measures to lessen epidemics, he wrote: "In this case economy is on the side of humanity, and the most expensive of all things is—to do nothing."[15] The expenses and losses caused by the neglect of sanitary measures included "A loss sustained by the state, in consequence of the diminished physical power and general liability to disease."[16] Shattuck estimated that the failure of the State of Massachusetts to adopt an efficient sanitary system resulted in 6000 unnecessary deaths, and that the average individual might have been productive for an additional eighteen years. Thus, society lost 108,000 years of labor at $50 per year, equalling $5.4 million. When this was added to the lost labor of the sick and the cost of sickness and of supporting widows and orphans, Shattuck estimated that the cost to the state was $7.5 million. Interestingly, he felt that this cost could be eliminated by an expenditure of only $3000 (largely in planning and what we would call today technical assistance).[17] Shattuck thus argued:

> According to the estimate above presented, the State suffers, from its imperfect sanitary condition, an unnecessary annual loss of more than 7½ millions of dollars! and this arises, partly at least, from the non-adoption of a measure which will cost but about $3,000. If saved, it would add that amount to the wealth of the State, besides the indefinite amount of increased happiness which would accompany it. Should any one consider this an extravagant estimate, let him reduce it to 3 millions, more than one half, and then the relation of expenditure to the savings, or to the income, will be as *one dollar to one thousand dollars*! And even if nine tenths of this latter sum be deducted, it will be like paying out *one* dollar, and receiving back again *ten*, as the return profit! What more wise expenditure of money can be desired![18]

In the latter half of the nineteenth century others were writing in much the same vein as Chadwick and applying the same concepts to a number of different fields. They would have accepted the statement by the Reverend J.E. Thorold Rogers: "It seems to me wholly un-philosophical to ignore capital in the person of a labourer, and to recognize it in a machine."[19] One writer, however, stands out above all others because of the method by which he calculated what he termed the "money value of a man," and because he applied the concept to general taxation problems as well as to social programs. William Farr, in a paper presented in 1853 discussing income and property taxes, used a method that is surprisingly close to the methods used today, since he did not base values on the costs of rearing the child (producing the machine), but rather on the wages that will be earned, on the future income stream."[20] In his volume *Vital Statistics*, Farr stated:

> Life has a pecuniary value. In its production and education a certain amount of capital is sunk for a longer or shorter time, and that capital, with its interest, as a general rule, reappears in the wages of the labourer, the pay of the officer, and the income of the professional man. At first it

is all expenditure, and a certain necessary expenditure goes on to the end to keep life in being, even when its economic results are negative.[21]

The sum of future earnings and the cost of future maintenance determines the value. Thus Farr estimates the following values for a Norfolk agricultural labourer: at birth £5; age 5, £56; age 10, £117; age 15, £192; age 20, £234; age 25, £246; age 30, £241, declining to £138 at age 55, and £1 at age 70, following which the values become negative (maintenance exceeds income). Thus, at age 80 the value is –£41. Farr uses these data to justify particular concern with those events that destroy lives at their prime—"fever, consumption, cholera, violence in all its forms, and childbirth."[22]

The estimates provided by Farr in *Vital Statistics*, that a human life was worth £770 a head were used by Gary Calkins in estimating that sanitation saved 856,804 lives with a value of $650 million from 1880 to 1890. This saving, he noted, exceeded the cost of sanitary improvements between 1875 and 1890, since the latter totalled $583.5 million.[23]

If Petty was the first to examine the concept of human capital and Chadwick the first to present detailed estimates and apply these quite carefully and extensively to justify various public expenditures, Farr deserves recognition as the first to analyze value in terms of future income streams, and to do this in relation to the general question of taxation rather than in a specific context of health (or other) expenditures.

In the period 1870-1920, the concept of human capital continued to be applied in a number of specific areas. The economic value of man entered into discussions on the cost of war (perhaps with the hope that war would be eliminated if it were recognized that when the loss in human capital was included in the "profit and loss statement" even the victor could be found to have made a poor investment). Detailed studies on the cost of the Franco-Prussian War of 1870 were undertaken (chiefly by Sir Robert Giffen). Additional studies on the South African War and the First World War included estimates of the production foregone during the war (because men were in the armed forces) as well as losses due to deaths and injuries.[24]

A second group of economists applied the concept of human capital to problems of emigration and immigration. British writers tended to focus on the loss that Britain was suffering because of emigration. Migration, it was felt, represented the loss of a capital asset (though the value of the asset was not always measured in terms of future income, but on occasion in terms of the cost of "creating" the asset; for example, the cost of upbringing and education). Archibald Hamilton, writing in 1877, noted that the value of an immigrant to the community has been estimated in the United States at £166. 13s. 4d. and "they have been computed to be worth £200 in New Zealand."[25] In response, Dr. Guy suggested that the value of an immigrant was £400 "and when it was remembered that an emigrant ... married and became the father of children who ... had families, it was difficult to say what the true value of an emigrant was."[26] There was general agreement, however, that the value of an immigrant depended upon the demand for labor in the place to which he emigrated. Thus Farr noted that the ex-prime minister of New Zealand, Sir Julius Vogel, had done "an admirable work ... to remove some of the agricultural labourers from a place where they were worth very little, to a place where they were worth a great deal."[27]

A third area of economic inquiry that utilized a capital concept of man dealt with health, and with the costs associated with specific diseases. Among the diseases studied were tuberculosis and typhoid fever.[28] These studies did not break new methodological ground, nor did they lead the general economist to a greater interest in the field of health. Just as the profession neglected the field of human resources in general, so too it neglected the area of health.

It is not clear why there was relatively little discussion of the economic value of human resources, except by scholars interested in applied specific problem areas. Economists, after all, have long referred to land, labor, and capital inputs and resources. They have devoted considerable analysis to the consequences derived from the observed fact that land is not homogeneous and from the observation that capital equipment differs in its productivity. Yet, to a considerable extent, much of economics has been written as if labor were all the same. Even when cognizance was taken of the obvious and observable differences in labor quality, there seemed to be little concern with analysis of the factors that brought about these differences, almost as if it were felt that the factors could not be controlled or were not amenable to change. It is significant, perhaps, that to the extent that human capital was considered (even by those in applied areas), greatest attention was paid to problems of mortality, total incapacity, or migration—issues involving the addition or subtraction of total productivity rather than an increase in productivity resulting from the individual's becoming more effective in his work.

We can only speculate why human capital was largely ignored by the main body of economics. In part it may be due to the fact that during the period of rapid economic growth (the period of rapid industrial growth and the period when economics was developing as an organized discipline), striking and rapid changes were taking place in the amount of capital equipment available to the society and at the disposal of the worker. The capital/labor ratio was increasing. It is, therefore, to be expected that capital equipment occupied the center of the stage and was the chief focus of interest. Higher standards of living were seen as the result of the process of industrialization. Industrialization, in turn, was seen as the consequence (synonomous with) investment in addition to the stock of capital equipment. Changes in the quality of human resources were not as obvious, certainly not as easy to measure or as dramatic, not as apparently the result of deliberate policies. Thus, they were given small parts in the chorus along with other actors called custom, organization, entrepreneurship, and so forth.

Second, capital and differences in capital could easily be measured in economic terms. Capital is traded in the market and no conversion to economic or monetary terms is required. The common denominator that expresses the value of capital equipment is there for all to see. One-time investments in capital yield future income streams. Labor, however, is not bought and sold. Only labor services are. In general (with exceptions in discussions of insurance), one did not think in terms of income streams when discussing labor.

Third, labor plays a dual role in the economic system: as input and as final consumer. Many of the things that increase the value and contribution of the worker as input (things that could be termed investments) are considered as part of consumption. They involve expenditures on goods and services that, in many cases, would be purchased even if they did nothing to improve the skill levels and productivity of the working force. Thus, the costs of recreation are classified as consumption expenditures even if they might be considered as part of the necessary costs required to maintain productivity. So, too, with health expenditures and with education expenditures. Surely people want health and education, and would purchase some of these two commodities, even in the absence of any impact on productivity and earning power? Surely, however, health and education do have such impacts and are not, therefore, entirely consumption expenditures? Some portion can be viewed (and in recent years this has been the case) as investment.

Fourth, the early orientation of economics failed to take account of the importance of "externalities." Expenditures on health and education that increased the productivity of the worker were viewed as private matters, since they increased the individual's income. It was not fully appreciated that all of us are the beneficiaries when some of us are more productive. Nor was it recognized that certain expenditures might make sound economic sense for society as a whole even though they did not do so for the individual. If externalities are ignored much of the rationale for public intervention disappears—much, but not all—and with a weaker rationale there was a lesser interest in such, clearly, private matters.

Fifth, economists, among others, failed to examine some expenditures as investments and failed to view human capital as capital, at least in part because the terminology was felt repellent when applied to man. Man is not a machine. How then could one use such terms as "human capital" or "investment in human beings"? The notion of man as something that can be assigned some dollar value reminds one of slavery. It seems to violate the concept of the sacredness of life. The notion is rejected as repugnant. Even when the ideas are explored and man is assigned an economic value, writers often felt it necessary to make disclaimers that man is much more than a robot merely embodying some set of skills. The fact that the writer felt that he might be misunderstood in the absence of such disclaimers is in itself significant.

In recent years, however, there has been a significant change in the place that human resources occupy in the literature of economics. The 1950s saw rekindled interest in health economics and the economics of education. This was built upon in the decade of the 1960s as economists turned their attention to a variety of issues relating to investment in human capital. No longer were these considered fringe areas. Today there is a field known as the economics of human resources. There are economists, courses, workshops, seminars, conferences, and a journal—perhaps the final evidence that a field exists—devoted to this area of inquiry. In little more than a decade the situation has changed from the case where individuals who had not yet succeeded in defining a field or having it accepted by their professional colleagues were working in relative isolation on problems that today would be defined as part of the "economics of human resources." In the course of this change, there has been an altered orientation to the questions that have been studied. It is to this altered orientation, particularly as it applies to questions in the health areas, that we now turn.

RECENT DEVELOPMENTS

We recall that many of the early contributions already referred to were designed to promote specific policies by demonstrating that funds expended for various social programs would bring economic returns. Economists or their analytical techniques were called upon "when the sentimentalist and the moralist" needed additional support. In this heavily investment-oriented approach one discovers little reference to programs that do not yield a high return. Nor do we find suggestions that expenditures for certain activities should be cut. This may be because economists chose not to address problems that might yield "negative" answers, because they chose not to publish "negative" results, or because there are few, if any, general social programs that have very low yields. While there may have been an element of the first two reasons—most of the articles, after all, were written by persons actively working in and dedicated to action in the particular applied field—the last reason is, perhaps, of even greater importance. The absence of low rates of return is particularly true if the analysis is cast in general and broad dimension rather than as an examination of a specific program, designed to accomplish a narrow and specific purpose in which the outcome can be measured. What was being evaluated was whether better health or more education had a substantial payoff, not whether this particular educational technique raised reading levels to a degree commensurate with the resources required to implement the technique or whether a particular health program in a particular location and designed to help a particular population group had a substantial payoff. Most of the literature spoke of health in general, education in general. Most of the literature did not describe the particular program that would be designed to alter the existing situation, and surely did not examine the likelihood that the program would accomplish its goals. The analysis was based on "average" data for large population groups, and did not concern itself with whether or not the population groups to be served by the expenditures which were being advocated would, in fact, exhibit an average response to the new program. Given the broad nature of the questions being addressed, it is not surprising that the returns were found to be high.

To be sure, part of the reason that one would expect to find high rates of return also relates to the methodology that was used to calculate the yields (the absence of discounting, for example). This, however, is not the critical element, for even today, when a more refined methodology (much of which works to lower the calculated rate of return) is utilized, rates remain high when one speaks of education in general (as contrasted with a particular program for particular students). Similarly with health.

Even during the 1950s, the decade in which the revival of interest in the economics of human resources began, elements of the older tradition were maintained. Much of the new work undertaken related to the economic rates of return to various levels of education and the economic costs of various diseases—not to the rate of return to specific education or health programs. The analysis did, of course, demonstrate that education had a high yield and that disease was costly. It did not ask, however, what specific programs could—in the real world—lower the incidence of disease and by how much. It did not ask what the rates of return would be for those programs. Similarly, it did not ask how learning could be increased and what the returns to new educational programs were likely to be. Yet, even the work that was done, limited as it was, was extremely important both in introducing economists to various applied fields in the social program areas and in introducing an economic dimension to the discussion of these kinds of activities.

The reasons for the revival of interest in the economics of health and education in the 1950s are many. Concern about rapidly increasing budgets for education (and to a smaller degree for health) led to attempts to "justify" those budgets by examination of the economic benefits of education and health activities. Concern about underdeveloped economies brought us face to face with the question of skills and productivity, with the costs to production that result from lack of adequate education and health. It was clear that plant, equipment, roads, and electric power were not enough to insure development, and that quality of the labor force also made a difference. In the United States, concern about Soviet scientific advances and the growth in Soviet Gross National Product led to attempts to put empirical content into the statements that a nation's richest resource was its skilled manpower, and that its wealth included its stock of engineers and scientists. Attempts to examine problems of economic growth in developed economies led to intensive examination of the sources of growth. United States Gross National Product, it is clear, has grown more rapidly than can be accounted for by increases in land, labor, and capital. There have, therefore, been attempts to provide more precise measurements and explanations of the part not accounted for, the residual element in growth. While primary emphasis has often been given to research and technology, a spillover effect has directed considerable attention to capital invested in men. Finally, economists have directed more and more attention not only to income differences between nations but also to differences between groups in the same nation, to the reasons for these differences and to socioeconomic policies that might narrow the differences. In the United States, the economic problems of blacks have been an important focus of interest for economists (and others), and many have attributed much of the income part of the problem to the underinvestment in education and health for this part of our population.

During the 1960s, however, the nature of much of the empirical effort in the economics of health (and of education) began to change. Increasingly, many felt that the work of economists on rates of return was interesting and illuminating, but not very helpful in guiding public policy and in choosing between public programs. High rates of return are encouraging to the practitioner in a given field and they make for fine banquet address material, but they do not answer two questions that government budgeteers raise: (1) are the specific programs for which support is sought "good" investments, i.e., what are the rates of return for the various proposals that come before the decision-maker; (2) which particular program should be favored over other programs, i.e., how does the rate of return for each program compare with rates of return for alternatives? In the government sector these are the kinds of questions that are asked and, particularly in the mid-1960s, the kinds of questions that United States government departments began asking of economists.

It should be remembered that there was a flavor, a "climate of opinion," in the early 1960s. Ideology, was "dead," and the problems were, to a considerable measure, viewed as technical ones that required "technical" solutions. The analyst was not only necessary but sufficient. Those were the days of "the whizz kids" in the Pentagon, those were the days when it was felt that hard intellectual effort, the power of logic, and rationality would provide the answers to the society. In such an atmosphere, the importance of economists in government grew considerably. Thus, economists were among those asking (and answering) the questions of allocation of budget resources.

The issue confronting the budget officer and other decision-makers, after all, is not whether there is or is not (which in terms of the analysis often means "has or has not been") a high rate of return (an economic payoff) to health activities in general. Government budgets do not allocate funds to health in general, but to specific programs and activities. The question, therefore, is and should be how specific programs and activities measure up and how they will do *in the future*, since the future may differ from the past (if only because the population groups to be served may become harder to reach). This is true whether one is conducting an economic analysis or any other type of evaluative effort. Furthermore, the decision-maker does not have free resources. He is subject to a budget constraint. He must *choose* between a large number of alternative programs. It is, therefore, necessary to compare the likely gains and costs of the various possible courses of action that are open to him. He needs to ask how a particular program compares with other programs, how an *incremental* expenditure in one area compares with others.

Thus, in the mid 1960s we witnessed a conscious attempt to utilize the economist's tools in behalf of the decision-maker. Economists, called upon to examine specific programs, had to shift their attention from the aggregative and macro aspects to the micro level. They were asked to compare programs and rank them in terms of the relationship between costs and benefits. These economists (and the data for analysis) were most often found in government rather than outside. They were at work for and at the behest of the decision-maker himself, not for persons in an applied area who were trying to influence the decisions in their favor.

It can be noted that the intervention of economists in the process was not without difficulties. There was some controversy whether the analytical effort could best proceed at the highest level, say in the Bureau of the Budget (i.e., the president's staff), in the office of the Secretary of a Department, or in the individual operating agencies. The problem of where to carry forward such work to insure that the analyst has access to data and to the experience of persons intimately acquainted with program operations and yet does not become a special pleader for the operating agency is important. Though we shall not discuss this at further length, we must note that success or failure in analysis and in influencing the decision-making process may hinge on the locational decision.

We speak of the economist's role in helping conduct *ex-ante* analysis of the consequences of decisions. This attempt often involved the application of quantitative methods to the analysis of the various alternatives open to the decision-maker. If it is granted that the essential characteristic of decision-making is that of choice as between alternatives (including, of course, the option of postponing the decision), then the process of choice involves some kind of a comparison of the likely gains and the likely costs of the various courses of action or inaction. This pattern of thought—though not necessarily in quantitative terms—is applicable to all facets of rational decision-making. Certainly it existed before 1965. What was new was the attempted quantification of costs and benefits, the attention to economic benefits, the involvement of economists, and the attempt to compare programs in an explicit way. It should be clear, however, that gains and costs need not be limited to or expressed in monetary terms. They must include any number of other considerations that are relevant to the problem or decision at hand: gains or costs in prestige, political fortune, satisfaction, good will, effort, energy, and so forth. What is important is that in the evaluation, the comparisons be made explicit. It is also helpful if they be made in units that are commensurable.[a]

---

[a]When the argument is cast in its broadest and most general terms it loses some of its operational significance, since it can presumably be argued that when comparisons are not

That economists were heavily involved thus does not mean that the only benefits that were or need to be considered are economic benefits, though, of course, there is the danger that a particular profession may tend to overlook the importance of things that lie outside its area of professional competence. Economists were involved for many reasons. They had developed a reputation in subjecting public decisions (particularly in the areas of water resources and defense) to analysis and in forcing the consideration of alternatives. They were used to empirical methods and to the pattern of thought that explicitly attempts to compare benefits and costs. They were conversant with the language of the men who prepare budgets. Finally, they were viewed as "objective," i.e., not special pleaders for a particular program or area.

Perhaps most important, economists had been most concerned with economic growth policies and with measures to increase the rate of growth. Many of the programs that were to be analyzed were examined from the perspective of growth. Furthermore, economists were concerned with the constraint of limited resources and the necessity for choice. The analysis was to involve the comparison of alternatives.

I do not propose to examine the details of the effort begun in the 1960s to bring the new type of analysis to bear on the governmental policy decision-making process. This is not the place to review that history. To do so would require that we move well beyond the area of our specific interests, since the analytical effort was tied in with a number of other new activities in the planning and budgeting process, all of them designed collectively to make for better decisions and for wider range of choice. Our purposes are better served by examination of some of the conceptual difficulties that are involved in the effort to assess costs and benefits of programs for people, particularly programs that are viewed as human investment programs. Let us, therefore, examine some of the issues that arise and that are involved in the quantitative analysis of benefits and costs.

CONCEPTUAL ISSUES

Basic to all considerations of programs is the need to specify the objectives of the program in question and to develop techniques and reporting systems that enable one to assess the degree to which the objectives are being met. It is clear that these are first and important steps. It is also clear that, in many cases, these steps entail great difficulty. The difficulties arise in part because the final objectives of many government programs are to produce outputs which, at least at the present time, cannot be measured directly. The difficulties also arise because, often, we know relatively little about the production process whereby

---

made—and decisions are arrived at on bases that, to some, may appear irrational—the individual making the decision felt that the benefits of undertaking more refined comparisons and of reaching decisions in a more deliberate and explicit manner were outweighed by the costs involved.)

these final outputs are created. I do not ignore the difficulties involved in creating data and reporting systems to measure the achievement of limited and well-defined goals (e.g., reduction in incidence of a particular disease). In no small measure our relative ignorance about many health matters relates to the fact that our data systems are underdeveloped and—in terms of funds and personnel—undernourished. Far too often we simply do not have the data we need for analytical purposes. These difficulties, however, are surmountable, and better reporting and data systems can be created. I refer instead to the even greater problems associated with the measurement of outputs that are amorphous in concept, outputs such as "higher levels of health," and that are contributed to by many factors (e.g., housing, income, nutrition, environment, medical care of all kinds), factors whose relative contribution may differ for different persons and whose relative contribution is largely unknown.

The difficulty of measuring the achievement of goals which lie on a continuum is apparent. We do not do as well in measuring pain, concern, or functional ability as we do in measuring states that are discontinuous, such as life and death. Two consequences arise as a result of the problem of measurement and of understanding how various states of health are or can be produced. First, our lack of understanding of the production process and our inability to measure outputs leads program administrators to define their goals in resource input terms: the goal is more hospital beds, more physicians, more patient visits, more examinations, more research, above all more money. It is an article of faith that good things are accomplished by more resources and that things will be even better if even more resources are utilized. This may indeed be the case, but it is not the issue, for the question must be, How much better? It is analogous to saying that a health program is effective because it produces a positive change. The argument that we present says that that is not a sufficient guideline to the policy-maker, since he must choose between different programs, and therefore must be concerned with levels of effectiveness. His concern cannot be with whether a form of treatment or a government program is likely to do some good, but rather with the amount of good accomplished per unit of resource input. He cannot be satisfied with a goal of more inputs unless he understands how inputs relate to outputs, in which case he might as well speak in output terms.

A second important consequence of our difficulty in measuring outputs arises most often in the development of new program alternatives. The pressure to quantify, to measure, to be able to assess whether the goal is being achieved and in what degree, creates a bias in favor of developing those programs that have output goals that can be measured, where data can be gathered, where the achievement of limited (but specified) goals can be documented. These, however, are not necessarily the most desirable, needed, or highest-yield programs. They may be, but they need not be.

The problem of measurement of output is a real one, and the consequences are real as well. There is no reason, however, to be totally pessimistic about their solution. First, we must recognize that except for the bias in selection of programs (a bias that I believe can be guarded against), these problems leave us no worse off than we are in the absence of the evaluation effort. It is not the attempt to calculate cost-benefit ratios that leaves us at sea, that makes us ignorant of production functions and forces us to speak of inputs rather than of outputs. These problems are with us all the time. Indeed, the cost-benefit analysis leads to a greater level of understanding of the deficiencies in our measurement techniques, of the vagueness of some of our goals. It does not make us ignorant, but makes us aware of our ignorance. It forces us to question the "conventional wisdom"—a discreet phrase that often really means well accepted, but not fully documented, professional judgments. In the long run—and because of the recognition of the inadequate state of our knowledge—many of the problems will be partially solved. Some of them, I believe, are not fully solvable, since they involve interpersonal comparisons and changing standards of need and adequacy, and thus changing measurements of the benefits derived from various programs. In the short run (and the short run may be a very long time indeed), we will be forced to find proxy measures for the outputs that are our ultimate interests. Thus, even if we are unable to develop a satisfactory index of health, there would be agreement that the absence of illness—while not a fully satisfactory measure of health—might serve as one of a number of proxy measures. It is necessary, of course, to be careful not to subvert the real aims of a program by adjusting it to serve the proxy measure—a program designed to improve the health of children with the consequence that they have fewer days of absence from school (the proxy measure) is different from a program that focuses so heavily on the proxy that its attempt to achieve success leads sick children to be sent to school, perhaps contributing to even more illness. The danger that new (and measurable) aims are substituted for the real ones can, however, be guarded against.

Let us assume that, alert to the difficulties and biases and the dangers that they entail, the goals of the programs have been specified and measures of the outputs have been developed. The difficulties are not yet over. Since the interest lies in the comparison of programs, there develops a need to find a common denominator for the different outputs, a way of translating different things into a common unit of measure, a way, for example, of comparing the value of a life saved with a case of blindness prevented, of the life of a ten-year-old with the life of a fifty-year-old, and so forth.

As has already been pointed out, such questions (e.g., the value of human life) are often found to be distasteful. Nonetheless, whether formulated explicitly or implicitly, they are being asked—and answered—all the time. Often, however, because they are not formulated explicitly, one may find that governments pursue expenditure policies that imply that some lives are worth much more than others (e.g., airplane passengers as contrasted with coal miners). Thus, distasteful as it may be to articulate this type of question, it is better to do so than to reach policy decisions without being explicitly aware of their value implications.

The search for a common unit of measurement is, however, fraught with danger. We are unable to measure units of satisfaction or of happiness generated by various government activities. Nor are we able to compare A's satisfaction with B's. Nonetheless, the climate of opinion places a premium on measurement. Since the evaluation of alternative programs is carried forward by economists who are responding to budget and treasury officials, themselves sensitive to data that are presented in financial terms, and since the evaluation of programs is being undertaken in an atmosphere that is investment and economic-growth oriented (while in the United States this atmosphere may be changing—one hopes that is the case—cost-benefit and program analysis is still too young to have outgrown its early and very recent history), the common denominator that is most often sought is a monetary unit and the benefits most often measured are monetary ones. The fact that the monetary benefits are measured does not imply that economists are less concerned about other benefits than are historians, philosophers, or the general public. It simply means that economists (among others) tend to measure that which is measurable and tend first to address their attention to those things that they are familiar with: dollar costs and dollar benefits. Thus, as with the writings of economists and others in an earlier period, benefits are often translated into dollars (more correctly, the benefits that are measured are those that can be cast in dollar terms). This is the case even though it is total benefits of all kinds that we are interested in. Monetary benefits are—at best—only a proxy for total benefits. They are only part (perhaps only a small part) of all benefits, and do not represent a stable or constant fraction of all benefits. The problems that may arise, therefore, are many.

In measuring the economic benefits of programs it has become traditional to assess the increase in earning power of the individual that results from the improved health brought about by the program under review. The increase in earning power is a measure of the gain to the economy, since the contribution to production is measured by wages and salary income. This is not different from the evaluation made by those whose writings we examined above. It will be recalled that in those writings the value of a human being was assessed in different ways at different times: sometimes in terms of the cost of rearing (of producing the "machine") but later—and as is still done today—in terms of future earnings, a measure of expected future productive contribution. Using this measure entails some decisions about conceptual problems: what value should be placed on productive contribution and work effort that does not receive monetary rewards through the market system, a problem not confined to but often found in the case of women; what adjustments, if any, should be made to the gross earnings figure to take account of the individual's consumption; should adjustment be made for the additional investments that the individual or that society might make in the future in order to increase the individual's skills and his productive contribution and his earning power; what account should be taken of unemployment at the national level and at the regional level (what assumptions are reasonable as regards mobility and migration); should the future earnings figures be adjusted when there is evidence that because of market imperfections the individual is being rewarded at too low a rate?[b] These and numerous other issues arise, and require a measure of agreement. Important as these issues are, we can only note them. Our discussion moves on to two matters that, it seems to me, are particularly troublesome.

The first issue, not unlike some of the difficulties that we have discussed earlier, relates to the problems and biases that may result from the inability to specify or measure the outputs that are sought. If only some of the outputs are measured, however eloquent the words concerning other outputs, a budget or treasury official may tend to focus on those outputs which have numbers (economic values) attached to them. Further, because of the investment orientation of the analysis, often reflecting the investment orientation of the policy-maker, we may come to overvalue programs that have an impact on future productivity and undervalue programs that relieve pain, distress, concern, and suffering but have little or no impact (or measurable impact) on productivity. It may, indeed, be that programs addressed to disabling conditions and to diseases involving mortality rather than to conditions that do not remove the person from economic activity should be favored. That conclusion, however, should not be reached primarily because some things can be measured while others cannot. The analyst may discount the nature of the difficulty and the likelihood that this might occur, believing that his description of the items (particularly benefits) that cannot be measured will suffice to alert the decision-maker to the inadequacy of the numbers. I suggest, however, that the analyst may underestimate the problem. He would do well to consider how compelling numbers are to finance officials and how high a rate of discount is applied to words, however well turned the phrases may be. There are those who feel that this danger is surmounted because all programs are likely to have nonmeasurable by-products. They therefore believe that there is value in assessing the part of the iceberg that is visible (even if one cannot do the same for the part that lies below the surface of the water). It is argued that it is, after all, better to know something than to know nothing (knowledge thus being equated with measurement and the inability to quantify equated with ignorance). Yet there is little reason to believe that the ratio of measured to nonmeasured is the same in all programs. If in some icebergs a higher proportion is visible than in others, how do we assess which icebergs are larger in total and

---

[b]Market imperfections arise in many areas. As early as 1861, it was suggested that '... the value of compulsory servitude in the Army ... (should include) ... the value between the market price of labour and the price paid for it by government ... '. This issue has, once again, arisen in the debates in the United States concerning the comparison of the cost of a volunteer and of a conscripted army.

which are smaller? It is better to know something than to know nothing, but we dare not minimize the danger that in knowing something we may behave as if we know everything.

In reference to quantification and its dangers, one cannot help but be impressed by the words of Charles Henry Hull. In his introduction to *The Economic Writings of Sir William Petty*, published in 1899, Hull noted that Petty was sometimes careless in his calculations. He indicated that Petty was aware of the conjectural character of his numbers, and pointed out that Petty had written: "I hope that no man takes what I say about the living and dyeing of men for a mathematical demonstration." Hull continued:

> But in the ardour of argument he was himself more than once mislead into fancying that his conclusions were accurate because their form was definite. His mistake is not without its modern analogies. Mathematical presentations of industrial facts, both symbolic and graphic, have by their definiteness, encouraged many an investigator in the false conceit that he now knew what he sought, whereas he had at most but a neat name for what he sought to know. Nevertheless the substitution of symbols for Petty's "terms of number" is an improvement in this, that calculations made in symbols must be consciously translated into the terms of actual life before any practical use—or misuse—can be made of them, whereas calculations in figures of number, weight, and measure are already concrete and appear to tell something intelligible even to a common man.[29]

The danger that Hull recognized is our concern. Almost three-quarters of a century has passed since then, but the problem has not been solved.

The second problem that arises when we concentrate our measurement on earnings is even more basic. The previous discussion addressed itself to difficulties that can, perhaps, be solved by acquainting the decision-maker with the inadequacy of the methodology, by requiring that all analysts be humble and all decision-makers be wise (requirements that are not easy to achieve). They can be solved by recognizing that *quantification is not a substitute for judgment*, but a contributor to it. The problem to which we now turn is, I believe, even more severe, for it asks the basic question whether programs are to be evaluated primarily on the basis of "investment criteria." Does the measurement of a person's worth in terms of his productive contribution really represent our social values?

I believe that it does not do so. In particular, it fails adequately to take account of equity and distributional considerations (which many believe to be one of the major functions of government). Note that the theory says that in instituting a program and measuring the benefits we ask what impact the program would have on the earning power of the individual. Because we cannot count *the* individual we tend, in our measurements, to deal with groups of individuals and with averages. Always, however, the theory would have us include as many characteristics of individuals as are relevant to the projection of future income and as are available to us: the sex and age of the people affected, their urban-rural and racial characteristics, their income and education levels, and so forth. A program directed at women would use the average income of women as a measure of benefit. A program directed at a specific age group should (and does) use the discounted value of future earnings of that age group (yielding different answers for persons 45-55 than for persons 25-35). Yet, taking account of the individual's characteristics (or classifying the individual as a member of a group that has certain average behavior patterns) could lead us to direct our health activities toward those with the highest potential incomes and away from those whose earning capacity would be low: away from those with less education and skills, from the poor (whose increase in potential income may also be low), from those in low productivity sectors such as agriculture, and so forth. It would also mean that programs directed at females would compete unfavorably with programs for males, that the old would compete unfavorably with the young. The latter two biases are offset because income is often imputed to women since the difficulty with using an earned income test is obvious and because in the case of the young the discount rate that is applied to future earnings has a very powerful effect in reducing the present value of future earnings. Nonetheless, the problem is clear and particularly so for the present poor, since their potential increase in earnings, however large in percentage terms, may be small in absolute terms, and it is the absolute that is measured.

It is apparent that the theory, and the results that would be obtained were the theory followed, stand in conflict with our value system. The victims, in many cases, of past discrimination would be discriminated against again because, as a result of past discrimination, they are "worth less" in economic terms—and this at a time when many feel that past discrimination justifies and necessitates compensation. In fact, the conflict does not arise because practice departs from theory. The analysis does not include all the information that it might. We are sufficiently sensitive to the problem of distributional equity that we do not include all the characteristics of the population to be affected in the projection of future income and thus in the benefit-cost calculation. In general, we ignore differences in education, in present income (at given ages), in occupation, and in other variables that might affect future earnings of different groups. The issue, therefore, is not raised because we are "getting the wrong answers" but, rather, in order to alert us to the fact that the conceptual and philosophical problems at issue have not been adequately addressed or resolved. These may not have been problems in earlier days when the arguments presented were cast in general terms and were in support of health, education, and other general programs. It is an issue when the analysis and arguments are addressed to problems of choice as between alternative programs *for alternative population groups*. Often the analytical issues are viewed as technical matters relating to how economists measure value. We must recognize that measurement is more than a matter of technical procedure, but that it carries with it an implicit value system and orientation. To suppose that economics is value free and that measurement is neutral is incorrect. Explicit discussion of the value system would be valuable, for the debate would illuminate matters that now are buried within jargon, regression equations, and technical considerations that few decision-makers are totally familiar with. Cost-benefit analysis is too important to be left to analysts or economists. It is more than regrettable that philosophers, historians, students of intellectual thought, and others have neglected this area of inquiry.

That the calculation of benefit-cost ratios entails other difficulties is well known. Many of these difficulties bear discussion. I propose, however, to address one remaining question, not technical in nature. It relates to the impact of the kind of analysis that we are reviewing. While much of the analytical effort stems from an attempt at rational decision-making and involves a pressure to depart from incremental budget-making. I would suggest that the (benefit-cost) analytical effort is likely to result in the development of small, innovative, experimental programs (all this is desirable) but likely to favor a "conservative" response toward bold, new, and large departures from existing policies, programs, and patterns of organization and funding. In my view this is undesirable. There are times when large changes are needed.

Social revolutions, bold new departures in social policy, and massive changes in the prevailing patterns of health financing or organization can probably not be subjected to rigorous benefit-cost analysis. Nor is it likely that when analysis could be undertaken, it could withstand the critics of the benefit-cost ratios that might offer support for such changes and departures. At the present time we do not know how much good is created by a physician visit, what benefits more medical care brings, what the contribution of other factors is to the level of health. If policies must be justified with quantitative arguments and economic data, we are likely to find that those who would delay the institution of new programs could argue that more experimental effort is required, that we are not quite ready, that the program is "good" but that it may not be "the best." I rather doubt that Britain would have a National Health Service had the decision involved the kind of analysis I describe. This is not because the analysis would have suggested that the NHS was undesirable (though since benefit-cost analysis would likely not have taken adequate account of one of the important objectives of the program, distributional equity, benefits would have been understated) but rather because the analysis would have revealed many "unknowns"—and would thus have favored the point of view of those who believed in more small experiments. The analytical effort is likely to reveal that there is much we do not know, and thus will favor marginal change in the status quo "until we know more." But there will always be more to know, more programs to analyze.

I do not argue that every revolution is good (though that may often be the case with social programs involving distributional equity). I simply argue that it is difficult to justify most revolutions on an *ex-ante* basis in the face of critics who are trying to avoid risks. In the analytical effort, after all, there is a climate of opinion that says that the program can be justified only when we are certain that there is no other program that is better. As I look at the social legislation enacted in the United States in recent years, I am forced to conclude that we have been well served by decision-makers who were willing to reach decisions and move on to new paths, battling for the answers given them by their ideological convictions. The programs might, of course, have been better constructed. Not all of them have been successes, and some of them have left much to be desired. It is not clear, however, that had the analyst been listened to the programs would have been better. They might simply not have existed ("Let's wait and do more research").

The reader will note that these comments are not based on the additional possibility that the benefit-cost ratio for a program that is massive in scope might differ greatly from the ratio for the small experiment. If this is the case then no experiment (other than one involving the massive change) can give us the right answer. This may well be the case with social programs that involve behavioral characteristics that are influenced by the fact that one is involved in an experiment, discontinuities, or long periods of time before their impacts can be fully assessed. The argument presented here is a more limited one, however. Here the issue is the flavor of the exercise, what I believe is a bias against big changes. Perhaps benefit-cost analysis has a nonincremental impact on the budget for existing programs and an incremental impact on experimentation. One may, therefore, favor it. It should be recognized, nonetheless, that incremental experiments are different from program changes, particularly major ones.

It should also be clear that I am not suggesting that all analysis is without value, and that major changes in programs should be supported by statements of faith. Our discussion relates to benefit-cost analysis, not to analysis in general. That economists (and others) can conduct useful analysis of the distributional impact of cash transfer programs, for example, should be evident. Their efforts at constructing more equitable, and more efficient transfer programs—some of them, indeed, representing major new departures—should not go unrecognized. Our discussion is not meant to detract from this type of analytical work. The ability to provide economic analysis of programs where the objective is simply distributional does not mean that there exists an equal ability to provide analysis of the ultimate benefits of programs whose aim is not solely distributional, or whose aim involves levels of performance via redistribution of services rather than money.

It is also useful to note one specific contribution to decision-making that can be derived from cost-effectiveness analysis, a mode of analysis close to, but not identical with, cost-benefit analysis. Let us assume that, in one way or another—perhaps through the political process responsive to and leading the electorate—a decision is reached to accomplish a certain purpose, to achieve a goal, to reach an objective, say in health. Whether it is the most worthwhile purpose, goal, or objective in terms of maximizing total satisfaction is no longer the issue. The particular output sought can usually be achieved in a variety of different ways, that is, with different combinations of resource inputs. In cost-effectiveness analysis we seek the optimal, economically efficient combination of these inputs so that resources are not wasted and so that they might, therefore, be available for other purposes. The object is to minimize cost per unit of output (or one may put it as maximizing output per unit cost). Because of the problems engendered by multiple outputs, each with different values and, thus, requiring some comparison of the values of the outputs (of the benefits), cost-effectiveness analysis does tend, at times, to move closer and closer to benefit-cost analysis. Nonetheless, the purpose to be served by the cost-effectiveness inquiry is different.

Cost-effectiveness analysis raises questions concerning tradeoffs (of inputs if not of inputs and outputs). Though more limited than benefit-cost analysis, it is valuable and reinforces our need to know more about the production function. It reminds us to consider quality considerations. Above all else, perhaps, it forces the professional to respond to the question whether the fact that things have been done in a particular way in the past means that that is the best way to do them in the future. Such questions, of course, are questions that the professional should be asking himself all the time, but the fact is that oftentimes it is the outsider who can question tradition more readily than the practitioner. There are many rewards to be derived in a wide variety of government programs from good cost-effectiveness analysis: rewards in the saving of resources in some instances, and in accomplishing much more good for people in others. Cost-effectiveness analysis, to some, seems to involve less exciting issues than is the case in benefit-cost analysis. Nonetheless, the benefit-cost ratio of this kind of work is likely to be extremely high. Major government stimulus of this kind of analysis is justified.

CONCLUSIONS

I have raised a number (though by no means all) of the problems that relate to the evaluation of the economic benefits of health (and other social) programs. Yet, earlier, I indicated the need for evaluation, for the kind of thinking that is involved in the comparison of programs, and for doing so in an explicit manner in order to improve decision-making. Where does that leave us? What contribution can the successors to Petty, Chadwick, and others make?

It should, I think, be clear that in my view we have not arrived at a stage where benefit-cost analysis can be as helpful as some (but not all) of its proponents believe to be the case in the allocation of scarce resources in public policy decisions. We are a long way (and will always remain a long way) from being able to allocate the total government budget as between competing priorities on the basis of this kind of analysis. Even more limited objectives are beyond our attainment. In the United States, major elements of the federal budget for health, education, and welfare fall within one department, the Department of Health, Education and Welfare. Yet, competing claims between the three major activities in that one department cannot be significantly illuminated and even partially resolved by benefit-cost analysis. Indeed, I rather doubt that, given the state of our data systems and the conceptual problems yet to be solved, the analytical effort can be more than only somewhat helpful in allocating scarce dollars within a single broad line of activity, say within the health arena. Helpful, yes, because it will force explicit statements about our ignorance, because it will help us to implement data and reporting systems, because it will provoke debate leading to questions and, in some cases, answers. The degree of usefulness will, however, depend on how wise the decision-maker is, how skeptical he is of measurement techniques even as he supports, encourages, and assists in their development.

Thus, we are not called upon to declare a moratorium on this type of analysis. To do so would, in my view, be an error. That we will find fewer answers than we seek is clear, but we will learn much in the formulation of the questions and in the seeking of the answers. Economists have until recently been underrepresented in departments and agencies concerned with social programs, and all of us, I believe, have paid a price for this underrepresentation. The economist's point of view, his questions, his perspective, are useful in forcing persons to examine a problem that they are professionally familiar with from another point of view. It leads, therefore, to a more intelligent debate concerning programs, issues, and goals. Since many of the programs referred to are concerned with human behavior and response, departments should also increase the number of behavioral and social scientists involved from disciplines other than economics. By focusing on the economist, I in no sense mean to ignore the potential contribution of the sociologist, anthropologist, psychologist, social psychologist, and others. My own background does permit me, however, to speak with more knowledge about the role that economic analysis and the thought process of the economist can play.

In my view the contribution of economists and analysts can be important. The skepticism that I have concerning some of the answers provided by cost-benefit analysis in no way detracts from my view about the potential contribution derived from the thought process, from the way of thinking about problems. Furthermore, Chadwick was correct when he stated that economists had a contribution to make. The contribution does not depend on the ability to measure whether removing persons from London during a plague yields a return of £84, or of £72, or £129 per pound expended. This will not often enable us to answer whether this or some other program is a "better" investment. But policy-makers and others need to be reminded that there are economic returns to health programs, that good health can be supported on investment grounds, that there are high costs (for the issue is total costs, both direct budget outlays and indirect costs associated with loss of production) as a consequence of poor health and inadequate education. Economics can help point up these issues. It can—and should—serve the protagonist (not only the decision-maker). The discipline is not debased by such analysis, nor is the public decision process harmed, for far too often health and education appropriations are insufficient not because other programs yield a higher rate of return, but because it is assumed that health and education appropriations are simply money down the drain, yielding no economic benefit. In a world oriented to economic benefits, this assumption becomes a difficult obstacle to surmount. Too many economists—perhaps afraid of being accused of being part sentimentalist and moralist, and because of their desire to assume the stance of "objectivity"—have been on the defensive too long. Too often we have said that health and education are valuable but that society must choose the most valuable program, and we cannot be certain which of the many possible activities are the most valuable. While this is true and important, we must recognize that in the political world those who would compete with health and education for funds often are far less objective and analytical. To subject health activities to analysis while, for example, leaving the military budget to emotional arguments is hardly to fight for scarce dollars on even terms. Surely I am not arguing for the end of the analytical effort, but rather for a greater willingness to do what Petty and Chadwick did: to bring supporting evidence for their point of view without that self-consciousness that some of us often have because we have not examined every alternative; to be willing to say that this is good even if we cannot yet say that this is best.

Earlier I noted that a major function of many government programs is to achieve a more equitable distribution of goods and services. The early history of economic analysis in the health field did not rest its case for an increased effort on the part of government on these grounds, nor, as has been indicated, does the present effort take due account of such considerations. Clearly, however, distributional equity does provide an important rationale for many health programs. To that extent, the task of the analyst and of the data and reporting system is made easier. If the objective of the legislature is to equalize services, to make available to certain population groups services that they would otherwise not be able to purchase in the market, services that people believe to be important (even if, in fact, they are less important or beneficial than is imagined), then the evaluation effort is much simpler. At present, in the United States, beset as we are by divisions and by tensions, distributional considerations lie at the heart of many of our problems. The healing of social wounds (not an unimportant objective even if its benefits cannot be quantified in monetary terms) may, today, be more readily accomplished by providing the services that people believe to be important than by providing that which the analyst has tentatively determined is most beneficial. The healing of social wounds is, at this moment, I believe more vital than the healing of disease. Though there is surely a relationship between the two efforts, and they need not be in conflict, there may well be a tradeoff between them. In that case, social harmony would, I suggest, be the overriding goal. It may, for example, be that certain medical procedures cannot be justified on economic grounds and, in fact, contribute very little to better health. If, however, they are available to many in the population and are utilized (even if this means that individuals are "wasting their money"), if the population believes them to be important, society may be compelled to make them available to all. This, though in many ways a more limited objective, is not a trivial one at all. We are a long way from its attainment and would do well to pursue it with vigor and commitment.

That distributional equity in the delivery of services is a limited goal should, nonetheless, be clear. An enlightened society will attempt to achieve a greater equity in outcomes rather than in inputs. In the United States, in the field of education there was a time when equality meant that children should attend schools with equal inputs. Difficult as it may be to achieve such goals, the formulas required for their attainment are easy to construct and require little knowledge of the educational process. Evaluation in such a context requires simple data. Today, however, equality of educational opportunity has come to mean that we should offer opportunities such that regardless of the circumstances of the child when he enters school and the environmental problems he faces while he attends school, the child should have equal opportunity to achieve a given level of education. Thus, the resources going to schools with a high proportion of poor children should be greater than the resources going to schools with more affluent children. The problem in evaluation when we are interested in unequal resource inputs and unequal provision of services so that we might have more equal outcomes is, of course, immensely more difficult, since it requires an understanding of the relationship between inputs and outputs and an understanding of the production process. Thus, an enlightened society can hardly avoid many of the analytical efforts we have discussed in this chapter. We cannot find an easy way out of the analytical difficulties.

We shall have to continue the kind of explorations begun by Petty and by others. We shall have to remember Chadwick's words. We shall, however, have to carry on this work with a certain modesty, remembering the words of Sir Arthur Newsholme: "There remains a further problem which must at least be mentioned. Is it possible in every instance to measure by means of statistics, influence and procedures benefiting the public health or improving social welfare?"[30]

Notes to Chapter Sixteen

1. E. Chadwick, "Opening Address as President of Section F (Economic Sciences and Statistics) of the British Association for the Advancement of Science," *Jl. Statist. Soc. Lond.* 25 (1862), 504, 509, 522.

2. Sir William Petty, *Political Arhithmetick*, (1690) in C.H. Hull, *The Economic Writings of Sir William Petty* (Cambridge: Cambridge University Press, 1899), p. 267.

3. Sir William Petty, *Verbum Sapienti* (1691), in Hull, p. 109.

4. Sir William Petty, "Magnalia Regni," in Marquis of Lansdowne, *The Petty Papers, Some Unpublished Writings of Sir William Petty*, edited from the Bowood Papers (London: Constable & Co., Ltd., 1927), pp. 265-67, 274.

5. Sir William Petty, "Of Lesening ye Plagues of London," (1667), in Hull, p. 109.

6. Petty, "Magnalia Regni."

7. Sir William Petty, "Anatomy Lecture" (1676), in Lansdowne, p. 176.

8. Petty, "Magnalia Regni."

9. E. Chadwick, *Sanitary Report* (1842), cited by the Right Honorable the Earl Fortescue, "Extracts from the Address of the President of Section F (Economic Sciences and Statistics) of the British Association for the Advancement of Science," *Jl. Statist. Soc. Lond.* 25 (1877), 558.

10. E. Chadwick, "On the Best Modes of Representing Accurately, by Statistical Returns, the Duration of Life, and the Pressure and Progress of the Causes of Mortality Amongst Different Classes of the Community, and Amongst the Populations of Different Districts and Countries," *Jl. Statist. Soc. Lond.* 7 (1844), 25, 30.

11. L. Shattuck, *Report of the Sanitary Commission of Massachusetts* (1850), Facsimile Edition (Cambridge: Harvard University Press, 1948), pp. 254, 257, 258-60.

12. E. Chadwick, "Results of Different Principles of Legislation and Administration in Europe; of Competition for the Field, as Compared with Competition Within the Field, of Service" *Jl. Statist. Soc. Lond.* 22, (1859), 405.

13. Chadwick, "Opening Address as President of Section F."

14. Ibid.

15. Shattuck.

16. Ibid.

17. Ibid.

18. Ibid.

19. Rev. J.E.T. Rogers, "On the Statistical and Fiscal Definitions of the Word 'Income,' " *Jl. Statist. Soc. Lond.* 28 (1865), 243.

20. W. Farr, "The Income and Property Tax," *Jl. Statist. Soc. Lond.* 16 (1853), 1-44.

21. W. Farr, *Vital Statistics*, ed. by N.A. Humphreys, (London: Offices of the Sanitary Institute, 1885), pp. 313, 314.

22. Ibid.

23. G.N. Calkins, "Some Results of Sanitary Legislation in England Since 1875," *Am. Statist. Ass.* 2 (1891), 297-303.

24. E.L. Bogart, Direct and Indirect Costs of the Great World War (New York: Oxford University Press, 1919); Sir Robert Giffen, "Some Economic Aspects of the War," *Econ. J.* 10 (1900), 194-207; Sir Robert Giffen, *Economic Inquiries and Studies* (London: George Bell & Sons, 1904), pp. 1-74; C.W. Guillebaud, "The Cost of the War in Germany," *Econ. J.* 27 (1927), 270-77.

25. Rogers.

26. Dr. Guy, "Discussion on Mr. Hamilton's Paper," *Jl. Statist. Soc. Lond.* 40 (1877), 40, 127, 129.

27. Ibid.

28. L.I. Dublin and J. Whitney, "On the Cost of Tuberculosis," *Am. Statist. Ass.* 17 (1920), 441-50; W.O. Mendenhall and E.W. Castle, "Vital and Monetary Losses in the United States Due to Typhoid Fever," *Am. Statist. Ass.* 12 (1911), 519-43.

29. Hull, p. lxviii.

30. Sir Arthur Newsholme, "The Measurement of Progress in Public Health," *Economica* (1923), 3, 201.

❈ *Chapter 17*

Community Participation in Health Care Decisions

Laurelyn Veatch

To whom should publicly financed hospitals be responsible? In the case of city hospitals the principle of accountability to city residents and taxpayers is at least given lip service. Yet translating the principle of public accountability into practice is always fraught with conflicting alternatives and difficult choices. For example, which "publics" are to be served and which are to govern, if any? What private influences are and should be involved in governing and receiving benefits?

The New York City municipal hospitals began, over one hundred years ago, as charity institutions supported by public funds for the direct benefit of the poor and the indirect benefit of the rich (who had the sick poor quarantined in the hospitals). New York City now has the largest municipal hospital system in the country. Nineteen municipal hospitals provide nearly one-half of the city's seven and one-half million residents with at least *part* of their medical care, and are the *primary* source of medical care for over a million and one-half persons, especially members of minority groups, the poor, the young, and the old.

Until 1970 the city government exercised nominal control over the city hospitals, which were, at first, directly governed by physicians who volunteered their time, and later increasingly by persons connected with medical schools and teaching hospitals. Influence was also exercised by hospital administrators, by Blue Cross, by politicians, and by others.

In 1970 the New York State Legislature established the Health and Hospitals Corporation (HHC) as a quasi-public benefit corporation, outside of the direct control of city hall. The new organizational scheme avoided some of the municipal bureaucratic regulations originally designed to insure public accountability, but more recently responsible for delays in the purchasing and construction of new facilities. The mayor and city council did retain influence in the

Health and Hospitals Corporation through their power to appoint members to its board of directors and through the city's financial contributions to the corporation. While the establishment of the corporation reduced formal accountability, at least at the city-wide level, to the people of New York City in the management of the city hospitals, at the same time a new accountability mechanism was introduced. "Community Advisory Boards" were to be established at each corporation hospital.[a]

Such an innovation raises questions about a series of competing claims to authority in hospital decision-making. It would be valuable (1) to analyze the bases upon which these claims have been made; (2) to relate these claims to the reasons for establishing community boards; and (3) to examine the community boards in action particularly as they function as a mechanism for patient and community participation in the city hospitals.[1]

FIVE CLAIMS TO POLICY-MAKING AUTHORITY

Claims for participation in the control of a hospital have been made on the basis of: (1) *money* contributed to the hospital; (2) *expertise*; (3) *work* (persons who work in or for a hospital); (4) *residence* in the geographical area served by the hospital; and (5) being a *patient* (an actual or potential consumer of health care at the hospital, or a close relative of a patient).

1. The assumption that contributing or paying *money* may carry with it a legitimate claim to participate in policy-making has a long history in the development of democratic government in the West. "No taxation without representation," was the cry of American colonists in the eighteenth century, and for a long time in many nations only taxpayers were allowed to vote. Philanthropists who supported early hospitals were generally allowed a major role on the hospitals' boards of directors, and later, important businessmen who were presumed to be able to raise or manage money were often placed on the boards of directors. Skill at managing money shades off into our next category, "expertise."

Individuals and groups who contribute money have not all had an equal influence over policy-making. Generally, the influential contributors have been those who have given large sums, have been able to withhold their money at their own discretion, and have been therefore recognized as legitimate policy-

---

[a]The establishment of community boards for municipal hospitals was part of a widespread movement toward community participation, community control, and decentralization which emerged in the 1960s. In New York City some of the forms for formal community participation are community planning boards, decentralized school boards, police precinct community councils, comprehensive health planning councils, mental health boards, consumer advisory boards of voluntary hospitals that participate in ghetto medicine programs, and the municipal hospital community boards. The district boundaries for the different kinds of community boards were drawn so as not to coincide, helping to prevent communities from effectively organizing around more than one issue. The State Charter Revision Commission recently proposed merging many of the district lines.

makers for the hospital. Some of the current contributors who influence hospital policies to varying degrees are the federal government, state government, city government, Blue Cross, insurance companies, fund-raisers, philanthropists (who maintain a great influence over voluntary hospitals more in line with past than with current contributions), and individuals who pay for services received (and at best have a minor, informal, diffuse impact).

2. Historically and currently, a second basis for participation in hospital policy-making has been *expertise* of a medical, administrative, or financial kind. Early hospitals were often run by the physicians who volunteered to practice in them. Initially as hospitals came to have full-time, paid administrators, they were most often physicians. Later, hospital administration became a specialized career, and a dual system of authority developed between the lay administrator and the medical board. Financial expertise found expression on the board of directors or in the hospital administrator. There are currently many kinds of authoritative experts sharing power in New York City municipal hospitals—the medical board, the hospital administrator, the affiliated medical school or hospital with its affiliation administrator, and the central Health and Hospitals Corporation with its administrative staff and board of directors.

3. The claim that *working* in or for a hospital entitles one to participate in hospital decision-making in some ways overlaps with and in other ways contradicts the expertise claim. Worker-control ideology has found greater acceptance in Italy, China, and Scandinavia than in the United States. In the United States, worker-community control has been espoused by some student and community groups and elements of organized labor. It is a central feature of the Dellums bill which will be proposed to Congress later this year.[2]

Some hospital workers, principally physicians but also social workers, nurses, and administrators have claimed and been granted power to influence hospital decision-making by virtue of their expertise. The worker-control claim has an egalitarian, antihierarchical, antiauthoritarian thrust within the organization. In this way worker control runs counter to the claim for power and authority based on medical or other expertise; at the same time, it absorbs physicians and administrators as some, but not all, of the workers.

4. Being a *resident* in the geographical areas served by and/or impinged upon by a hospital is the fourth basis we have identified for a claim to participate in the control of a hospital. Participation in decision-making on the basis of geographical residence was the next step in Western democracy after voting by taxpayers only. Participation in the policies of a local institution by the residents has been well established in the case of many school districts in the United States. "Community control," going beyond the schools, has been part of two recent movements, one decentralizing decision-making in city government, the other giving ethnic and lower-income groups a greater voice in the institutions that serve them.

5. The fifth basis for a claim to participate in hospital policy-making is being

a *patient* in the hospital, a potential patient, or the close relative of a patient—especially the spouse, parent, or child of a patient. The claim that patients are legitimate policy-makers draws much of its strength and ideology from the consumer movement. The underlying assumption here is that as consumers of health care, patients should be able both to make informed choices regarding the health care they consume and also to be in a position to decide priorities in the kinds of health care available (for instance, readily accessible preventive health care rather than highly specialized clinics for exotic diseases).

In what ways are the five claims recognized as legitimate and given institutionalization for policy-making in hospitals, particularly New York City municipal hospitals?

Claim number one is based on money contributed. This claim finds institutionalization for the federal government in regulations governing Medicare and Medicaid: in federal aid for hospital construction, medical education, and medical research; and in the annual appropriations that budget the money available for federal health programs. New York State's influence is institutionalized in the legislation establishing and regulating the Health and Hospitals Corporation; in laws governing hospital accreditation; and in the power to appropriate state aid for health care. New York City has some control over city funds appropriated for the municipal hospitals and over appointments to the Board of Directors of the Health and Hospitals Corporation. Since third-party payments are largely governmental in New York City municipal hospitals, other common financial sources like Blue Cross have little influence.[3]

Patients who pay for services received have little influence over health policy-making. Their sole recourse is withdrawal of patronage—an indirect, inexact, and unorganized means of influencing policy. The power of free choice in purchasing health care is limited by many factors. There may be only one hospital within reasonable distance of the patient. The patient may not have adequate knowledge with which to judge the quality of services received, or may be able to judge only after major medical care has been received unsuccessfully but in a manner in which a refund cannot be adequately given (e.g., a leg has already been cut off). And in emergency medical situations the patient does not have the time or ability to "shop around."

Expertise is the second claim to legitimate influence and is institutionalized in the dual system of authority within hospitals—the administrative hierarchy culminating in the executive director and the "medical" hierarchy culminating in the chiefs of service and the medical board. The fact that there are parallel, potentially conflicting authority systems within hospitals opens opportunities for a third force to ally with one side or the other.

As already noted, social workers, nurses, and medical schools also make claims to authority based on their expertise. Recognition of some of these claims is institutionalized for social workers and nurses in the authority they are given over some of the other hospital workers, over patients, and in the token representation they are given in New York City municipal hospital community boards. The affiliation contracts that New York City municipal hospitals have with medical schools, teaching hospitals, and some voluntary hospitals are, in part, a legitimation of the authority of the presumed expertise of these institutions. In addition they are one method of recruiting physicians for the municipal hospitals. The affiliation contracts give the affiliated voluntary hospital or medical school a great deal of control over money, allocation of health-care priorities, and authority in decision-making.

Working in or for a hospital is a third basis for a claim to participate in decision-making regarding the hospital. Most New York City hospital community boards give one seat on the board to a hospital employee who is not a physician or nurse. The seats designated by type of employment fit primarily into the expertise category rather than into the category based on work which would grant equal decision-making power to *all* those who work in or for a hospital.

Compared to claims one and two (money and expertise), claims three, four, and five (work, residence in the community, and being a patient) have received little recognition as legitimate bases for authority in hospital decision-making. Establishing community boards for the New York City municipal hospitals, for hospitals participating in ghetto medicine programs, and elsewhere, has been one attempt to offer community residents and patients participation in hospital policy-making. While these boards now have formal authority for only marginal participation in policy-making, they are institutionalized as a pressure group and they are a source of demands for increased consumer and community influence.

THE BEGINNINGS OF THE COMMUNITY BOARDS

According to one of its architects, among the purposes of the Health and Hospitals Corporation was "controlled decentralization of decision-making." Yet the extent to which local citizens have participated in decision-making has been an unsettled question since 1970. The legal basis for the corporation hospital community boards was a provision in the legislation which established the Health and Hospitals Corporation. The state legislature stipulated that:

> The corporation shall establish a community advisory board for each of its hospitals to consider and advise the corporation and the hospital upon matters concerning the development of any plans or programs of the corporation, and may establish rules and regulations with respect to such boards. The members of such advisory boards shall be representatives of the community served by the hospital.[4]

Before 1970 and the establishment of the Health and Hospitals Corporation, few hospitals had community advisory boards. Those that did exist were called into being by the hospital administration either as a lobbying group to gain more city funds for the hospital or as an advisory group on noncontroversial areas of patient care. Some of the old community advisory boards became the planning boards for the new community boards. The executive director of each hospital was responsible for establishing a community board for his hospital within the guidelines drawn up by the corporation.

The preamble to the corporation's "Interim Policy and Guidelines," in giving reasons for establishing community boards, implies that they must be more than advisory; yet the only clearly stated power that goes beyond advice is concurrence in the selection of an executive director for the hospital. The preamble states that the corporation seeks to forge a partnership with communities, that the corporation is committed "to involve the total community as participants in the development of plans and programs of the corporation." Within each hospital, community boards are to participate in establishing priorities, allocating funds, judging the acceptability of services to patients, and area-wide planning. "In their advisory capacity" they have a right to "full discussion on issues ... consult with responsible officials ... make specific recommendations." The extent of "participation" is left unclear in the corporation guidelines, but even the limited functions indicated for community boards can make a significant difference in hospital administration and planning. Most of the boards have not been able to exercise all the "rights" given them in the 1970 "Interim Policy and Guidelines," particularly the right to information controlled by the executive director.

The community boards are required by law to have consumers as a majority of members. Community representatives are the next largest category of members on most boards. And hospital employees, either as experts or workers, have some representation on the boards. The method of selecting community board members varies from hospital to hospital. It also varies for each type of representative. Consumers are almost always elected; community representatives are usually elected by geographical areas but sometimes by community groups; the medical board representative may be elected by his peers or the medical board president may be designated a permanent member.

The Health and Hospitals Corporation defined a consumer as a person using the hospital as his or her primary source of health services. This was interpreted in different ways. Bellevue defined "consumer" as anyone who had a patient record. Morrisania Hospital required a clinic card, an in-patient stay of at least three days in the last two years, at least four emergency room visits in the last two years, and no equivalent care elsewhere. Community representatives can be residents of the hospital's service area. Sometimes they can be employees in the area.

While the state legislation establishing the corporation mandated "community *advisory* boards," most of the boards have themselves dropped the word "advisory" from their titles and hope eventually to obtain final authority for policy-making in their own hospitals—authority analogous to that of the board of directors in a voluntary hospital. One of the sources of strain in the operation of the boards is ambiguity and conflict over the amount of authority they should have, an issue springing from the wider uncertainty about how much power community residents and patients should have in hospitals.

In practice the community boards act more like interest groups than like decision-making bodies. They have difficulty obtaining information; they consider what comes before them, make recommendations, and attempt to influence policies in the direction of their recommendations. They act as consumer advocates to the hospital and hospital advocates to the corporation and the city government. They make the hospital administration aware of patient needs. They join with the executive director and medical board in trying to get more resources for their hospital, to get a new hospital opened, or to prevent the closing of an old one with no replacement.

There are common threads but also differences in the practices of various community boards. Following are differences in emphasis that have developed at some of the New York City hospitals.

A MIDDLE-CLASS COMMUNITY BOARD

The service area for Elmhurst Hospital includes 900,000 persons in the northwest corner of Queens. The population is primarily white and middle class or working class. Many residents have lived in the area for a long time. There is a disproportionate number of persons over sixty-five; 14.6 percent in the service area as compared to 12.4 percent in Queens as a whole, 12 percent in New York City, and 10 percent in the nation in 1970. The area is changing. In 1960 there were 94 percent whites, 5 percent nonwhites, and 1 percent Puerto Ricans. In 1970 these figures were 91 percent, 7 percent, and 2 percent. Among whites there are many ethnic groups.[5]

The Elmhurst community board is composed of thirty-one elected members and four non-voting, ex officio members from the hospital staff. The voting members include four other hospital staff members elected by their respective groups (medical staff, nursing staff, nonmedical staff, and the department of social service); sixteen consumers and nine nonconsumers from four election districts in the community; and two members-at-large (one under twenty-one, one over sixty-five) who may be either consumers, or nonconsumer residents of the area.[6]

In the spring of 1973 the community board was elected. It began to meet during the summer and spent the remainder of the year writing the constitution and by-laws and participating in orientation sessions related to various aspects of the hospital. At the end of the year elections were held for permanent officers. In January a new executive committee began to function and the committees were reconstituted.

The community board, like the residential area, is largely white. There are a few black and Hispanic persons on the board. A larger proportion of Spanish-speaking and black persons are hospital users than is reflected in the demographic statistics for the "catchment area," the area the hospital serves. The board does not reflect the social characteristics of hospital consumers as well as it reflects the social groups who live in the area. Many of the nonuser members of the board are motivated by a desire to participate in a community service organization.[7]

The Elmhurst community board has obtained representation on the medical board of the hospital. The chairman of the community board together with other hospital personnel has met with Queens politicians to try to obtain more money for the hospital. The board has been approached for assistance by various groups and persons including social workers (seeking to remain under an affiliation rather than corporation contract), a nurse (seeking decorations for a part of the hospital), and the three hospital chaplains (seeking support to keep three separate chapels at the hospital). The board has discussed but not taken action on these requests.

The community board's patient-care committee has picked a pamphlet on patients' rights to give to all patients who come to the hospital. The community relations committee is working on a blood bank program in which participants and their families would be insured against future blood needs. They are also working on an open-house day for the hospital, an open community board meeting, and health fairs, which would include information about the community board.

According to the corporation's "Kerz Report," Elmhurst is underfunded compared to other municipal hospitals.[8] The community board sent a letter to Lowell Bellin, chairman of the board of the corporation, regarding the financing of Elmhurst Hospital, but at last report had received no answer.

Compared to other community boards, the Elmhurst community board considers itself to be relatively conservative. It uses little ideological rhetoric; yet some of its members hold the long-term goal of having their board evolve into a board of directors for the hospital. Although many of the other municipal hospital community boards favor abolishing the affiliation system, the Elmhurst community board does not want to terminate its affiliation contract.[9]

A CHRONIC-CARE FACILITY

Goldwater Memorial Hospital on Roosevelt Island is a chronic care institution in which the patients call themselves patient-residents. Most of the patient-residents, who make up 51 percent of the community board, are able to give a good deal of time to community board activities and are always present in the hospital. They know what has been happening over a period of time and have little difficulty getting together.

Goldwater has had patient councils since the 1950s. The patient councils focus on personal and ward situations and make nominations for the Community Advisory Board. The community board works on overall policy. The community board and hospital staff held a joint rally attended by five hundred people to protest the bad road conditions on the island. This influenced the development corporation to improve the roads and lighting. The community board started a patient-managed and -operated tailor shop. It started a once-a-week social club; obtained a cut in the curb for wheelchairs and an outing-bus better suited to handicapped persons; instigated an overhaul of the library by a patient-resident; and checked the operation of all the hospital call boards. The community advisory board was able to obtain a new canteen for the hospital and a drop service from the New York City library. It started the hospital newspaper.

The community advisory board communicates with patient-residents through the hospital newspaper, in the one open meeting a year, by posting minutes on bulletin boards, and through overlapping membership of the community board and the patient councils. It communicates outside the hospital through membership on committees around the city, including the Mayor's Advocacy Committee, Planning Board Eight, and the health task forces on Roosevelt Island. It has recently been very active in organizing demonstrations and political opposition to closing Goldwater for economy reasons.

A COMMUNITY BOARD WITH STAFF

Kings County Hospital had the first executive assistant hired by a community board. The community boards of other hospitals have been dependent for staff support on their hospital's executive director, the director of community affairs, and whatever secretarial assistance is made available through one of those two persons. Future executive directors must have the concurrence of community boards for their appointments by the corporation. The directors of community affairs have been hired by the executive directors. In Kings County Hospital the community board hired an executive assistant, a secretary, an ombudsman, and another staff member. Money for these positions was provided by the executive director out of general hospital funds.

The catchment area for Kings County Hospital includes the East New York, Brownsville, Bedford-Stuyvesant, Crown Heights, and East Flatbush sections of Brooklyn. The population is primarily black and Hispanic. The community board was established in 1970, but was not installed by the corporation until 1972. This board has more selection and less election than most community boards.

When the corporation attempted to fire the executive director at Kings County without consulting the community board, the community board supported him in retaining his office. This cooperation probably helped the community board gain some of its goals within the hospital.

The executive assistant feels that the board has increased hospital accountability to residents and patients. "Some people know there is someone here." The Kings County community board has had some employees reinstated and some "rude and uncouth" *per diem* physicians fired. It provided the impetus to get seating and numbers for the pharmacy. In the future the community board will participate in the hiring of all persons above the assistant director's level, and other personnel if it wishes. Two community board members are voting members of the medical board.

PATRONAGE

The chairperson of one community board has great influence at the hospital with regard to hiring. His interests are patronage rather than patient care. He is charismatic, autocratic, demogogic, and in control of the community board. Most of the board members are of one ethnic group which has recently become numerically dominant in the area. The chairperson gets patronage for his ethnic group. There are ethnic conflicts at the hospital, which previously served a primarily black patient population. The lower-level employees used to be black; physicians have always been primarily white. During the 1960s this hospital was the focus of a great deal of community group and employee activism. The current focus on patronage by the community board illustrates a perennial problem facing a "democratic" or "representative" system.

BOARD MEMBERS' ROLES

In general, the lay members of community boards do not see themselves as having much power, although many of them hope that their power will increase with an increase in their knowledge and with a possible rise in demand for accountability to the public in the expenditure of public funds. Some boards do not envision an increase in their power. Rather they see their role as primarily providing information to the professionals, who can thereby increase the quality of patient care. Some laypersons expect to use their community board to further their own goals or those of their constituency as a first step in a political or health-care career. Many of the lay members of community boards are attempting to perform a humanitarian service: they are (1) trying to increase the quality of the technical care within the city hospitals and (2) trying to improve human relationships within the hospitals, particularly to assure the patients' dignity and a recognition of their human rights.

Many lay members of community boards are working to make the boards an integral part of decision-making in their hospitals. They would like the community boards to give concurrent approval to important policy decisions. At present some community boards are asked to ratify plans already made. The board at one hospital, for example, was asked to approve a television series about the hospital after it already had been approved by the hospital administration and the Health and Hospitals Corporation. In general, community boards are far from exercising equal authority with hospital administrations in decision-making. In some cases the community board is not consulted at all. Frequently it is given partial information only a short time before action must be taken. Executive directors often give community boards proposed budgets shortly before they must be sent on to the corporation.

During the last two years there seems to have been an increased recognition by some of the physicians on the boards of the legitimate need for community boards. This is apparent in the mutual respect generally shown in the verbal interchanges at meetings. It was also expressed in the recent formation of the Joint Action Committee of medical boards and community boards of the municipal hospitals. Despite some increased communication between health providers and health consumers, large differences in ability to influence decisions still exist. Laypersons on community boards are most at ease and most vocal at the meetings of their own boards and their committees. At meetings of the Health and Hospitals Corporation Board of Directors or its committees, community board members are more passive than are representatives of medical boards and of executive directors of the hospitals.

ISSUES

In spite of the fact that the power of community boards has been very limited compared to that of medical boards and administrators, community boards have at times had an impact on events and institutions.

This year the first community board member was selected to fill an opening on the Health and Hospitals Corporation Board of Directors by the New York City Council. Subsequently the state legislature was presented with a bill requiring that at least five members of this board of directors be community board members. Though this bill failed passage, the mere proposal indicates a change in people's expectations as to appropriate membership on the board of directors.

Even before the recent selection of a community board chairperson as a member of the Corporation Board of Directors, the Council of Community Boards was able to get observer status at board of directors meetings and on board committees. The community boards are an important element in a current proposal for a New York City public medical school based in the municipal hospitals and with prospective students chosen on the basis of prior community service related to the municipal hospitals. At one point in New York City's 1975 fiscal crisis, after the Health and Hospitals Corporation refused the mayor's request to cut 551 persons from the corporation payroll, the Council of Community Boards and the Joint Action Committee (community boards and medical boards) organized a demonstration in support of no layoffs.

The Council of Community Boards strengthened accountability mechanisms in the contracts which the corporation is currently offering affiliated medical schools and voluntary hospitals. Community groups have long criticized the lack of affiliates' accountability in their expenditure of public money and their use of municipal hospital patients for teaching and research.

ACHIEVING GOALS

Health and Hospitals Corporation goals for community boards have been vaguely defined, and the means to attain the goals have not been explicitly granted. In addition, community board members work on an essentially volunteer basis. To attain their goals they must influence full-time health professionals.

The four functions in which the corporation expects the community boards to participate (establishing planning priorities, allocating funds, judging the acceptability of services to patients, and area-wide planning) require information. Acquiring information is a common problem for laypersons. The lay members of community boards are essentially volunteers (they receive a small compensation) who have other jobs and commitments. They are up against health professionals who have training in, daily contact with, and control over information that would be useful to community board members. The Health and Hospitals Corporation "Interim Guidelines" give community boards "the right to consult with responsible officials and outside authorities"; but "consulting with" does not assure full disclosure. Most of the community boards are dependent primarily on the executive director of the hospital for information, and secondarily (in New York City municipal hospitals) on the director of community affairs, who is usually hired by and responsible to the executive director.

The struggle and ultimate failure of a consumer advisory board of one Manhattan voluntary hospital illustrates some of the difficulties lay boards face, particularly in gaining access to information. This hospital, which we shall refer to as "Voluntary," was formerly supported by religious philanthropy. In accepting state funds from the ghetto medicine program, the hospital was required to set up a consumer advisory board to monitor the funds and provide a vehicle for community viewpoints. Ghetto medicine funds were intended to expand services for the poor, particularly clinic services; but many voluntary hospitals, caught in a budget squeeze, used the money for budget deficits and maintenance of current programs.

The consumer advisory board at Voluntary had seventeen members. Nine were consumers and eight were from the hospital. The eight hospital members were all chosen by the hospital administration. Various organizations, chosen by the public at a public meeting substantially controlled by the hospital (which packed the meeting, according to a community informant), picked the consumer slate after interviewing various candidates and volunteers. Despite these formal procedures, which would doom most consumer boards before they began, the nine consumer members of this particular board stuck together and elected as chairperson a member who had been through similar fights in the schools, knew how to bring a lawsuit, knew how to issue a press release, and had friends in the press.

Before the first meeting of the consumer advisory board, none of the nine consumers knew any of the other nine. The first six months were spent consolidating the consumers. At first the meetings were held in the hospital. The chairperson said that the meetings should be held elsewhere. Lacking other suggestions, they were moved to his office and other community places such as a local settlement house. The chairperson offered to have his secretary take minutes (for which he paid her overtime). The consumers then had control of some information. Many other consumer advisory boards continued to meet at the voluntary hospitals and allowed their minutes to be taken and kept by the hospital administration.

Voluntary Hospital had planned to build a nurses' residence with walk-in clinics and emergency services on the lower floors. The board was able to participate in the planning, urging that care not be fragmented into specialty clinics. They also saw that the waiting rooms would not be big enough nor was there enough room for waiting children. The consumer board wanted an open public meeting to present architectural plans to the community for discussion. The hospital administration resisted. The consumer board chairperson threatened a press conference over withholding plans from the community. The hospital then said they were going to have to postpone building for lack of money. The consumer chairperson responded by saying that they had a common cause, and should join together in a press conference revealing that the state was reneging on promised funds. The administration was delighted. At the next meeting the chairperson said that the first thing the press would want to know were the facts. The administration was not prepared to disclose facts; they continued giving partial information. Throughout these negotiations, the administration was saying damaging things, and minutes were being taken.

The chairperson called a meeting of the nine community people and said they should sue the hospital for the information. A public-interest lawyer filed a suit for them. They called a press conference. The hospital was represented by a big Wall Street firm. Arguing that the law that created the consumer advisory board gave the board no powers, the hospital moved to have the suit dismissed. The consumers countered that the consumer advisory board had a right to information, otherwise creating such a board would have been pointless. The judge accepted that argument and denied the motion to dismiss the complaint.

By that time a new election was near for the consumer advisory board. Fighting both the election and the lawsuit would take enormous time. The consumers decided not to continue the fight. They resigned en masse, releasing their reason to the press.[10]

In spite of the fact that the consumer board of Voluntary failed in its immediate objectives, it did take some actions from which others can learn. The consumer members were in effect granted standing to sue for information. (Their lawsuit was not dismissed for lack of standing.) They showed the value of several kinds of actions: holding meetings on their own turf, keeping their own records, having their own secretary, having access to the media, knowing how to bring a lawsuit, and having (or, in their case, the negative importance of lacking) the time, energy, and resources to follow through on a lawsuit or whatever action is taken.

THE FUTURE OF COMMUNITY BOARDS

Neither money nor expertise, I would argue, ought to be recognized as valid grounds for allocating authority in hospital decision-making. Whatever the legitimate influence wielded by money in a competitive, free-market situation, in the monopolistic or oligopolistic conditions of U.S. health services, money is not a just basis for determining authority. Contributions, especially when they provide large sums that can be withheld at the discretion of the giver, almost inevitably possess undue power and influence. It follows that making health care delivery responsive to the general public through democratic institutions virtually requires that health services be publicly supported from tax moneys.

Expertise, of course, is as powerful a source of authority in practice as it is invalid in theory.[11] In theory, technical expertise should be at the service of policy-makers legitimated on other grounds, a tool to be controlled by public policy and the individuals, namely patients, who are potentially most harmed and benefited.

On the other hand, those who have traditionally based their power on the authority of expertise do have a new basis on which legitimately to share in decision-making—but not dominate it. That basis is work. To what extent does the claim to decision-making authority on the basis of work in a hospital imply an equal participation in decisions by all health care workers? To what extent should there remain hierarchies of authority based on expertise? To what extent is the claim to decision-making authority on the grounds of work simply superseded by the claims of others—community residents, taxpayers, citizens, or patients? The leverage of hospital workers, vis-à-vis those wielding the traditional sources of power—money and expertise—has been increased recently through unionization. The claims of residents and patients, in theory perhaps the strongest of all claims, have till now found the least institutional expression.

In New York City, the Health and Hospitals Corporation community boards were designed to meet these last categories of claims, to give patients and community residents a voice in their hospitals. The question remains, *how can community boards be more effective in giving advice and in influencing decisions?*

Access to information is one of the most significant problems community boards face. This problem can be alleviated through legislation, education, the cooperation of enlightened health care providers, and the change of consciousness that seems to be occurring in the United States regarding the rights of people to open information.

The community board itself needs explicitly authorized access to nearly all hospital and corporation information, including budget planning at all stages, research presently going on in the hospital or being contemplated, hospital rules, hospital practices, affiliation contracts, employee and patient grievances, financial audits, service evaluations, and employee recruitment. It should also have the authority to hire its own consultants and to conduct audits and evaluations of health care services.

The volunteer nature of community board work can be partially overcome by giving the boards a full-time staff responsible to the community board, hired by it, fired by it, and possessing the authority to get the information it needs in order to take necessary action. Full-time staff is an important element in the success of community boards; the one community board that has had its own staff for more than a year has been one of the most effective. Other community boards have recently begun to hire staffs.

Community boards not only need increased communication with those who currently have more power than they do, they also need to be responsive and responsible to their constituencies. *Communication with communities and health care consumers* can be increased by: (1) holding open meetings; (2) publishing a newsletter; (3) placing suggestion boxes in hospitals; (4) being responsive to constituents' requests; (5) developing access to the local press; (6) helping to educate patients and community members about their hospital, their rights, and their responsibilities; (7) promoting health fairs and other services to constituents; (8) encouraging communication and cooperation with other groups and individuals who are interested in health care; and (9) planning well-run and -publicized elections for the boards.

Community boards can fight for and/or be given *increased* powers. Additional powers could include the selection of new hospital personnel, budget planning, formulation and approval of affiliation and other contracts, increased membership on the Health and Hospitals Corporation Board of Directors (in the case of the New York City Corporation hospitals), and acquisition of the powers of the board of directors for their own hospital.

Community boards can increase their knowledge and power by forming local, regional, and national organizations. New York City municipal hospital boards have established the Council of Municipal Hospital Boards, which has served a coordinating function for demonstrations and exchange of information. This council could be further strengthened by making use of the executive assistants whom some hospital boards have as staff members.

In some hospitals and some cities, community boards can take advantage of the duality or multiplicity of lines of authority to form *alliances* with whichever professionals have goals most in line with their own. The establishment of community advisory boards is powered by a number of trends in contemporary American society. This review of their genesis, the contexts in which they operate, and their experiences was undertaken in an effort to explore their potency as an idea and a fact, and the policy conflicts such groups inevitably encounter.

Notes to Chapter Seventeen

1. Research for this study included (1) *interviews* with members (usually several members) and/or staff of six community boards, with other hospital staff persons, Health and Hospitals Corporation (HHC) staff, members of health activist groups, and a former member of a ghetto medicine community board; (2) *attending meetings* (at least one each of the following): Council of Municipal Hospital Boards (most of the members are chairpersons of their community boards); Bellevue Community Board; Elmhurst Community Board; the Community Relations Committee of the HHC; staff meetings of the office of Community Relations of the HHC; an HHC senior staff meeting; and demonstrations at HHC during meetings of the board of directors; (3) *working in the office of community relations*, HHC, as a volunteer, primarily on new guidelines for community boards and on an educational workshop program being planned for community board members; (4) reading many *articles, reports, and books*.

2. The "National Health Rights and Community Health Services" bill which Congressman Dellums has considered proposing would ensure the rights of citizens to health services and put the burden of health planning and policy-making on health workers and community residents, in effect combining community and worker control of health care. New York City municipal hospital community boards combine community and consumer members as the two principal groups represented on the community boards.

3. For an analysis of the role of Blue Cross as a financing organization for American hospitals, see Sylvia A. Law, *Blue Cross: What Went Wrong?* (New Haven: Yale University Press, 1974).

4. New York City Health and Hospitals Corporation Act, 5301-A.

5. Michael M. Stewart, "Report from the Department of Ambulatory Care and Community Medicine, City Hospital Center at Elmhurst," January 1974; also, City Hospital Center at Elmhurst, "A Proposed Plan to Establish a Community Advisory Board at the City Hospital Center at Elmhurst," pp. 23-24.

6. City Hospital Center at Elmhurst Community Advisory Board, *Constitution and By-Laws*, pp. 5-8.

7. Personal interviews with Elmhurst community board nonconsumers (community members) indicated a strong commitment to maintain the quality of the neighborhood and if possible improve health services (as a secondary goal); while interviews with Elmhurst consumer community board members focused on the need to upgrade particular hospital services and the general level of care at the hospital.

8. Barbara Yuncker, "Report Cites Bias in Funding of Hospitals," New York *Post* (January 30, 1974), p. 12.

9. A majority of community boards agreed in substance with the affiliation statement in the "Council of Municipal Hospitals Community Boards: Draft" (later revised). The draft statement read: "the Council of Community Boards calls for the phasing out of the affiliation contracts as fast as it is practicable to do so. We are convinced that affiliation contracts represent a drainage on the resources of the corporation and believe that it should be replaced with competitive salaries offered by the Health and Hospitals Corporation institutions in order to attract doctors and other professionals it needs. We believe that physicians and all employees of an institution must be accountable to the institution where they render services," p. 6.

10. Private communication, Ira Glasser, New York Civil Liberties Union.

11. For a discussion of the problem of experts being given authority to make value decisions beyond the competence of their expertise, see Robert M. Veatch, "Generalization of Expertise," *Hastings Center Studies*, 1 [2] (1973), 29-40.

Chapter 18

Technology Assessment and Genetics

LeRoy Walters

No one—not even the most brilliant scientist alive today—really knows where science is taking us. We are aboard a train which is gathering speed, racing down a track on which there are an unknown number of switches leading to unknown destinations. No single scientist is in the engine cab, and there may be demons at the switch.[1]

There can be no question that many of the benefits of modern life are the direct result of scientific research and technological development.[2] During the past decade, however, it has become increasingly apparent that technology is not an unmixed blessing. One attempt to cope with the mixed character of technological development is the technology-assessment movement.

CONCEPT OF TECHNOLOGY ASSESSMENT

The term "technology assessment" (TA) seems to have been coined in a report of the House Subcommittee on Science, Research, and Development.[3] Due primarily to the tireless efforts of the subcommittee and its chairman, Emilio Q. Daddario, the concept of TA gradually spread into the academic world, where it was picked up in particular by engineers and physicists. During the year 1969 a scholarly literature on the subject of TA began to develop; indeed, it is possible to identify ten recent reports of books which have achieved almost-canonical status within the movement.[4] Late in 1971 an International Society for Technology Assessment was formed to "contribute to the structuring, study, control and resolution of the world's technological challenges and dilemmas."[5] The Society, in turn, began publishing a quarterly journal, *Technology Assessment*, in the summer of 1972.

What precisely is meant by the term TA? Joseph F. Coates, a program manager in the National Science Foundation, offers the following concise explanation: "Technology assessment may be defined as the systematic study of the effects on society that may occur when a technology is introduced, extended, or modified, with special emphasis on the impacts that are unintended, indirect, and delayed."[6]

Two phrases in Coates's definition merit brief elaboration. Practitioners of TA generally construe the idea of "effects on society" in rather broad terms. Their particular concern is to take into account environmental and other social consequences of technology and to avoid an exclusive focus on economic profit and loss. When Coates employs the terms "unintended, indirect, and delayed" to describe certain of these consequences, he alludes to another major emphasis within the TA movement, namely, second-order consequences. Immediate, direct, and intended effects of technological change are generally termed first-order consequences. The primary focus of TA is on the less obvious social impacts of technology, that is, on second-, third-, and higher-order consequences.[7]

Writers on TA have distinguished several subtypes of assessment. For example, an obvious distinction can be drawn between retrospective and prospective analyses, between studies of the past and of the future. Closely related is the distinction between problem-initiated and technology-initiated assessments. The former type surveys currently available technologies in quest of a solution to a specific problem; the latter mode of assessment attempts to follow through time "the inherently proliferating set of impacts" of a particular technology.[8]

If the above definitions and classifications indicate the general contours of TA, they do not yet give a clear picture of its methodology. There is, in fact, no single universally accepted method for performing TA. Perhaps the most thorough and systematic attempt to formulate such a methodology is a study written by Martin V. Jones, an economist at the MITRE Corporation.[9] In his programmatic essay Jones lists seven major steps to be taken in performing a comprehensive technology assessment:

Step 1. Define the assessment task: establish the scope of the inquiry.
Step 2. Describe relevant technologies: outline the state of the art in the major technology being assessed as well as in related technologies.
Step 3. Develop state-of-society assumptions: identify and describe the major nontechnological factors influencing the application of the relevant techniques.
Step 4. Identify impact areas: list the societal characteristics that will be most influenced by the application of the assessed technology.
Step 5. Make preliminary impact analysis: trace and integrate the various specific impacts of the assessed technology upon society.

Step 6. Identify possible action options: develop and analyze various programs of obtaining maximum public benefit from the assessed technologies.

Step 7. Complete impact analysis: analyze the degree to which each action option would alter the specific societal impacts (listed in Step 5) of the assessed technology.[10]

In taking Step 1 the assessor decides whether to attempt a total-impact assessment or whether to be content with a partial assessment. Having made that choice, he proceeds to Step 2, a precise description of the technology under consideration. According to Jones, this description should answer the following questions: (1) What is the current state of the art in the assessed technology? (2) What is the current state of the art in related or supporting technologies? (3) What technical breakthroughs are needed? (4) What future developments in the state of the art are anticipated and within what time frame? (5) What are the current and prospective uses and applications of the assessed technology?[11]

Steps 3 and 4 refer to the complex reciprocal relationships between society and technology. In Step 3 the assessor of technology attempts to project general trends in the society of the future and to predict how these social phenomena might accelerate or retard the development and application of the technology in question. In Step 4 the process is reversed: one seeks to identify the general spheres of human life that are most likely to be affected by future developments in the assessed technology. These general spheres, or major impact categories, include personal and community values, the environment, demographic trends, social goals and problems, economic factors, and institutions.[12]

Steps 1-4 are preparatory to Step 5, which is the primary goal of the assessment. Here the assessor attempts to anticipate and describe specific consequences of technological development. A helpful framework for this impact-analysis is provided by Jones in his methodological essay:

Table 18-1. Key Impact Questions[13]

Questions	Types of Answers
Technology	
Development	Describe the initial effect of the development: to lower cost, to improve performance, etc.
Application	Describe the use to which this development is put.
Social	
Social Impact	Identify the first level impact of the application.

Table 18-1. (continued)

Questions	Types of Answers
Impact Characteristics	
Affected Group	What social group will be most affected: old or young, rich or poor, workers or managers, the sick or well, etc?
How Affected	For better or worse, and in what specific way?
Likelihood	E.g., 50-50 chance.
Timing	Estimate dates both for initial impact and later widespread effect.
Magnitude	Preferably in dollars, percentage increase, number affected, etc., rather than adjectives like "large," "small," etc.
Duration	Indicate whether initial impact will improve or worsen, and for how long.
Diffusion	Breadth and depth of impact. An unfavorable impact of equal total magnitude (e.g., dollar volume) that is concentrated on a few people will cause more social distress than if it were diffused through many people.
Source	Indicate the source (industry, federal government, foreign source, etc.) from which the development leading up to this impact originates.
Controllability	Is it likely that a public program could heighten or dampen the impact generated by the technology?

The final two steps in a technology assessment consider whether various types of monitoring- or control-mechanisms could modify the rate or direction of technological development and thus alter its social impact. Among possible action options the most important are methods of allocating research and development funds; other financial incentives, including taxes; legislation; court action; mass-media publicity; education; and the construction of new systems or facilities.[14]

In addition to the How of TA it is necessary to consider the Who question: Who should participate in the complex process of assessing technology? Much of the current initiative for systematic TA comes from the Congress, some of whose members fear that the executive branch is gaining a monopoly over scientific information. Currently under debate is a bill that would establish a Congressional Office of Technology Assessment, modeled on the pattern of the General Accounting Office.[15] Other possible forums for TA include departments and administrative agencies in the executive branch, the courts, industry, international organizations, professional societies, ad hoc task forces, research institutes, and university-based interdisciplinary research teams.[16]

Perhaps equal in importance to the locus of TA is the composition of the group that makes the assessment. Self-evidently, research scientists from the relevant physical or life sciences must be involved. The presence of engineers on the assessment team frequently serves to bridge the gap between research and application. During recent years there has also been increasing sentiment in favor of including social scientists in the assessment process. In addition, some advocates of TA have ventured to suggest participation by "concerned individuals outside science: industrial executives, lawyers, clergymen, and journalists."[17]

Even if TA sounds plausible as a proposal and a theory, one must raise the practical question: Has TA been tried, and, if so, with what degree of success? The answer, in brief, is that until now very few full-scale assessments have been attempted. Pilot studies have made partial assessments of the following present or future technologies: sea farming, mechanized teaching aids, computer-communications networks, industrial enzymes, microwave diodes, and the supersonic transport.[18] Problems that have been assessed in a preliminary way include automotive emissions, water pollution through domestic wastes, the Alaska pipeline, and a snow-enhancement project for the Colorado River Valley.[19] Only in a few cases—for example, the Jamaica Bay-Kennedy Airport Study—can one speak of a comprehensive or total-impact assessment.[20]

ASSESSMENT OF BIOMEDICAL TECHNOLOGY

As the foregoing examples illustrate, TA has until now been concentrated on two major areas: environmental problems and developments in the physical sciences. The field of biomedical technology has been almost totally ignored.[21] In her comprehensive review of TA in the federal government Vary T. Coates noticed this gap in current TA studies, and voiced concern about the possible long-term consequences of such neglect:

> Biomedical technologies, especially bioengineering and pharmacology, are producing or are likely to produce some of the most profound effects on social mores and behavior of the future. It is likely that public policy issues will soon arise from this area in great numbers, and that these policy issues will be profoundly interwoven with religious, social, economic, cultural, and ideological factors. Very little anticipatory assessment is being done and almost none by the federal agencies which are financially supporting much of the scientific research driving this technological development, or which may be called upon to exercise whatever regulatory authority society may choose to impose. Public opinion and political leadership will therefore lack a firm base of information and issue analysis to guide public discussion, and action will very likely be taken in a crisis situation, with a corresponding plethora of irrational and uninformed charges and countercharges. Or no action at all will be taken, until social change is irreversible and irremediable. Therefore the opportunity for positive social direction of a burgeoning but still rudimentary technology

will be lost, and with it the opportunity to identify societal options and the opportunity to influence developments along socially and individually desirable paths.[22]

A partial explanation for the lack of TA in the biomedical field may be that there are significant differences between the physical sciences and the life sciences. For example, technologies based on research in the life sciences are usually applied to human beings by licensed medical practitioners, that is, by a unique social group with a distinctive tradition and code of ethics. Successful TA in the biomedical field is thus heavily dependent on active cooperation by the medical profession. In addition, developments in biomedical technology are supported primarily by public funds; according to one estimate, approximately two-thirds of all money spent on research and development in biomedicine and health comes from the federal government. Thus, advances in biomedical technology already reflect public-policy decisions to a much greater extent than do technical advances in the field of physics and physical engineering.[23]

A third distinction between the physical and life sciences is somewhat more elusive. It could perhaps be called a difference in the intimacy of effects. The development of new products and devices has always had a profound impact upon society. However, when biomedical technology is applied directly to man, to human flesh, the stakes seem to be higher, and human concern is correspondingly greater. Hans Jonas has captured the significance of this difference in a few terse lines:

> Among the sciences that progressively contributed to the technological revolution, *biology* has so far not figured. Are we perhaps on the verge of another—conceivably the last—stage of that revolution, based on biological knowledge and wielding an engineering art which, this time, has man himself for an object? This has become a theoretical possibility with the advent of molecular biology and its understanding of genetic programming.[24]

These differences between the physical and life sciences raise a fundamental question: Can a single methodology be employed to evaluate technological developments in both fields? To rephrase the issue, can the TA methodology that was outlined earlier be applied to biomedical technologies?

The thesis of this chapter is that the same methodology, with minor adjustments, is applicable to the biomedical field. Preliminary evidence in support of this thesis is contained in a study performed by the Committee on the Life Sciences and Social Policy of the National Research Council.[25] This study, coordinated by Dr. Leon R. Kass, investigates present and potential developments in four biomedical technologies. The committee considered the following set of issues in selecting the technologies and in making its assessments: (1) stage of development of the technology; (2) scale of use; (3) relation to other technologies; (4) ease of monitoring and control; (5) reversibility; (6) nature and scope of social consequences; and (7) implications for decision-making.[26] On the whole, the committee's method of study parallels precisely the progression of thought in the TA methodology outlined above. More specifically, the seven issues discussed in the committee report are virtually identical to those raised in Steps 2, 5, and 6 of the proposed TA methodology.

There are numerous developments in biomedical technology that could be made the subject of assessments. The pioneering study of the Committee on the Life Sciences and Social Policy concentrates on four technologies: in vitro fertilization; techniques for predetermining the sex of children; techniques to slow the biological process of aging; and techniques for the modification and control of the nervous system and behavior.[27] Other innovations predicted by experts in biomedicine include the following: implantable artificial hearts and other mechanical organs; safe, inexpensive contraceptive agents capable of being administered on a mass scale; asexual reproduction, or cloning, of human beings; chemotherapeutic cures for various types of cancer; an artificial placenta, which would allow extrauterine development of the fetus; methods for stimulating the regeneration of the central nervous system, organs, or limbs; and techniques for the repair or alteration of specific genes.[28]

ASSESSMENT OF GENETIC TECHNOLOGY

A significant subcategory of biomedical technology is based on the science of human genetics and allied disciplines. Indeed, it can be argued that recent developments in the general field of genetics are comparable in importance to the discovery and utilization of atomic energy a generation ago. In the words of Dr. Bentley Glass:

> The discoveries of molecular biology and genetics during the past twenty years are now generally acclaimed to be the most significant basic scientific advances of our present generation, just as the understanding of the focus of nuclear energy in the atom was that of the preceding generation. Like the application of nuclear energy to both destructive and constructive uses, the application of the spectacular finding that deoxyribonucleic acid (DNA) is the chemical basis of heredity offers man a magnificent extension of power over nature and at the same time lays on his conscience a frightening responsibility in the use of that power.[29]

Strictly defined, the term "genetic technology" includes the following present or potential developments: the detection of genetic defects in the unborn through amniocentesis; techniques for identifying, or screening, heterozygous carriers and homozygous victims of genetic disease; and gene repair through DNA therapy.[30] A somewhat broader definition of genetic technology might encompass as well the techniques of in vitro fertilization and cloning, both of which have obvious eugenic applications.[31] In the ensuing paragraphs, this second, more comprehensive definition of genetic technology is employed.

Until now, no published study has attempted a comprehensive assessment of any of the five genetic technologies noted above.[32] However, numerous books and articles have discussed the possible long-term impact of genetic technology in a mode *akin to* that of TA. In my view, these studies—which might be called partial assessments—constitute important building blocks for future efforts to provide comprehensive assessments in the field of genetic technology.[33]

Two examples will serve to illustrate the close resemblance between these studies and the seven-step TA methodology outlined above. In a lecture given at the Kennedy Foundation's International Symposium on Human Rights, Retardation, and Research and subsequently published in the *Journal of the American Medical Association*, Paul Ramsey discusses the issue of in vitro fertilization.[34] After defining the scope of his topic and briefly sketching the current state of the art, Ramsey notes a major nontechnological factor which in his view should inhibit the application of this particular genetic technology to human beings, namely, certain generally accepted rules or codes concerning human experimentation. In the second part of his essay Ramsey turns from this deontological argument to a more teleological mode of analysis, arguing that the general impact of in vitro fertilization in human beings would be to replace reproduction with manufacture and to pervert the traditional function of the medical profession.[35]

More specific social impacts are discussed by Professor Ramsey under the rubric of the "thin end of the wedge" argument. In an eloquent passage Ramsey argues that the application of in vitro fertilization to human beings would have serious detrimental second-order consequences:

> To be valid ... the wedge argument need not, like my reasons drawn from medical ethics, attempt to show the inherent immorality of a given sort of action of practice. It need only show that if we do this particular action or permit or encourage a particular practice (perhaps because of undeniable immediate values, e.g., enabling a woman to have a child) we will influence others and cause ourselves to take following steps that in foreseeable succession add up to immense disvalue for the human community. So we shall have to assess in vitro fertilization as a long step toward Hatcheries, i.e., extra-corporeal gestation, and [toward] the introduction of unlimited genetic changes into human germinal material while it is being cultured by the Conditioners and Predestinators of the future.[36]

Ramsey does not propose the adoption of any specific action option to forestall such possible developments, but the very publication of his essay in a leading medical journal constitutes an effort to educate a significant group of decision-makers and thus to alter or avert the potential impact of in vitro fertilization on society.

A second example of partial TA in the field of genetics is contained in a recent article by Bentley Glass entitled "Human Heredity and Ethical Problems."[37] Again in this essay one can easily discover the seven steps of Martin Jones's suggested TA methodology. After defining the scope of his study, Dr. Glass devotes a great deal of attention to describing the state of the art in genetics and molecular biology. According to Glass, the techniques of tranduction, amniocentesis, and genetic screening have made possible significant advances in euphenics[38] and negative eugenics. Such methods pale, however, in comparison with Glass's list of potential developments in positive eugenics, or genetic engineering: selective breeding, in vitro fertilization, embryo transfer, gestation in an artificial placenta, laboratory cultivation of human reproductive organs, cloning, genetic surgery, and gene transfer.[39]

Glass notes that several nontechnological factors affect the development or application of the various genetic technologies. Inhibiting factors are the expense of currently available tests, ethical objections to abortion, the small number of scholars in certain critical disciplines, and society's lack of unanimity on a definition of genetic superiority. On the other hand, Glass observes, the economic cost of caring for persons afflicted with genetic disease tends to push society toward more rapid adoption of available genetic techniques.[40]

In the opinion of Glass, the general impact of employing genetic-engineering techniques would be to help mankind avoid global disaster. Without such techniques, he argues, the human race would at best suffer gradual genetic deterioration; at worst, "if in the aftermath of dreadful nuclear war, survivors are unable to provide the necessary artifices—drugs, surgery, and prosthetic devices—to maintain life in spite of their genetic burdens, mankind may perish."[41] Glass also lists several specific impacts that would probably result from the widespread application of present and future genetic technology: "A complete liberation of the sexual life from its relationship to reproduction"; "greater freedom of choice in new respects"; and recognition of the "right of every person to be born physically and mentally sound, capable of developing fully into a mature individual."[42]

Certain possible action steps are mentioned or recommended during the course of Glass's essay; these include mandatory sterilization for retinoblastoma patients, obligatory abortion of seriously defective fetuses, routine genetic testing of all newborn infants, and a licensing procedure to limit the number of children born to each couple.[43] The intent of these measures would not be to alter the societal impacts of genetic technology. Rather, if I understand Glass correctly, their purpose would be to insure that the desired impacts did in fact occur.

In the concluding paragraph of "Human Heredity and Ethical Problems," Glass issues a ringing appeal for broad, interdisciplinary involvement in the assessment of technology.

I have asked many questions which cannot at present be answered. I predict a future in which many cherished values of our society and many ethical standards will be questioned or superseded. It is not sufficient to have a few scientists raise such issues. . . . Only a prolonged and profound attention by many of the wisest men of our times, men of philosophy and religion, students of society and of government, and representatives of the common interests of men throughout the world, together with teachers and scientists, may achieve a wise and sober solution of the crisis of values evoked in our world by scientific discoveries and their applications.[44]

The foregoing analysis of the essays by Ramsey and Glass tends to confirm the thesis that the TA methodology is applicable, at least in principle, to the assessment of biomedical technology. The diametrically opposed conclusions of Ramsey and Glass serve to underline the relatively modest role of the TA methodology: it functions as a formal aid to systematic analysis; in no sense, however, does it predetermine the assessor's final evaluation of a particular technology.

A THEORETICAL PERSPECTIVE ON TECHNOLOGY ASSESSMENT

Without question, I think, the intellectual roots of the TA movement are to be found in the ethical tradition known as utilitarianism.[45] This heritage can be traced both generally and specifically. The general connection of the TA movement to utilitarianism has perhaps been mediated through social scientists, several of whom have been deeply involved in developing the theoretical foundations of TA.[46] For a variety of reasons, scholars in the social sciences generally tend toward a utilitarian normative theory. In the words of Braybrooke and Lindblom:

> Utilitarianism, at least in the English-speaking world, is the school toward which most social scientists are inclined, if they are inclined toward any. There are historical reasons for this inclination: Important branches of social science, among them economics and sociology, grew out of utilitarian preoccupations. There is also a natural convergence in preoccupations between utilitarianism and social science. Utilitarianism, after all, insists more strongly than any other ethical theory on forcing moral judgments to the test of facts—the facts of social science.[47]

To this general connection between TA and utilitarianism a more specific link can be added. When it focuses on the second-order consequences or social effects or impacts of technology, the TA movement clearly identifies itself as a utilitarian school of thought. At times the very words employed in assessing social consequences are reminiscent of classical utilitarianism. For example, the key impact questions listed by Martin Jones (Table 18-1) are virtually identical to Jeremy Bentham's categories for measuring the effects of an action. According to Bentham, seven circumstances must always be taken into account: intensity, duration, certainty or uncertainty, propinquity or remoteness, fecundity, purity, and extent.[48]

The type of utilitarianism espoused by the TA movement is both comprehensive and rather sophisticated. Unlike Bentham, who tended to reduce all ethical argument to a calculus of pleasure and pain,[49] theoreticians of TA are willing to take into account a wide variety of consequences—economic, social, political, environmental, legal, and moral.[50] To phrase the same point in more general terms, the TA movement is not necessarily committed to any particular theory of nonmoral value; rather, it seems willing to accept the positive worth of a plurality of values.[51] Advocates of TA also realize full well the complexity of the task that is to be accomplished. In its final report the Panel on Technology Assessment of the National Academy of Sciences listed numerous "problems and pitfalls" of the TA enterprise, including shortcomings of modes of analysis, failures of imagination, deficiencies in the data base, and institutional constraints.[52]

One can, I think, be profoundly grateful for the positive contributions of the TA movement. In the first place, it has introduced a broadened perspective into the analysis of technological development. Most traditional assessments of technology have been focused almost exclusively on internal costs and benefits. In the words of the National Academy of Sciences panel, "With few exceptions the central question asked of a technology is what it would do (or is doing) to the economic or institutional interests of those who are deciding whether or how to exploit it."[53] In contrast, the TA movement urges that this traditional calculus be supplemented by a humane evaluation of external social consequences.

The flexibility of the TA methodology is also a point in its favor. As noted above, the employment of this method does not commit the assessor either to a particular value theory or to a predetermined evaluation of a particular technology. The methodology acknowledges a reciprocal influence of technology and society, thus avoiding any commitment to a partisan ideological position.[54] It is also sufficiently comprehensive to allow for consideration of a variety of nontechnological factors, such as values, institutions, education, and political action.[55]

Third, the TA methodology lays the foundation for an expanded concept of moral responsibility. Its overall thrust is to hold men accountable for the remote, as well as the immediate, consequences of their decisions and actions. Spatially interpreted, this concept of responsibility could easily include members of the human community living in other nations.[56] Temporally extended, TA would serve to protect the interests of future generations.[57] To rephrase the point in theological terms, the TA methodology calls to our attention a whole new group of neighbors, toward whom concern and love can and should be directed.

318 *Ethics and Health Policy*

Without denying these positive contributions of TA, one can, in my view, also raise certain fundamental questions about the TA methodology. First, to what extent should policy or morality be based on an assessment of possible consequences? Practitioners of TA are already keenly aware of this problem; in fact, one study of TA explicitly warns that projections that attempt to see more than five years into the future are likely to contain gross inaccuracies.[58] The great German philosopher Kant was even more pessimistic about man's ability to predict the consequences of his acts. Arguing that omniscience would be required to insure accurate prediction, Kant wrote off the entire enterprise of hypothetical ethical analysis and turned his attention instead to the formulation of categorical imperatives.[59] Even if one rejects Kant's extreme position, there remains the question whether ethics or policy should be based solely on a comprehensive assessment of consequences.

This problem can be formulated more precisely with the help of an illustration. Let us assume what Kant would have denied, namely, that in a given case the social consequences of a particular technology could be comprehensively and accurately assessed. One might proceed to record the results of one's analysis on a bar graph as follows:

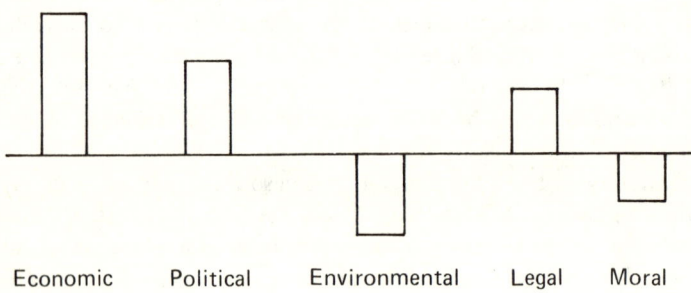

Figure 18-1. Overall Impacts of an Assessed Technology.

Several questions can be raised about this hypothetical result: (1) How can the various kinds of impacts be compared? Is there a common denominator? (2) Which impact, if any, takes precedence over other possible impacts? Does a negative impact within a particular category, e.g., a negative moral impact, automatically lead to a negative assessment of the technology? (3) How are the various impacts distributed among members of the society? Would a serious negative impact on a few persons be outweighed by a slight positive impact on many persons?[60]

Because of such inherent difficulties in consequential analysis, many moral philosophers and Christian ethicists have suggested that utilitarianism should be supplemented by a second ethical dimension. William Frankena and John Rawls, for example, emphasize the principle of justice or fairness.[61] For Charles Curran, the concept of human dignity serves to limit what may be done, even for the sake of good consequences.[62] Paul Ramsey has repeatedly expressed the view that the Christian ethic is primarily an ethic of means, not of ends.[63] In the theology of Karl Barth, the religious obligation to obey the command of God virtually supplants the duty to calculate consequences.[64]

A final, somewhat more theoretical question can be raised concerning TA: Does the general perspective of TA tend to overlook or obscure certain phenomena of human life? The meaning of this question can be illustrated in two ways. As we have noted, the TA methodology can be applied either to a particular technology or to a particular social problem. Would the same methodology be applicable to philosophical questions like the following: What goals should we adopt as a nation or an international community? or, What is the end of human life?[65] If the methodology could not address such questions directly, would it allow one's answers to the same questions to affect in a significant way one's overall assessment of a technology or a problem?

The thrust of this final question can also be illustrated metaphorically. In his book *The Responsible Self*, H. Richard Niebuhr distinguished three images of man: man-the-maker, man-the-citizen, and man-the-answerer. The first image depicts man as a producer of ideas, actions, and things. In the second image, man's duty to obey the civil and moral law predominates. The third image focuses on "man engaged in dialogue, man acting in response to action upon him."[66] It is quite clear that the TA movement emphasizes the first of these three images, the metaphor of man-the-maker. In so doing, it inevitably tends to neglect other important aspects of human experience.

In summary, the technology-assessment methodology provides a coherent framework for analyzing the social impact of technological change. Although the method was devised primarily in response to environmental problems and developments in the physical sciences, it is in principle applicable to advances in biomedical technology. In fact, several studies of biomedical technology in general, and of genetic technology in particular, have employed analytical categories which parallel precisely the various steps of the TA methodology.

Because of its intellectual rootage in utilitarianism, the TA movement tends to focus primary attention on man-the-maker. However, the formal character and inclusive categories of the TA methodology allow for a significant degree of flexibility in the assessment process. One hopes that in the future this useful analytical tool will be systematically applied to a wide variety of technologies and particularly to the series of complex problems arising in the field of human genetics.

Notes to Chapter Eighteen

1. Ralph E. Lapp, *The New Priesthood: The Scientific Elite and the Uses of Power* (New York: Harper & Row, 1965), p. 29.

2. In this essay science, whether basic or applied, is defined as an information function. Technology, on the other hand, is conceived as the development and social use of scientific information. In practice it is not always possible to draw a clear line between science and technology. See U.S. Congress, House, Committee on Science and Astronautics, "Science Policy: A Working Glossary," Prepared for the Subcommittee on Science, Research, and Development by the Science Policy Research Division, Congressional Research Service, Library of Congress (Washington, D.C.: U.S. Government Printing Office, 1972), p. 53.

3. U.S. Congress, House, Committee on Science and Astronautics, "Inquiries, Legislation, Policy Studies Re: Science and Technology," Second Progress Report of the Subcommittee on Science, Research, and Development, 89th Congress, second session (Washington, D.C.: U.S. Government Printing Office, 1966), pp. 27-28. Mr. Philip B. Yeager, Counsel to the Subcommittee, is generally given credit for having coined the term "technology assessment."

4. The most important works on TA are the following: (A) Four reports to the Subcommittee on Science, Research, and Development of the House Committee on Science and Astronautics: (1) Science Policy Research Division, Congressional Research Service, Library of Congress, *Technical Information for Congress* (April 25, 1969; revised, April 15, 1971); (2) National Academy of Sciences, *Technology: Processes of Assessment and Choice* (July 1969); (3) Committee on Public Engineering Policy, National Academy of Engineering, *A Study of Technology Assessment* (July 1969); (4) National Academy of Public Administration, *A Technology Assessment System for the Executive Branch* (July 1970). (B) Two volumes of hearings before the same Subcommittee: (5) *Technology Assessment* [1969] and (6) *Technology Assessment–1970*. (C) Two books: (7) Raymond A. Bauer, *Second-Order Consequences: A Methodological Essay on the Impact of Technology* (Cambridge, Mass.: M.I.T. Press, 1969); (8) Raphael G. Kasper, ed., *Technology Assessment: Understanding the Social Consequences of Technological Applications* (New York: Praeger, 1972). (D) Two other studies: (9) Martin V. Jones et al., *A Technology Assessment Methodology* (7 vols.; Washington, D.C.: MITRE Corporation, 1971); (10) Vary T. Coates, *Technology and Public Policy: The Process of Technology Assessment in the Federal Government* (2 vols.; Washington, D.C.: Program of Policy Studies in Science and Technology, George Washington University, 1972). The best and most comprehensive bibliographical essay on TA appears in the first issue of the journal *Technology Assessment:* Genevieve J. Knezo, "Technology Assessment: A Bibliographic Review," *Technology Assessment* 1 (1972), 62-83.

5. This quotation is taken from a descriptive brochure entitled "The International Society for Technology Assessment." The American office of I.S.T.A. is located in Suite 5038, 1629 K Street, NW, Washington, D.C. 20006.

6. "Technology Assessment: The Benefits ... the Costs ... the Consequences," *Futurist* 5 (1971), 225.

7. Bauer, *Second-Order Consequences*, passim.

8. Committee on Public Engineering Policy, National Academy of Engineering, *A Study of Technology Assessment*, p. 5.

9. *A Technology Assessment Methodology 1: Some Basic Propositions* (hereafter cited as *TAM* 1).

10. Adapted from Jones, *TAM* 1, 26.

11. Adapted from ibid., pp. 29, 46.

12. Ibid., p. 67.

13. Ibid., p. 82 (slightly revised). Reprinted by permission of the author.

14. Adapted from ibid., 1, 102.

15. Deborah Shapley, "Office of Technology Assessment: Congress Smiles, Scientists Wince," *Science* 175 (March 3, 1972), 970-73.

16. Emilio Q. Daddario, "Technology and the Democratic Process," *Technology Review* 73 (July-August, 1971), 19-23; Don E. Kash and Irvin L. White, "Technology Assessment: Harnessing Genius," *Chemical and Engineering News* (November 29, 1971), pp. 40-41.

17. John Lear, "Predicting the Consequences of Technology," *Saturday Review* (March 28, 1970), p. 44; cf. Committee on Public Engineering Policy, National Academy of Engineering, *A Study of Technology Assessment*, p. 4.

18. Jones et al. *TAM*, Vols. 3, 4, and 5; Committee on Public Engineering Policy, National Academy of Engineering, *A Study of Technology Assessment*, pp. 37-75, 107-42; Raymond Bowers and Jeffrey Frey, "Technology Assessment and Microwave Diodes," *Scientific American* 226 (February 1972), 13-21; George N. Chatham, "The Supersonic Transport," in Science Policy Research Division, Congressional Research Service, Library of Congress, *Technical Information for Congress*, 2nd ed., pp. 685-748.

19. Jones et al., *TAM*, Vols. 2 and 6; J. Coates, "Technology Assessment," p. 229.

20. Steven Ebbin, "The Jamaica Bay Study: A Case History," *Futurist* 6 (February 1972), 27-28.

21. Of 206 citations in Genevieve J. Knezo's bibliographical essay, only three (nos. 140, 169, and 190) refer to articles that discuss biomedical technology ("Technology Assessment: A Bibliographic Review," pp. 80-82). In her study of TA and the federal government Vary T. Coates was able to discover only three examples of already completed assessments in biology or medicine; the studies dealt with cardiac replacement, abortion, and the use of drugs in the treatment of behaviorally disturbed children (*Technology and Public Policy* 1, chap. 3, pp. 17-22). A general attempt to anticipate the social impact of future developments in both biology and physics is: Theodore J. Gordon and Robert H. Ament, *Forecasts of Some Technological Developments and Their Societal Consequences*, IFF Report R-6 (Middletown, Conn.: Institute for the Future, 1969).

22. *Technology and Public Policy*, 1, 26-27.

23. For the distinctions and information contained in this paragraph I am indebted to a personal communication from Dr. Leon R. Kass.

24. "The Scientific and Technological Revolutions: Their History and Meaning," *Philosophy Today* 15 (1971), 99.

25. *Assessing Biomedical Technologies: An Inquiry into the Nature of the Process* (A Study by the Committee on the Life Sciences and Social Policy, Assembly of Behavioral and Social Sciences, National Research Council), Washington, D.C.: National Academy of Sciences, 1975.

26. Ibid., pp. 5-9.
27. Ibid., p. 5.
28. Gordon and Ament, *Forecasts*, pp. 24-28.
29. "Human Heredity and Ethical Problems," *Perspectives in Biology and Medicine* 15 (Winter 1972), 237.
30. Richard Roblin, "Some Recent Developments in Genetics," *Theological Studies* 33 (September 1972), 403-10.
31. Of these five technologies the first two, amniocentesis and genetic screening, are currently in use. Technically speaking, in vitro fertilization in humans seems to await only the solution of certain minor difficulties. The application of cloning and DNA therapy to man, on the other hand, faces major technical obstacles; these techniques should therefore be regarded as future possibilities rather than as imminent developments.
32. The study of the Committee on the Life Sciences and Social Policy, published subsequent to the completion of this chapter, includes an extended, systematic analysis of in vitro fertilization. See n. 25 above.
33. The following are among the most important currently available studies in this field: the series of articles which appeared in the September, 1972, issue of *Theological Studies*; Peter G. Condliffe et al., eds., *Ethical Issues in Genetic Counseling and the Use of Genetic Knowledge* (New York: Plenum, 1972); Charles E. Curran, "Theology and Genetics: A Multi-Faceted Dialogue," *Journal of Ecumenical Studies* 7 (1970), 61-89; Robert G. Edwards and David J. Sharpe, "Social Values and Research in Human Embryology," *Nature* 231 (May 14, 1971), 87-91; Glass, "Human Heredity" (see n. 29 above); James M. Gustafson, Richard Roblin, Marc Lappé, et al., "Ethical and Social Issues in Screening for Genetic Disease," *New England Journal of Medicine* 286 (May 25, 1972), 1129-32; Michael Hamilton, ed., *The New Genetics and the Future of Man* (Grand Rapids, Mich.: Eerdmans, 1972); Maureen Harris, ed., *Early Diagnosis of Human Genetic Defects: Scientific and Ethical Considerations*, Fogarty International Center Proceedings, no. 6 (Washington, D.C.: U.S. Government Printing Office, 1971); Leon R. Kass, "Babies by Means of In Vitro Fertilization: Unethical Experiments on the Unborn?" *New England Journal of Medicine* 285 (November 18, 1971), 1174-79; Leon R. Kass, "Making Babies—the New Biology and the 'Old' Morality," *Public Interest*, no. 26 (Winter 1972), 18-56; Paul Ramsey, "Shall We 'Reproduce'? I. The Medical Ethics of In Vitro Fertilization; II. Rejoinders and Future Forecast," *Journal of the American Medical Association* 220 (June 5, 1972), 1346-50; (June 12, 1972), 1480-85; Paul Ramsey, *Fabricated Man: The Ethics of Genetic Control* (New Haven: Yale Univ. Press, 1970); James R. Sorenson, *Social Aspects of Applied Human Genetics*, Social Science Frontiers, no. 3 (New York: Russell Sage Foundation, 1971). For further bibliography and penetrating analysis of several of the works cited above, see the essay of Richard A. McCormick in the September 1972 issue of *Theological Studies*.
34. "Shall We 'Reproduce'?" (see n. 33 above).
35. Ibid., pp. 1347-49, 1480-82.
36. Ibid., p. 1481.
37. See n. 29 above.
38. Euphenics can be defined as the effort to compensate for a genetic defect

by controlling the phenotype rather than the genotype; for example, diabetics use insulin as a compensatory measure.

39. Glass, "Human Heredity," pp. 238-43, 246-49.
40. Ibid., pp. 240-242, 247, 251-52.
41. Ibid., p. 246.
42. Ibid., pp. 253, 252.
43. Ibid., pp. 242, 252, 240, 250-51.
44. Ibid., p. 253.
45. For a succinct characterization of classical utilitarianism, see John Rawls, *A Theory of Justice* (Cambridge, Mass.: Harvard University Press, 1971), pp. 22-27.
46. For example, of the seventeen members who participated in the National Academy of Sciences' study of TA, seven were social scientists (*Technology: Processes of Assessment and Choice*, pp. 151-63). Martin Jones, who developed the comprehensive TA methodology surveyed above, is an economist.
47. David Braybrooke and Charles E. Lindblom, *A Strategy of Decision: Policy Evaluation as a Social Process* (New York: Free Press, 1963), pp. 205-6.
48. *An Introduction to the Principles of Morals and Legislation*, chap. 4, par. 4.
49. Ibid., chaps. 1 and 3.
50. National Academy of Sciences, *Technology: Processes of Assessment and Choice*, pp. 29-30.
51. For general discussions of value theory, see William K. Frankena, *Ethics* (Englewood Cliffs, N.J.: Prentice-Hall, 1963), pp. 63-77; and G.E. Moore, *Ethics* (New York: Oxford University Press, 1965), pp. 96-108.
52. *Technology: Processes of Assessment and Choice*, pp. 43-71; cf. pp. 29-32.
53. Ibid., p. 26 (italics removed); cf. pp. 53-54, 67.
54. See Steps 2 and 3 in Jones's methodology.
55. See Steps 3 and 6.
56. Dennis Livingstone, "International Technology Assessment and the United Nations System," *American Journal of International Law* 64 (September 1970), 163-71; cf. Edward Weisband and Thomas M. Franck, "A Rationale for International Technology Assessment: Towards an Ethical Science," New York University Center for International Studies, Policy Papers, Vol. 4, 1971. The importance of extending TA spatially is already apparent in current discussions of the ocean-pollution problem.
57. On this topic see the following companion essays: Daniel Callahan, "What Obligations Do We Have to Future Generations?" *American Ecclesiastical Review* 164 (1971), 265-80; and M.P. Golding, "Obligations to Future Generations," *Monist* 56 (January 1972), 85-99.
58. Committee on Public Engineering Policy, National Academy of Engineering, *A Study of Technology Assessment*, p. 5.
59. Immanuel Kant, *Groundwork of the Metaphysic of Morals*, tr. H.J. Paton (New York: Harper & Row, 1964), pp. 82-86.
60. Martin Jones argues that "An unfavorable impact of equal total magnitude ... that is concentrated on a few people will cause more social distress than if it were diffused through many people" (see the explanation of the term

"Diffusion" on the chart cited in n. 13 above). In order to justify this argument, Jones would have to introduce some nonutilitarian, or nonconsequential, ethical principle. For a discussion of this point, see Frankena, *Ethics*, p. 32.

61. Frankena, *Ethics*, pp. 38-42; Rawls, *Theory of Justice*, pp. 3-22.

62. "Theology and Genetics," pp. 83-85.

63. See, e.g., *Fabricated Man*, pp. 29-30; cf. *Deeds and Rules in Christian Ethics* (New York: Scribner, 1967), pp. 108-9.

64. *Church Dogmatics* (English tr.) 2/2, 650. Barth accepts the legitimacy of considering consequences but argues that obedience to the divine command is "not merely the highest duty but also the highest good" (ibid., p. 652).

65. Leon R. Kass, "The New Biology: What Price Relieving Man's Estate?" *Science* 174 (November 19, 1971), 779, 785-786.

66. *The Responsible Self: An Essay in Christian Moral Philosophy* (New York: Harper & Row, 1963), pp. 49-56.

Index

Abortion, 23, 25, 101, 157, 170, 200, 315; in China, 65; "genetic," 42-43; "indirect," 24; reform movement, 160; therapeutic, 200
Abram, Harry, 208
Acupuncture, 61, 62
Addiction, drug, 191
Admonita, 21
Aesculapius, 101
Agape, 82, 90-92
Aging, 313
Aiken, S.C., 17
Alaska Pipeline, 311
Alcoholism, 191
Alopecia, 141
American Hospital Association, 101, 148
American Medical Association, 6, 17, 103, 148, 179, 180, 236
American Medical Machine, The, 190
Amniocentesis, 157, 163, 170
Anemia, 105; sickle cell, 42, 170
Anopheles mosquito, 106
Antigone, 107
Aristotle, 21, 36-37, 102
Arrow, Kenneth, 121, 179, 183
Arthritis, acupuncture and, 62
Artificial heart, *see* Heart, artificial
Artificial Heart Assessment Panel, National Heart and Lung Institute, 43-46, 219-46, 247-55
Artificial insemination, 200
Ashbrook bill (HR 288), 148
Atherosclerosis, 226

Barefoot doctors, China, 70
Barnard, Christiaan, 207
Barry, Brian, 191, 192
Barth, Karl, 319
Battery-operated artificial heart, *see* Heart, artificial
Bedridden, 172
Beecher, Henry K., 49-50
Beinecke Rare Book Library, Yale University, 47-48
Bellevue Hospital, NYC, 294
Bellin, Lowell, 296
Bentham, Jeremy, 105, 173, 317
Bethune, Norman, 67
Bible, Hebrew, 47
"Bioethical Creed for individuals," 7
Bioethics, 3, 5-16
Biological fuel cell, artificial heart, 221, 235
"Biomedical Progress and the Limits of Human Health," 157-65
Biomedicine: "progress" in, 157-65, 167-74; technology of, 311-13
Biostatistics, 28
Birth control, in China, 62, 64-65
Blood, human, sale or donation of, 178, 182-85
Blue Cross, 291, 292
"Blueprint for Survival," 166
Bonum communum, 50
Boulding, Kenneth, 104, 107
Brothers Karamazov, 107
Branson, Roy, 3, 5-16
Braybrooke, and Lindblom, 316

325

Brock bill (S 3670), 148
Buncher, Charles Ralph, 41-42
Burleson-McIntyre bill (HR 5200, S 1100), 148
Bureau of the Budget, 272

Cahn, Edmond, 201, 205
Calabresi, Guido, 255
Calkins, Gary, 266
Callahan, Daniel, 7, 14-15, 104, 156, 157-65, 167-74
Cancer, 17, 234, 313
Capitalism and Freedom, 190
Catholicism, medical ethics and, 23-25
Central nervous system, regeneration of, 313
Ceylon, 106
Chadwick, Edwin, 261, 264, 265, 266, 281, 283, 284, 285
Chamber of Commerce, national health insurance proposal, 150, 151
Chang Cheng-yu, 61-62
Chao Huan-ching, 61
Chesterfield, Lord, 20
Chicago, Ill., 17
Childbirth: Lamaze method of, 101; psychoprophylactic method of, 101
Childress, James, 11, 197, 199-212, 213-18
China, medicine in, 4, 57-75
China's Medicine, 70, 71
Chronic-care facility, NYC, 296-297
Civil defense policy, U.S., 105
Clarke, Edwin C., 5
Cleft palate, 163, 170
Cloning, 313-14, 315
Club of Rome, 106
Coates, Joseph F., 308
Coates, Vary T., 311-12
Code ethics, 19-22
Colorado River Valley, 311
Commission on Medical Malpractice, HEW, 10-11
Committee on Life Sciences and Social Policy, 312-13
Common good, doctrine of, 27, 37, 40
Community boards, NYC municipal hospitals, 293-98
"Community Participation in Health Care Decisions," 289-305
Compensatory justice, *see* Justice, compensatory
Comprehensive Health Insurance Act of 1974 (HR 12684), 148
Comprehensive Health Insurance Plan (CHIP), 103, 143, 149, 150
"Conceptual Foundations for an Ethics of Medical Care," 17-34

"Conceptual Foundations for an Ethics of Medical Care: A Response," 35-55
Congress, 93rd, 142, 143
Congressional Office of Technology Assessment, 310
Consent, highway accident victims and, 52
Contract theory perspective, health care and justice and, 111-26
Contraception, 62, 101
Corneal transplant, 200
Cosmetic surgery, 23, 141; *and see* Face-lifts
Council of Community Boards, NYC, 299-300
Council of Municipal Hospital Boards, NYC, 303
County Medical Society, Prince George County, Md., 179-80
Cryogenics, 121
Cultural Revolution, China, 59, 70, 71, 72
Curran, Charles, 319

DDT, 106
DNA therapy, 29, 313
Daddario, Emilio Q., 307
Death, quality of, 224-26
Defects, genetic, 157, 234
Defense Department, xx
Deformation, infant, 157
Dehumanization, 29
Del Vecchio, Georgio, 29
Dental care, insurance and, 149
Department of Health, Education and Welfare, 283
Diagnosis, prenatal, 42, 157
Dialysis, 86, 105, 121, 162, 203, 208, 214, 215, 227
Diabetes, 73, 141
Dingell, 143
Diphtheria, 63
Diseases, priorities of, 141-42
Divine dominion, 23
Doctor's Dilemma, The, 199
Dogmatists, Cult of, 101
Dorfman, Robert, 107-8
Dostoievski, Fyodor, 107
Down's Syndrome, 159, 163, 170
Drug therapy, 158; psychoactive, 29
Duchenne muscular dystrophy, 42
Duties and *Character of the Physician*, 21

East Harlem, NYC, 105
Ecologist, 106
"Econometrics," 108
"economic ethic," 107
Economic Writings of Sir William Petty, 278
Ectopic pregnancy, 23-24
Edwards, Jonathan, 48

Egalitarianism, 133-34
Electrical system, artificial heart, 221
Elmhurst Hospital, NYC, 295-96
Embryo transfer, 315
Empedocles, 101
Encephalitis, 63
Energy systems, artificial heart, 221-22
England, 185, 262-63, 264
Entralgo, Leon de, 22
Epidemiology, 28
Epistulae, 21
"Ethical arithmetic," 99
Ethical Principles of the American Medical Association, 19-20
"Ethics and Allocating Scarce Medical Resources," 195-255
"Ethics of Health Care Delivery: Computers and Distributive Justice," 99-109
"Ethics and Health Policy Planning," 257-324
"Ethometrics," 108
Etiology, 101
Etiquette, 20-21
Eugenics, 314, 315
Euthanasia, 23, 25, 200
Evil, intrinsic, 178
Exotic Lifesaving Therapy (ELT), 208
Expenditures, national health, 80
Extensivity, 27-28

Face-lifts, 163, 170, 172
Family planning, 64-66
Fannin bill (S3353), 148
Farr, William, 265-66, 267
Federal Trade Commission, 182
Fees, physicians', 177-80, 181
Fein, Rashi, 259, 261-88
Fengsheng, 8, 60, 61
Fertilization, in vitro, 43, 141, 149, 170, 313-14
Fetus: death of, 23-24; extrauterine development of, 313
"First come, first served," 208-9, 216
First World War, 266
Fletcher, Joseph, 23, 77
Forrester, Jay, 108
Franco-Prussian War, 1870, 266
Frankena, William, and John Rawls, 319
Freedom, 57-58, 178-86
"Freedom and Utilities in the Distribution of Health Care," 175-93
Freidson, Eliot, 6
Freud, Sigmund, 173
Freund, Paul, 206
Fried, Charles, 207
Friedman, Milton, 178, 190-91
Frigidity, 102

Fulton-Broyhill-Hartke bill (S 444, HR 2222), 148
"From each according to his ability, to each according to his need," 177
Fuqua bill (HR 4349), 148

Gambling, 191
Gene transfer, 315
General Accounting Office, 310
"Genetic" abortion, *see* Abortion
Genetic control, 29
Genetic disease, 313
Genetic engineering, 157
Genetic surgery, 315
Genetics, 171; technology and, 307-24
Genomes, defective, elimination of, 29
Giffen, Sir Robert, 266
"Giving the Patient His Medical Record: A Proposal to Improve the System," 10
Glass, Bentley, et al., 163, 313, 315-16
Goldwater Memorial Hospital, NYC, 296-97
Goodby, Mr. Rosewater, 22
Graft rejection, 215
Great Britain, 106, 189, 192, 266; blood donation in, 182, 184, 185, 186, 187; malpractice lawsuits in, 180-81; national health service in, 188, 189, 192; *and see* England; Ireland; National Health Service; Wales
Great Proletarian Cultural Revolution, 61
"Greater good for the greater number," 30, 44, 77, 132; *and see* Utilitarianism
Green, Felix, 71, 229n
Green, Ronald M., 77, 111-26
Greene, John C., 6
Griffiths-Kennedy "Health Security Act" (HR 22, 53), 148
Gurley, John G., 73-74
Guy, 266-67

HEW, *see* Department of Health, Education and Welfare
Hair transplants, 149
Hamilton, Archibald, 266
Han Suyin, 64, 66
Hangchow, 59, 64, 67-68, 70
Hardin, Garrett, 109
Hartmann, 21
Havighurst, Clark C., 43, 45, 46, 197, 244n, 247-55
Hayek, F.A., 178
Health (defined), 100, 160-61, 169-70; biomedical progress and, 157-65
Health care: in China, 59-66; in contract theory perspective, 111-26; decisions, community participation in, 289-305; delivery, ethical conflicts and, 1-75; equal

328 Index

Health care (cont.)
  access to, 13-14, 28, 79-98; justice and, 77-153; policy, military, 105; right to, 155-93; national, *see* National health care
"Health Care and Justice in Contract Theory Perspective," 111-26
Health goods, distribution of, 128-36; *and see* Selection criteria, health goods recipients
Health and Hospitals Corporation (HHC), NYC, 289-90, 291, 293, 299, 300, 302, 303
Health Insurance Association of America, 148, 150, 237
Health maintenance organizations (HMOs), 95, 102
Health programs, measuring economic benefits of, 261-88
Heart, artificial, 11, 12-13, 162, 197, 219-46, 247-55, 313; advantages and disadvantages, measuring, 229-31; availability of, government role in, 227-28, 254-55; benefits of, 226-27; biological fuel cell, 221, 235; allocation and regulation, 236-45; candidates for, 222-24, 227; costs of, 226-27, 231-32; electric-battery-powered, 43, 44, 45-46, 233, 234; electrical system, 221; insurance and, 236-37, 238; mortality rate with, 225-26; nuclear-powered, 12, 29, 43-44, 45, 141, 197, 233-36, 238, 242, 243, 245, 250-53; Plutonium-238 system, 221-22, 234; population impacts of, 228; power sources, alternative, 232-36; selection of recipients of, 12, 253-55
Heart disease, 44
Heart transplants, 11, 200, 207; *and see* Heart, artificial
Hegel, 107
Heilungkiang Province, 70
Hellegers, André, and Albert Jonsen, 3, 7, 8, 13, 17-33, 35, 37-38, 39-41, 46-47, 53-55
Hemodialysis, 50, 141, 200, 213
Hemophilia, 42, 162
Herb medicines, 62, 63
"Herd immunity," 63-64
Hippocrates, 6, 101
Hippocratic Oath, *xix, xx*, 19-20, 21, 170
Hobbes, 172, 173
Holmes, 200-202, 205
Hormone therapy, 101
Horn, Joshua, 68-69, 70, 73
Hospitals, municipal, NYC, 289-305
House Subcommittee on Science, Research, and Development, 307
"How We Have Struggled against Unstable Diabetes Mellitus in the Light of Mao Tse-Tung's Thought," 73

Hsu, Francis L.K., 57-58
Hull, Charles Henry, 278
"Human Heredity and Ethical Problems," 315
Hygeia, Cult of, 101
Hypertension, 62

Immunization in China, 63, 74
Impartiality, 29-30, 114
Implantation, heart, candidates for, 222-24, 227
Impotence, 102
In vitro fertilization, *see* Fertilization, in vitro
Indigenous health personnel, China, 70-71
Individualism, 57-58
Informed consent, 11
Institute of Society, Ethics and the Life Sciences, *xx*, 7
Insulin, 141
Insurance: and artificial heart, 236-37, 238; malpractice, 11; national health, 88, 93-94, 142-53, 178-79
Integration, 191-92
International Code of Medical Ethics, 48
International Society for Technology Assessment, 307
International Symposium on Human Rights, Retardation, and Research, 314
Ireland, 264

Jamaica Bay-Kennedy Airport Study, 311
Japan, blood availability in, 185-87
Javits bill (S 915), 143-48, 150
Jesus, 104, 107
Johns Hopkins Institute of the History of Medicine, 5
Jonas, Hans, 312
Jones, Martin V., 308-10, 315, 316-17
Jonsen, Albert, 12-13, 105, 229; André Hellegers and, 3, 7, 8, 13, 17-33, 35, 37-38, 39-41, 46-47, 53-55
Journal of the American Medical Association, 314
Journal of Health and Social Behavior, 6
"Just medicine," 26, 30-31
Justice, 26, 28, 29-30, 31; compensatory, 140-41; distributive, 101-4, 177-78; and health care, in contract theory perspective, 111-26; health care delivery and, 77-153; theories of in health care, 128-36; utilitarianism and, 248-50

Kaiser-Permanente Medical Care Program, 95
Kansas City, Ks., 182
Kant, Immanuel, 21, 46, 318

Kaplan, 229n, 238n
Katz, 229n
Kass, Leon R., 312
Kennedy Foundation, 314
Kennedy-Griffiths proposal (SR 22-23), 148, 149, 150
Kennedy Institute Center for Bioethics, 9
Kennedy-Mills bill, 103, 150
"Kerz Report," 296
Kiangsi Province, 69
Kidney, artificial, 204
Kidney disease, 214, 227
Kidney machine, 50, 56, 105, 162, 208
Kidney-sharing programs, 215
Kidney transplants, 200, 203, 213, 214, 227
Kierkegaard, 102
Kings County Hospital, NYC, 297-98
Knowles, John, 100
Kolff, Wilhelm, 204
Korea, 185
Kung Chiang New Village, 65-66

Lamaze method, childbirth, 101
Latin America, blood availability in, 187
Lawsuits, malpractice, 180
Lead poisoning, 105
Leake, Chauncey, 20
Least well off, 137-39
Leukemia, 43, 234
Life expectancy, 98n
Life, quality of, 224
Limits of Growth, 106
Long-Ribicoff-Wagonner bill (S 2513, HR 14709), 148, 149
Long Stanton bill (S 1416, HR 8380), 148, 149
Ligation: tubal, 64; vas deferens, 64
Liverpool, Eng., 200
Locke, John, 171, 172, 173
London, Eng., 188, 283
Lottery selection, *see* Selection criteria, health goods recipients
Lujan bill (HR 15006), 148, 151
Luther, Martin, 37, 102

MITRE Corporation, 308
Malaria, 106
Malthus, 173
Malpractice, 10-11; insurance, 11, 180; lawsuits, 180-81
Ma Hai-teh, 71
Mao Tse-tung, 61, 63, 64, 66-67, 69, 72-73
Maoist principles, 66-67
Marriage law, 1950, China, 64
Marx, Karl, 177, 187
Massachusetts, 103
Massachusetts General Hospital, 103

Massachusetts Institute of Technology, 108
"Mathematics of mercy," 106
"Maximin" reasoning, 115, 120-21, 134-36
Mayor's Advocacy Committee, NYC, 297
McCormick, Richard, 8
McNamara, Robert, *xx*
Meadows, 106
Measles, 63
Medical care, equal access to, 13-14, 28, 79-98
"Medical Care as a Right: A Refutation," 87-89
Medical Defence Union (Great Britain), 180
Medical resources, scarce, allocating, 195-255
Medicaid, 169
Medicare, 98n, 143, 169, 227; artificial heart and, 238
Medicine: in China, 57-75; dehumanization of, 29; history of, 5-6; "just," 26, 30; justice and, 26, 28, 29-30, 31; law and, 30-31; sociology of, 6; society and, 3
Medicredit, 103, 148
Medicus Politicus, 21
Meningitis, 63
Merit, to each according to, 81-85, 139-40
"Metaethical theories," 135
Middle Ages, 21
Mill, John Stuart, 106, 172, 173
Mills-Kennedy plan, 148
Modern Methods in the History of Medicine, 5-6
Mongoloidism, 159
Montana Supreme Court, 101
Moral Decision, The, 201
Morrisania Hospital, NYC, 294
Mortality, infant, 158-59
Mortality rate with artificial heart, 225-26
Moses, 104
Muscular dystrophy, 42

Nader, Ralph, 179-80
National Academy of Sciences, 317
National Blood Resource Program, 42
National Blood Transfusion Board, Great Britain, 185, 188
National Comprehensive Health Benefits Act, 1973, 143
National health care, 178-79
National Health Care Act, 150
National health insurance, 88, 93-94, 178-79; proposals, 142-53
National Health Insurance Act, 151
National Health Planning Council, 131-32
National Health Standards Act, 150
National Health Service, Great Britain, 184, 188, 189, 192

National Heart and Lung Institute, 12, 43, 219
National Institutes of Health, xx, 43, 237
National Research Council, 312
National Science Foundation, 308
Natural law, 23, 46-47
"Natural primary goods," 112, 114
Nazis, 50
Neoplatonists, 101
Neurosurgery, 171
New China News Agency, 68
New England Journal of Medicine, 10, 87
New York City, 17, 105, 185, 259; municipal hospitals in, 289-305
New York City Council, 299
New York State, malpractice insurance in, 180
New York State Legislature 289
New Yorker, 57
New Zealand, 266, 267
Newfoundland, 200
Newsholme, Sir Arthur, 285
Niebuhr, H. Richard, 319
Night soil, China, 70
Nixon-Weinberger proposal, 103
North, 99
Nuclear-powered heart, 12, 29, 43-44, 45, 141, 197, 233-36
Nuremberg Medical Code, 48-49, 50
Nursing, 172

Obstetrical techniques, 23
O'Connor, T.P., 99-100
"On Measuring Economic Benefits of Health Programs," 261-88
"On Practice," 66
Open-heart surgery, 222
Open market, health care on, 175, 177, 178, 180
Orleans, Leo A., and Richard P. Suttmeir, 68
Othello, 107
Outka, Gene, 13-14, 77, 79-98, 133-34

PPBS, 131
Pacemaker, 172
Panel on Technology Assessment, National Academy of Sciences, 317
Paternalism, 190
"Paper tiger" theory, 69, 73
Pareto optimality, 137
Patient: bedridden, 172; right of to medical records, 10-11; role of in China, 72-74; selection of, 11-12; social worth of, 11; *and see* Selection criteria, health goods recipients
Patient as Person, The, 7-8, 79
Patient-physician relationship, 21-22, 54

Patient's Bill of Rights, 101
Patriotic Health Campaign, China, 66, 67
Peking, 59, 60-63
Peking Third Hospital, 72-73
Pell-Mondale proposal (S 2796), 143
Penicillin, 105, 141, 199
People's Liberation Army, 59, 68
Percival's Medical Ethics, 20, 21
Perpetuity, 27-28, 30
Pertussis, 63
Petty, Sir William, 99, 262-64, 266, 278, 281, 284, 285
Pharmaceutical cosmetics, ownership of stock in, 17
Pharmacological psychiatry, 171
Philadelphia, Pa., 200
Physicians: fees, 179-80, 181; importation of to U.S., 13; income of, 98n
Ping-Pong, 58
Pius XII, Pope, 23
Placenta, artificial, 313, 315
Planning Board Eight, NYC, 297
Plutonium-238 system, artificial heart, 221-22, 234, 238
Pneumonia, 141
Policy-making, 290-93
Poliomyelitis, 58-59, 63
Political Arithmetick, 262-64
Pollution, China, 68, 70
Potter, Van Rens selaer, 7
Poverty, 190-91
Power sources, alternative, artificial heart, 232-36
"Preciousness of life," 47-48
Pregnancy, ectopic, 23-24
prenatal diagnosis, 42
Prince George County, Md., 179-80
Principles of Medical Ethics of the American Medical Association, 6
Principles of Morals and Legislation, 105
Professional Standards Review Organizations (PSROs), 103
Professionals, role of in China, 71-72
Progress, biomedical, 157-65
Promises, making and keeping, 49
Prostheses, dental, 141
"Protection of Human Subjects: Policies and Procedures," 43
Psychiatry, 100, 149, 170; pharmacological, 171
Psychoanalysis, 141
Psychoprophylactic method of childbirth, 101
Psychosurgery, 29, 158
Pythagoras, 101

Quantifying qualities, 106-9

Radiation, from nuclear-powered artificial heart, 12, 45, 234-36, 243, 250-51
Railsback bill (HR 2618), 143, 150, 151
Ramsey, Paul, 3, 7-8, 9, 11-12, 13, 14, 22, 35-55, 79, 80, 86, 206, 314, 316, 319
Rand, Ayn, 82
Rawls, John, 14, 77-78, 111-26, 134-37, 248; and William Frankena, 319
Red Medical Workers, China, 61, 62-63, 64, 65-66, 70
Renaissance, 21
Renal failure, 208, 214
Report of a General Plan for the Promotion of Public and Personal Health, 264-65
Reproduction, asexual, 313
"reproductive engineering," 43
"Requests for Proposals RFP NHLI-71-18, Prenatal Diagnosis of Inherited Hematologic Diseases," 42
Rescher, Nicholas, 208
Research Group on Ethics and Health Policy, Institute of Social Ethics and the Life Sciences, *xx*
Responsible Self, The, 319
Retinoblastoma, 315
Ribicoff, Abraham, 176, 190
"Right to health care," 128, 155-93
"Right to Health Care and the Anxiety of Liberalism: A Reply to Daniel Callahan," 167-74
Robert Wood Johnson Foundation, *xx*
Rockefeller Foundation, 100
Roe-Beall bill (HR 1054, S 587), 148, 151
Rogers, Rev. J.E., 265

Sade, Robert M., 87-89
Salpingectomy, 23-24
Samuelson, Paul, 107-8
Sanitation, China, 67-68, 70
Sapolsky, 244n-245n
Saylor bill (HR 1916), 148
Scarce Life-Saving Medical Resources (SLMR), 200, 201-2, criteria of selection of recipients, 202-5; random selection of recipients, 205-10
Schistosomiasis, 58, 69 70
"Scope of Bioethics: Individual and Social, The," 5-16
Scott-Percy bill (S 2756), 148
Scriptures, Christian, 47
Seattle, Wash., 204
Seattle Artificial Kidney Center, 204, 240
Selection criteria, health goods recipients: for artificial heart, 238-45; for SLMR, 11, 202-10, 213-18; and *see* Social worth
Selective breeding, 315
"Selection Process as Viewed from Within:

A Reply to Childress," 213-18
"Self-Reliance and the Collective Good: Medicine in China," 57-75
"Separate Views on the Artificial Heart," 247-55
Septicemia, 67
Sex chromatin tests, 42
Sex problems, 102
Shakespeare, 107
Shanghai, 59, 65, 66, 67
Shanghai Mental Hospital, 73
Shanghai Municipal Revolutionary Committee, 68
Shatin, Leo, 203-4, 240
Shattuck, Lemuel, 264-65
Shaw, George Bernard, 199
Shenkin, Budd, and David Warner, 10-11
Shinn, Roger, 106, 107
Sickle cell disease, 42, 170
Sidel, Victor and Ruth, 4, 57-75
Sigerist, Henry, 5
Silvery Lane health station, 64-65, 70
"Similar treatment for similar cases," 77, 91-96
Singer, Peter, 155-56, 175-93
Sleuth, 26
Smallpox, China, 63
Smith, Adam, 172, 173
Smythe, 229n, 231n
Snow, Edgar, 71
Social-contract theory, 111-26
"Social Justice and Equal Access to Health Care," 79
"Social primary goods," 111-12, 114, 116, 117
Social worth, as criterion for SLMR, 203-4, 208, 209, 210, 213-18, 240-41
Soochow Creek, 68
Sophocles, 107
South African War, 266
Spina bifida, 159
Sri Lanka, 106
Staggers, 143
Steinfels, Peter, 155, 167-74
Sterilization, 17, 24, 43, 101, 315
Steroid contraceptive pill, 106
Summum bonum, 101
"Supplementary judgment," 43
Surgery: cosmetic, 23, 141, 164; genetic, 315; open-heart, 222
Surrogate therapy, 102
Survival, 161
Swedish Hospital, Seattle, 86, 240
Sydenham Society, 18
Syphilis, China, 71

Tay Sachs disease, 163, 170

Taylor, Gordon Rattray, 106
Technology: biomedical, 311-13; culture and, dialectic between, 158; genetic, 313-16; genetics and, 307-24
Technology Assessment, 307
"Technology Assessment and Genetics," 307-24
Terminal disease, 51
Tetanus, 63
Theobald, Robert, 105
Theory of Justice, A, 248, 14, 111, 112
Thielicke, Helmut, 204-5
Thoreau, Henry David, 86, 204
Throat culture, fees for, 180
Titmuss, Richard, 175n, 182, 183, 184, 185, 186, 187
Totality, 23-25
"Totally Implantable Artificial Heart: Economic, Legal, Medical, Psychiatric, and Social Implications, The," 219-46
"To each according to his contribution in satisfying whatever is freely desired by others in the open marketplace of supply and demand," 87-89
"To each according to his merit or desert," 81-85
"To each according to his needs," 89-91, 130
"To each according to his societal contribution," 85-87
Toulmin, 108
Transplants, 11, 23; corneal, 200; heart, 11, 200, 207; hair, 149; kidney, 200, 203, 213, 214, 215
Triage decisions, 105, 213
Tuberculosis, 63
Tyranny of Survival, The, 171

U.S. v. Holmes, 200-202, 205, 206
U.S.-Kuomintang alliance, 69
"Uncertainty and the Welfare Economics of Medical Care," 179
Union Seminary, 106
United States: blood availability in, 182-88; civil defense policy of, 105; importation of physicians to, 13; malpractice lawsuits in, 180-81; military health care policy, 105; sociology of medicine in, 6

University of Virginia Law School, 209
University of Virginia Hospital Renal Unit, 208
Utilitarianism, 14, 30, 44, 46, 50, 114, 131-33, 209, 248-50
Utility, 186-88

Vaccination, in China, 63-64, 74
Values, quantifying, 106-9
Vanderbilt University, 105
Veatch, Laurelyn, 259, 289-305
Veatch, Robert, 78, 127-53
"Veil of ignorance," 113-14, 135
Venereal disease, 199; in China, 70-71
Vital Statistics, 265-66
Vogel, Sir Julius, 267
Vonnegut, Kurt, 22

Wales, 185
Walters, LeRoy, 259, 307-24
Walton, Isaac, 21
Warner, David, and Budd Shenkin, 10-11
Ways and Means Committee, 103
Weaver, Warren, 106-7
Westervelt, Frederic B., 197, 213-18
Whangpoo River, 68
"What Is a 'Just' Health Care Delivery?" 127-53
"Who Shall Live When Not All Can Live?" 199-212
William Brown, 200
Williams, Bernard, 83-84, 133, 154
Willrich, Mason, 209
Wittgenstein, Ludwig, 99, 102
Wolin, Sheldon S., 172
Women, heart disease in, 44
World Health Organization, 100, 106, 160, 169-70
World Medical Association, 48
Wu Ting station, 61

X-rays, 181

Yale Law School, 255
Yang Hsio-hua, 61-62
Yang Pu District, 65
Yenan, 69
Yukian County, 69-70